Edited by
Paul H. Skinner
University of Arizona
Ralph L. Shelton
University of Arizona

Speech, Language, and Hearing: Normal Processes and Disorders

ADDISON-WESLEY PUBLISHING COMPANY

Reading, Massachusetts
Menlo Park, California • London • Amsterdam
Don Mills, Ontario • Sydney

This book is in the Addison-Wesley Series in
Speech Pathology and Audiology

Consulting Editor
Ira Ventry

Second printing, May 1978
Copyright © 1978 by Addison-Wesley Publishing Company, Inc. Philippines copyright 1978
by Addison-Wesley Publishing Company, Inc.

ISBN 0-201-07461-3
ABCDEFGHIJK-HA-798

To Fritzie and Abe

PREFACE

The purpose of this text is to provide an introductory survey of normal processes and disorders in speech, language, and hearing for beginning students in speech and hearing and in related professions, such as education, special education, nursing, dentistry, medicine, psychology, rehabilitation, social work, counseling, and speech communication or arts. The text is intended to provide a general understanding and perspective of normal communication processes and disorders, but not to provide the student with research competencies or clinical skills. The development of scientific or clinical competence requires the accumulation of extensive knowledge and use of that knowledge in problem-solving situations. Clinical training involves a variety of practicum experiences.

Speech and hearing evolved in this country as a behavioral discipline essentially out of interest and concern for speech and hearing disorders. Scholars interested in the etiology, diagnosis, and treatment of disorders learned that knowledge of anatomy and physiology, acoustics, psychology, and linguistics provided a framework for interpretation of scientifically founded applied knowledge about the disorders themselves. Moreover, it became apparent that study of normal processes in speech, language, and hearing should precede the study of disorders or at least should be presented concurrently. One must have a fundamental understanding of "normal" in order to understand, describe, and treat that which is abnormal. Study of normal processes enhances the study of disorders, and vice versa. In this regard, it should be understood that the value of the clinician in the marketplace is based on the scientific principles which underlie diagnosis and treatment. It should be understood also that interest and concern for disorders have given the scientific study of speech and hearing its greatest impetus and resource.

Persons studying both normal and disordered aspects of human communication have formed an integrated discipline which encompasses speech, language, and hearing. This discipline is known as speech and hearing science or speech pathology and audiology. This discipline, however, is not the only field concerned with human communication. Scientists, artists, and professional workers from many fields are intently and uniquely involved in human communication. This text endeavors to place speech and hearing in perspective as a unique and vital process in communication, to describe the normal processes in speech and hearing, and to discuss the disorders of speech and hearing and their evaluation and treatment.

Part One deals with normal processes; Part Two, with disorders. Persons using the text may choose to cover the material as presented or focus on either part of the book. The subjects covered in the two parts are as follows: *general and professional* (Chapters 1 and 7); *speech* (Chapters 3, 4, 8, 9, and 10); *language* (Chapters 2, 11, and 12); and *hearing* (Chapters 5, 6, and 13).

Tucson, Arizona   P.H.S.
August 1977   R.L.S.

PART ONE

**Normal Processes
in Speech, Language,
and Hearing**

CONTENTS

CONTENTS

PART TWO

Disorders in Speech, Language, and Hearing

CONTENTS

13

**Disorders
of Hearing**

William R. Hodgson
University of Arizona

Normal Processes in Speech, Language, and Hearing

CHAPTER 1
Overview

Chapter 1, "Speech and Hearing in Communication," is intended to provide you with an understanding of communication and how it is accomplished. We define communication as the transmission and exchange of information through coded symbols which form languages. Communication through biological processes, machines, mass media, and social and personal interaction is discussed.

Speech, language, and hearing are viewed as a special system of communication in which human language is distinguished from a more general concept of language. Speech, or spoken language, is described as a body of words with rules for combining and using them. Thus speech and hearing, as used in this context, include language. Speech and hearing are described as encoding and decoding processes of spoken language. The essential physiological processes of speech are reviewed: respiration, phonation (voicing), resonation (vocal quality), and articulation (speech sound formation). Also, the processes in hearing are described as the conversion of sound to neural impulses which form the physiological bases of perception and comprehension of speech.

In order to provide a better understanding of speech production and hearing, several theories of speech and hearing as a system are presented. The first theory provides an elementary overview of the processes involved in the interaction between a speaker and a listener. A second theory emphasizes the role of the ear as a component of the speaking system. This stresses the importance of hearing

Speech and Hearing in Communication

one's own speech. A third theory of speech and hearing deals with speech production and reception as dyadic communication, in which the listener and speaker are components of a single system.

These theories introduce you to the study of normal processes in speech and hearing to enhance your understanding of how these aspects of communication are accomplished. Reference is also made to disorders that occur in speech, language, and hearing and to their evaluation and treatment. Thus speech and hearing are introduced as a professional area of interest which involves both scientific and clinical pursuits. The role of the scientist is discussed in terms of questions and developments in basic and applied research. The role of the clinician is discussed, including interaction with related professions.

Paul H. Skinner, Ph.D.
University of Arizona

Introduction

The term **communication*** is often used to include only the spoken word and its perception; however, **speech** and **hearing** comprise only one of the many aspects of communication. Communication, or communication theory, involves numerous fields, not only the speech and hearing process. Students interested in speech and hearing or related areas should gain an awareness of the broad realm of communication in order to place speech and hearing in proper perspective. This chapter is intended to provide that perspective. In addition, we will try to provide an understanding and appreciation of speech and hearing as a unique and dynamic form of communication. This chapter is also intended to introduce you to the normal processes and disorders of speech and hearing and to related scientific and clinical endeavors.

Communication

Let us proceed, then, to see what is meant by the term "communication," to survey its vast domain, and to see how speech and hearing emerge as a communicative process. Communication is the transmission and exchange of information. Communication is accomplished through an astounding variety of media which pervade all aspects of life. Communication is fundamental to basic life processes in the biological world; it transcends human experience and knowledge over the ages; it is the cohesive, compelling force which is essential for society and human culture; it is the dominant influence in our personal lives. To ensure that the obvious does not elude us, it should be said that the ultimate purpose of communication is knowledge. Communication facilitates the creation, preservation, advancement, and utilization of all knowledge. Knowledge is preserved and transmitted through publications, books, films, and recordings. Libraries are the reservoirs for these resources which can be stored and utilized to share the wisdom and knowledge obtained by men and women over the ages.

How is communication accomplished? Communication requires the use of signs or symbols, which may be coded to form **languages** in a progression or hierarchy of communication. It is clear that communication can be accomplished simply by isolated signs or symbols: a car horn or flashing light may be a sign of warning; a hen's clucking is a symbol that sets her brood scurrying to her. The human expressions also surely are revealing: a sigh, a yawn, a tear. Clearly, we humans, as well as animals, have our instinctive set of signs or symbols to express hunger, fear, love, and they are important in communication. We would not equate these expressions with language, however; certainly "human lan-

---

*   Terms in boldface type are defined in the glossary at the end of the chapter.

guage is vastly more than a complicated system of clucking" (Cherry, 1957).

Communication can be enhanced or refined by **codification** of symbols. A code is an organized set of symbols arbitrarily used to represent words or concepts to convey meaning. Codes may vary in complexity from a set of hand signals used by automobile drivers to mathematical symbols used to express concepts in a very rigorous form of logic. In fact, speech may be thought of as a coded set or system of sounds, undoubtedly a definition which lacks the eloquence that some of us may prefer to associate with our speech. Coded symbols may be integrated and transmitted through various media: sound waves carry the sound patterns of speech; electrical pulses (dots and dashes) are used to represent letters in telegraphy known as Morse code; letters form words, and numbers form equations to provide written codification of information. In a general sense, each of these sets of coded symbols may be considered a form of language.

How does communication occur? Many kinds of communication are an integral part of nature; many kinds have been developed by humans; and many kinds no doubt remain to be discovered or developed. Communication can be classified in a number of ways although these classifications may be somewhat arbitrary and redundant. Even so, the use of general classifications is warranted for the added insights afforded.

Biological communication   Some interesting examples of biocommunication are genetic communication, sensory communication; later, we shall consider speech and hearing as bioacoustical communication. Genetic communication is fundamental to basic life processes. Recently, biochemists and biophysicists have isolated the elements (nucleic acids DNA and RNA) that transmit information that has determined all species and specific characteristics within each specie since the beginning of biological creation. This information is transmitted from generation to generation by a genetic code "encapsulated" in the chains of molecules which form the microstructure of genes. Scientists who study these elements are not commonly thought of as communication scientists; however, such scientists are employed by large communication industries and laboratories. A focal point of their research is genetic communication.

The surrounding world and immediate environment become reality through sensory communication, or input to the brain by hearing, seeing, or feeling. Humans depend essentially on vision for orientation; also, hearing is important for localization of various sounds. Localization by hearing may be critical for the pedestrian in traffic to avoid an approaching car or for animals to avoid predators. Some bats rely entirely on sonar (echo location) for orientation to their environment and to seek out their prey (insects) for food. A species of moth, in turn, is able to produce "jamming" signals to interfere with the bat's "sonar system," thereby avoiding their predator. More primitive life forms, such as certain fishes, rely primarily on a sensation analogous to touch or feeling. Indeed, sensory communication is a fundamental medium for survival in the animal kingdom and our complex, mechanistic society as well.

Machine communication Physicists, historically, have been concerned with communication through the transmission of sound, light, and radio waves. These properties of nature have been sufficiently well understood and described by scientists that engineers have been able to develop the technology for useful communication systems: sonar (sound waves), laser (light waves), and radar (radio waves). These systems have been highly and successfully developed to transmit information with or without a human intermediary. Sonar is a valuable technique for underwater navigation and radar for aeronautical navigation. Sound and radio waves are generated, reflected from objects, and detected in a surrounding field. Laser has become important for long-distance communication, e.g., earth to satellites and distant planets. Humans have achieved phenomenal success in recent years in developing these forms of communication.

Mass communication Mass communication encompasses many forms of communication: newspapers, books, movies, radio, and television. Although movies, radio, and television could be viewed as machine communication, they are usually considered to be forms of mass communication. The influence of mass communication no doubt exceeds our awareness. Mass communication influences our personal and social behavior, philosophical bases, and aesthetic, cultural, and political attitudes.

Social communication Social communication is the process by which our society conducts its business of everyday living. Letters from home, telephone calls, conversation among individuals and groups in meetings, campus debates, legislative proceedings, the special vernacular of cults or groups—all are forms of social communication.

Personal communication A discussion of communication surely would be incomplete without reference to interpersonal communication. The effectiveness of one's communicative skills provides an index of success in countless personal endeavors. Communication skills influence one's self-concept, psychological and social adjustment and well-being, success in establishing and maintaining relationships, and gainful employment. This topic will be pursued further as speech and hearing in communication are considered.

Speech, Language, and Hearing

Speech and hearing comprise but one aspect of communication, yet the speech and hearing function is dynamic and unique. Speech and hearing are the foundation and primary medium of most human communication. This system permits communication of subtleties and abstractions; it is the basis for written language, and it is the dominant medium in mass, social, and personal communication.

It may be debated whether speech is a manifestation of human language or language a manifestation of speech, or whether speech and language are interdependent systems (Cutting and Kavanagh, 1975). Language may be defined in a very general sense as any means, vocal or other, of expressing or understanding thoughts, ideas, or feelings. It is true that human language may be expressed and understood in forms other than speech. Deaf persons commonly communicate by sign language; a tribe of cliff dwellers in Africa relies on a language system of whistles. Since human language provides expression of feelings and thoughts, speech may be considered a medium for expression of language. Spoken language may be described as a set of methods and rules for combining and using words. (Considerably more attention will be given to the acquisition and structure of language in Chapter 2.) Speech is often used to mean spoken language or as a term that encompasses spoken language. This is the case when the expression "speech and hearing" is used in this chapter.

Speech and hearing may be thought of as encoding and decoding processes in communication. Speech, of course, involves the process of encoding a linguistic message, and speech production requires four primary biological functions: respiration, phonation (voicing), resonation (vocal quality), and articulation (sound formation). These processes will be discussed in Chapter 3, which covers the speech mechanism and speech production. The speech signal is transmitted acoustically in coded sound patterns which vary over time and carry information. Speech acoustics and perception will be covered in Chapter 4. Hearing involves decoding the linguistic message for the perception and comprehension of speech and is based on two processes—**transduction** and auditory perception. Transduction is a process by which the acoustic energy of speech is changed in form to nerve impulses in the auditory nervous system. The hearing mechanism and the transduction process are discussed in Chapter 5. Auditory perception is the reception and comprehension of the neural impulses at the brain that occur as a result of transduction. Auditory perception is a complex phenomenon, and although much is known about the ear's perceptive abilities, little is known about how the ear and higher nervous systems synthesize and comprehend the neural patterns that represent speech (Chapter 6).

The speech and hearing mechanisms are anatomically separate biological structures. In the production of speech, however, the hearing mechanism becomes an integral component of the speaking system. In speech production, then, we describe the speech and hearing mechanisms as a single system—the speech and hearing system. The integrated roles of speech and hearing in the production and perception of speech provide a biocommunication system. Let us proceed to discover how the speech and hearing system functions.

The Speech and Hearing System

In seeking to understand and explain the function of various systems of nature, e.g., the solar system, nervous system, or the speech and hearing system, scientists develop theories. A **theory** is structured on available factual information and reliance on hypothetical constructs. Scientists commonly use theories to help them understand complex models or systems. Many theories and explanatory models have been developed to explain the function of the speech and hearing system, so our discussion must be selective. A very general theory will be presented initially which depicts the communication act between a speaker and listener. Next, we will describe a more specific theory which involves speech production by a single speaker. This theory emphasizes the role of auditory feedback in speech production. Finally a verbal-behavioral theory of two-way communication will be presented. These three theories have been selected because they provide views of speech and hearing as a physiological and a behavioral system in communication. Other, more complicated theories that involve problems of listening in noise or listening to competing messages have been omitted, since they exceed the scope of this introductory text.

Simplified Version of Speech Production and Reception

The first theory and model, described by scientists at Bell Telephone Laboratories (1968), illustrate in a general manner how a speaker develops and produces speech, how speech is transmitted to a listener, and how a listener perceives and comprehends the speech signal (see Fig. 1.1). In short, it depicts what happens when two people talk to each other. The speech process originates at the linguistic level in the brain of the speaker. The speaker formulates the message, the thoughts or feelings to be expressed. The message is put into linguistic form through the selection of appropriate words and sequences of words and word groups as dictated by the grammatical rules of the language. Then the brain lays down the instructions for the speech mechanism to encode the message.

The message is transduced, or changed, from the neurolinguistic to the physiologic level by neural impulses sent by the brain through motor nerves to the respiratory mechanism and the vocal folds of the larynx and the articulators such as the lips and tongue. Neuromuscle action and air pressure from the lungs produce vocal-fold vibration, which causes small pressure changes in the surrounding air in the throat and oral cavities. These pressure changes, or sound waves, are modified by the articulatory action of the tongue, palate, and lips, and speech sounds are transmitted as pressure changes in the air (sound waves) which travel from the mouth of the speaker to the ear of the listener.

The resultant sound waves impinge on the conductive mechanism of the ear. Specifically, the eardrum (tympanic membrane) is set into vibration by sound

9

Figure 1.1

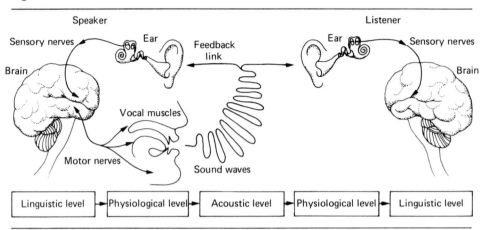

The speech chain. (*Adapted from* The Speech Chain *by Peter B. Denes and Elliot Pinson. Copyright © 1963 by Bell Telephone Laboratories, Inc. Reprinted by permission of Doubleday & Company, Inc.*)

waves and in turn displaces three tiny bones (ossicles) in the middle ear. The ossicular vibrations set up pressure waves in the fluid of the inner ear, thereby stimulating the fibers of the auditory nerve. Neural impulses travel to the brain of the listener and are decoded in ways which scientists do not completely understand. That is, the speech sounds are perceived and comprehended, and communication has taken place. The processes of speech, language, and hearing that produce human communication (as described) are discussed more fully in Part I of this text (Chapters 1–6). Disorders that may occur in speech production, linguistic processing, or hearing are discussed in Part II (Chapters 7–13).

It should be noted that speech sounds are perceived by the ear of not only the listener, but also the speaker. Both the speaker and listener hear the speech as it is transmitted. Hearing one's own speech is a critical part of developing speech. In fact, this aspect of speech development and production is the focus of our second theory and model.

Speech and Hearing as a Servosystem

It was noted earlier that the speech and hearing mechanisms function as a system, although this concept was not made explicit in the initial theory. This concept is important in understanding how speech is produced. In the speech and hearing system, hearing provides feedback of the speech message to the brain. This permits the system to function as a **servosystem,** namely, one that is self-regulating or self-controlling.

A servosystem is a device that automatically operates and controls various machines. There are two types of automatic control devices—open loop and closed loop. Open-loop systems carry out a series of operations based on preset controls, but do not have the capacity to modify or regulate those operations. Examples of open-loop automatic control devices are alarm clocks and traffic lights. We all have had first-hand experience with such devices and know only too well that once programmed or preset, they will function accordingly. The alarm clock will not delay its starting signal because you experienced insomnia; the red traffic light will not turn green even though no other car is in sight.

The closed-loop system is sensitive to errors, self-adjusts to correct errors, and controls its own output or operation. Thermostatically controlled heating or cooling systems used to regulate home temperatures and missile guidance systems used to search out and strike targets are two examples of closed-loop systems. To describe the concept further, the temperature-sensitive device in thermostats controls a furnace or refrigerator by starting or stopping heating or cooling to maintain a preset temperature range. The human body utilizes numerous servosystems to regulate body temperature, blood circulation, and metabolism. In fact, the speech and hearing system is another example of a bodily servosystem, or automatic control device. Since we now have some general understanding of such systems, let us explore just how the speech and hearing mechanisms function as a self-regulating system.

Speech sounds are a series of acoustical patterns produced by biological action. Thus the speaking systems may be described as a bioacoustical system. Early theories and models often viewed the role of hearing in speech production as auditory monitoring and interpreted this function to be a "checking up" on what the speech mechanism had produced. The role of hearing is more extensive, however, since the function of "self-hearing" during speaking is to modify and control speech. The monitoring interpretation suggests that the ear functions only as a receiver, when in fact it is a component of the speaking system. Thus the speech and hearing system functions like a closed-loop system. The brain programs thoughts and feelings into words and orders the words grammatically. Motor actions are developed for the vocal organs to produce the speech signals as formulated. The speech signals are perceived by the ear, which provides feedback to the brain for a comparison of the desired and the actual speech signals. In other words, a comparison is made between what actually was said and what was intended to be said. If the feedback is positive, that is, if no errors occurred, speech production proceeds without interruption; if the feedback is negative, that is, if errors are perceived, the speech signal is modified to correct the errors.

Actually, function of the speech and hearing system is considerably more complex than the other closed-loop systems noted earlier. Whereas the only function of a closed-loop, or thermostatically controlled, heating system is to maintain a preset range of temperatures, the speaking system continuously varies its output over time according to the instruction laid down by the speaker's brain. Speech consists of qualitatively different units which must be selected and ordered in advance and presented in a time sequence that is unique. The speaking system could be likened to a tape recorder in which instructions are stored and the tape drive is alternately started and stopped. Also, presumably because it receives somaesthetic **sensory feedback** (e.g., sensitivity of the joints, muscle sense), the brain is able to predict the occurrence of some errors during the act of speaking and to modify the speech before it reaches the acoustic level.

In Fig. 1.2, a simplified model of an electronic servosystem is compared to speech and hearing as a servosystem. The *controller* establishes operation through three components: storage unit, mixer, and comparator. Information retained by the storage unit is sent to the mixer for processing and action. The comparator receives feedback of the output or speech signal and compares the actual to the desired output. These components are analogous to different areas of the brain. For example, the storage unit may be likened to the recall and association functions of the brain. The mixer might be compared to the motor cortex, which

Figure 1.2

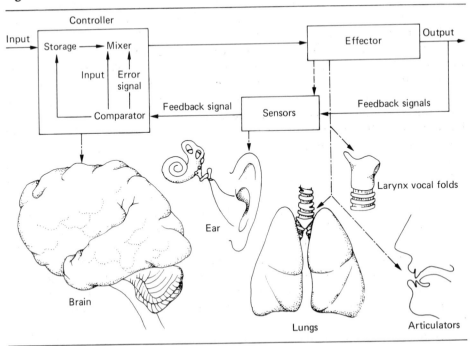

*Speech and hearing as a servosystem. (Adapted from G. Fairbanks, "A Theory of the Speech Mechanism as a Servo-System," J. Speech Hearing Dis. **19** (1954): 133–139.*

controls the encoding of speech through neural impulses to the vocal organs. The role of the comparator will be discussed further in conjunction with the feedback mechanism.

The *effector* produces the output or speech signal. In the speaking system, the effector comprises the lungs, larynx, resonators (throat, mouth, and nose), and articulators (tongue, lips, and soft palate).

The *comparator* receives both the feedback from the sensors of the output or speech signal and an intended speech signal from the storage unit. Thus the comparator is able to provide a comparison between the actual and desired speech signals. Any difference between the two is termed the "error signal."

The *error signal* is transmitted continuously by the comparator to the mixer. If the error signal is zero or positive, the speech signal continues without interruption; if it is negative, the speech signal is corrected.

The concept that speech and hearing function as a servosystem not only enhances our understanding of normal speech production, but has considerable practical importance in the management of speech and language disorders as well. Mysak (1966), for example, dedicated an entire text to the implications of feedback theory for normal processes and disorders in speech and language. Each of us depends to some extent on the feedback provided by the ear to control the speed or rate at which we talk, articulation, and the pitch and loudness of our voice. If feedback of one's own voice during continuous speech is delayed (through use of a special tape recorder and earphones), dramatic changes usually result in the rate, loudness, and fluency of speech. A very simple example of the effect of feedback on loudness can be experienced merely by plugging both ears with your fingertips while talking. This changes the mode of hearing from air conduction or transmission to bone or body conduction, and therefore your voice will immediately sound louder; to compensate, you will probably reduce the loudness of your voice.

It is intuitively clear, then, that persons who have language disorders (impaired use of symbols or words), voice disorders (abnormal pitch, loudness, or quality), or faulty articulation must utilize sensory feedback as part of their treatment or remediation. This modality has been stressed as a part of treatment by Van Riper and Irwin (1958) and McDonald (1964), as well as by Mysak, and also in several of the chapters on disorders in the second part of this text.

Our first theory focused on language, speech production, and auditory perception for the purpose of providing a basic overview of the speech and hearing system. The second theory emphasized the speech and hearing mechanisms as a single, integrated system that is particularly dependent on sensory feedback. It is important to explore at least one more perspective of speech and hearing in communication. We recognize, of course, that communication through speech and hearing is a behavioral phenomenon and in this respect differs from many other forms of communication. For example, in what was described earlier as machine communication, information is encoded, transmitted, and received, but no other type of interaction occurs between transmitter and receiver. We know from our own experience in human communication, however, that not only what we say, but also how we say it is influenced greatly by how a listener reacts or in the anticipation of what a listener will think. Clearly, communication through speech and hearing involves behavioral interaction. The last theory to be presented will consider this point of view.

Interpersonal, or Dyadic, Communication

Communication between a speaker and a listener is referred to as interpersonal or **dyadic** (two units treated as one) **communication.** A model for dyadic communication describes the interaction which integrates two communication units into a single system. The simplified model presented in Fig. 1.3 merely illus-

Figure 1.3

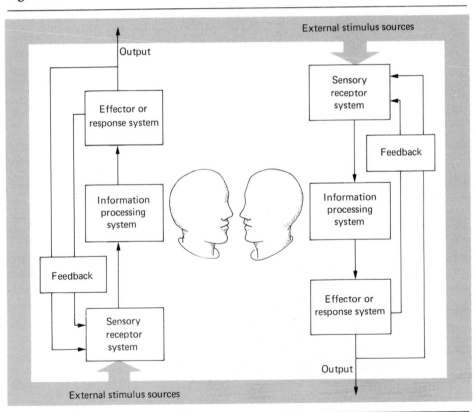

Dyadic communication.

trates the concept of a behavioral-interaction model. Although visual interaction may be significant in the general model, our discussion will be restricted to verbal behavior, that is, speech and hearing.

A dyadic model of communication involves extremely complex interactions, such as the speaker's intent, the listener's interpretation, and the effects of interaction. The speaker attempts to communicate a message by word choice, intonation and inflection of the voice, and visual, gestural, and other auditory cues. Interpretation of the message may depend on the listener's preconceived ideas, differences in connotative meaning of words, or even the mood of the listener. Perhaps the most serious inefficiency of speech and hearing as a medium of communication is the lack of precision in the meaning of spoken language. It also is a most intriguing and fascinating aspect of speech. How many tales have you heard about embarrassing incidents which arose from misinterpretation? You no doubt have had your own experiences which you may or may not choose to recall.

Verbal behavior is formulated by the information-processing system as a result of internal thought processes or in direct response to external stimulation. The effector, or response system, produces verbal behavior. The sensory receptor system, of course, receives information from the environment or from another speaker and transmits this information back to the information-processing system. The feedback loop shown earlier in the servosystem model is included here to permit "self-hearing." The significance of this model is that the listener is an integral component of this communication and may exercise some control over the verbal behavior of the speaker.

A primary purpose of speech is to establish interaction with other persons, and it is important to study speech and hearing in terms of the interaction between speaker and listener. That is, verbal behavior is behavior in which reinforcement, be it positive or negative, can be mediated by another—the listener. This realization is of importance in the normal acquisition or development of speech and language as well as in the habilitation of persons with speech and language problems.

The relationship between adult and child influences the development of the child's verbal behavior. Encouragement of misarticulated sounds in infant speech development (baby talk) as cute behavior may produce mild articulation problems to poorly intelligible speech in the otherwise mature child or adult, as described in Chapter 8. It has been hypothesized that an overly critical or demanding attitude toward a young child's speech development may lead to disorders of fluency (stuttering), as described in Chapter 10. Negative or inadequate response to children's language may seriously retard their language acquisition, as discussed in Chapter 11.

Parents, elementary and special education teachers, pediatricians, and psychologists, as well as speech clinicians (speech pathologists) should be aware of speech and hearing as a behavioral phenomenon. This is particularly important

15

for the speech pathologist, who must depend on behavioral interaction in providing remediation for speech and language problems.

Theories and models aid in understanding the biological and behavioral phenomena of speech and hearing and provide insight regarding the unitary function of speech and hearing as a system in the production of speech. It is clear that normal speech production requires adequate hearing. "We speak as we hear."

It is hoped that the introductory theories and models have given you a better understanding and appreciation for speech and hearing in communication and created an interest to gain further information about normal processes and disorders of speech and hearing. Communication and spoken languages are areas of human behavior which are not fully understood. Many clinical problems exist that are associated with speech, hearing, and language. These interests and concerns led to the development of speech and hearing as a profession.

Speech and Hearing as a Profession

The speech and hearing profession includes scientific and clinical pursuits, and their interaction provides mutual enhancement. The scientist can better understand normal function by studying the effects of disorders; in turn, the clinician can better understand disorders by studying normal function.

What is involved in the scientific study of speech and hearing? Investigation of the normal processes and the disorders of speech and hearing may be described as a communicative science. Obviously, many disciplines are involved in different aspects of communicative sciences: audiology and speech pathology, biology, medicine and surgery, physiology, psychology, special education, and others as well. A common starting place for all, however, is to study basic function—normal processes.

What is meant by normal processes of speech, language, and hearing—what is involved? Reflection on the first general theory will reveal a number of processes that occur in spoken language and its reception. Included are (1) linguistics —how language is acquired and structured for speech; (2) speech physiology— the production of speech; (3) speech acoustics—the physical characteristics of speech and how sound travels; (4) auditory physiology—how sound stimulates the ear and how the ear works; and (5) psychoacoustics—what and how we hear. All of these processes are involved in communication by speech and hearing; they are the normal processes.

It is apparent that these topics may be of interest to scientists, but what do they mean to clinicians or teachers? Clinicians or clinical students often say, "I am interested in disorders and what I can do to help people with problems. How will studying the basic sciences (normal processes) make me a better clinician?"

Perhaps a good response is to ask, "What is normal?" or, for that matter, "What is abnormal?" Do not respond too quickly.

The experienced clinician or scientist will be the most cautious in responding. That which is commonly observed is taken as normal; obvious, yet normal function may become surprisingly elusive to rigorously quantify or even qualify. Although normality and abnormality may be a continuum rather than a dichotomy, the ability to determine what is abnormal clearly is dependent on the ability to establish what is normal. The situation is reminiscent of the humorous anecdote of the cynical husband who responded to the question, "How's your wife?" with another question: "Compared to what?"

The understanding and description of "normal" provides a fundamental reference for the speech pathologist and **audiologist,** both of whom deal with speech and hearing problems. "Is the pitch of my voice too high?" "Does my son stutter?" "Does my child have a hearing loss?" Other clinicians and teachers face similar problems. The answers to all of these questions is: Compared to what? How can one hope to approach or achieve adjustment to "normal" without a clear understanding of what is normal?

The Role of the Scientist

The scientist must have an awareness and intellectual curiosity to understand the obvious—that which is taken for granted, e.g., light and vision, sound and hearing, speech production and perception, language. The communicative scientist must possess special knowledge in physical, biological, and behavioral sciences and in quantitative and experimental methods. When facts are incomplete, the scientist utilizes theory to help understand systems or behavior and its modification.

Basic scientists explore fundamental questions in an effort to comprehend normal processes. How is speech produced and understood? What are the processes by which information is transduced from neurolinguistic to physiologic levels? What are the processes by which the ear transduces speech sounds to neural impulses (encoded)? How are the neural impulses perceived as speech (decoded)? Even though speakers do not produce identical sound patterns when they pronounce the same words and their vocal quality and accents differ, the words are, nonetheless, usually understood.

Scientists and engineers have "taught" machines to speak. Although this synthetic speech characteristically might be associated with "robot" speech as heard on TV science fiction programs, it is intelligible. Machines thus far have not been "taught" to understand speech, with the exception of very limited aplications. In fact, this would appear to be an impossible task had it not been demonstrated in a workable model—the human brain. The brain has a capacity, which existing machines lack, to use linguistic and other clues stored in its "memory bank" to understand speech.

Answers to these questions are important for the communications industry as well as for understanding speech and hearing and related disorders in humans. There is no shortage of research questions. Unfortunately, solutions often are lacking. Even so, communicative scientists have expanded horizons through basic research and have provided necessary understanding to investigate and solve practical problems.

Clinical, or applied, scientists and engineers must bridge the gap between the basic scientist and the practicing clinician if communicatively handicapped persons are to benefit. The clinical scientist must understand the pursuits and techniques of the basic scientist and clinician and have the knowledge and insight to meet the needs of the communicatively impaired. The task of the clinical scientist is to advance diagnosis and treatment through research. What can be done to restore vocal ability to persons who lose their larynx (laryngectomy) as a result of cancer? At present, artificial larynges sound harsh and mechanical. Applied scientists hope to develop an artificial larynx with a natural sound. (It should be noted that speech pathologists have developed techniques for teaching many laryngectomies how to speak, a topic discussed in Chapter 9.) Speech scientists and engineers have developed speech-compression devices which speed up the rate of speech by eliminating unessential acoustic information. Teachers of the blind have found that "compressed speech" recordings facilitate the presentation of information more so than Braille does. "Speech expansion," which slows the rate of speech, may be helpful for mentally retarded or persons with language problems. The work of applied scientists has led to improved diagnosis and treatment of articulation- and language-impaired persons through linguistic, behavioral, and physiologic research.

Parents and pediatricians, psychologists and teachers, as well as speech pathologists and audiologists, know how important it is to identify any special problems early in the life of a child. Children with sensory impairments must receive appropriate educational placement and training as early as possible. How can hearing problems be detected and quantified in infants? Communicative scientists have made great advances in their computer analyses of nerve and brain waves to determine which parts of the auditory system respond to sound. The hope is that this research eventually will permit early diagnosis and quantification of hearing problems in infants. What is the effect of noise or amplified music (rock and roll) on hearing? Scientists have established damage-risk criteria to indicate what intensities and kinds of noise may be damaging to the ear. Even though advances have been made, countless areas of research remain to be investigated. Much research has been done, much is in progress, and much remains to be done.

It is apparent that much of the work of basic as well as applied scientists has been motivated out of concern for persons who suffer communicative disorders. By example, it might be noted that Alexander Graham Bell (whose wife was deaf) developed the telephone from his efforts to construct an electronic amplification device for deaf persons. These concerns are shared by teachers and clinicians in speech and hearing, medicine, and psychology. Many clinical specialties and interdisciplinary activities have been developed in behalf of the communicatively handicapped.

The Role of the Clinician

The clinician must have an awareness and concern and the appropriate personality traits to assist fellow human beings. These human traits alone, however, will not provide the assistance needed by the communicatively handicapped. What are the special skills and knowledge that the speech or hearing clinician must have?

Speech and hearing involve physiological, neurological, and behavioral processes, any or all of which may be involved in a speech, language, or hearing disorder. These processes often are associated with other disorders; thus the clinician must have the knowledge and tools to distinguish among potential causal factors. To do so, the clinician must have knowledge of the anatomy, physiology, and neurology of all the mechanisms involved in speech, language, and hearing and how disorders or pathology of these mechanisms affect associated behaviors. Does the child with an articulation problem have a hearing loss, and if so, what effect might certain hearing losses have on speech? What effects do certain disorders of the speech mechanism, such as cleft palate (incomplete closure of the roof of the mouth), have on voice quality and articulation? What effect does brain damage have on language and speech production? What effect does middle-ear infection or a tumor of the auditory nerve have on hearing?

Clinicians from several professions must provide special expertise in answering these questions and planning appropriate treatment. The speech pathologist and the audiologist work closely to ascertain possible effects of hearing loss on speech. The speech pathologist also works closely with otolaryngologists (ear and throat physicians), oral and plastic surgeons, orthodontists, and others in diagnosing and treating disorders of the speech mechanism that affect voice and articulation. The speech pathologist's evaluation may be a determining factor in a decision on whether surgical or speech therapy procedures are necessary. The speech clinician may need to inform the orthodontist or oral surgeon of the effects of orofacial problems on speech production and must consult with laryngologists regarding voice production and laryngeal pathology. The speech or language pathologist must work in consultation with neurologists regarding patients with adult aphasia (loss of language function) associated with brain damage as a result of injury or stroke. The audiologist often works closely with the otologist and neurologist in determining the cause and treatment of hearing disorders. Often no medical treatment is possible, so the audiologist must provide for other types of rehabilitative measures. Numerous problems exist which involve many

19

clinicians interested in different aspects of speech and hearing. Nurses, parents, psychologists, and teachers also commonly encounter these problems and need to be aware of their causes and treatment.

As noted earlier, speech, language, and hearing disorders involve behavioral as well as physiological processes and anatomical structure. Since spoken language and its perception pervade most aspects of our educational and social pursuits, parents, teachers, psychologists as well as speech pathologists and audiologists need to understand speech and hearing as a behavioral phenomenon. To do so, speech and hearing clinicians and those in related professions must have knowledge of sensory and developmental psychology, principles of motivation and learning, and abnormal psychology. In addition to this background, special clinical skills and knowledge are required to evaluate these behavioral phenomena as they pertain to speech, language, and hearing problems. Does the child with an articulation or voice problem have inadequate intelligence to develop language normally? Does the child have a poor speech model, imitating someone with poor speech? What is the child's level of maturity; is she or he motivated or encouraged to develop good speech?

The same questions may be considered in assessing the child with a language problem. What is the child's vocabulary and other language abilities, and how do they compare to those of other children of the same age (normal)? Is language a necessary and rewarded activity in the child's environment? What are the effects of rehabilitative measures and teaching on speech and language in the hearing-impaired individual? Is the child or aged person motivated to use a hearing aid? Behavioral aspects are important to the evaluation and treatment of adults as well as children with communicative disorders.

Parents as well as speech and hearing clinicians, psychologists, and teachers must provide special knowledge and skills in answering these questions and planning appropriate training. The role of the parent is particularly important in providing an appropriate environment and providing motivation to the child. The speech and hearing clinician must consult with the psychologist and teacher to assess intelligence, educational level, and achievement. The psychologist may need to evaluate the emotional and psychological status of the child. Interaction among the various specialists and a child's parents often is necessary to overcome behavioral problems associated with communicative disorders.

Conclusion

The educational and training demands for professionals to serve the communicatively impaired are great, but so are the rewards. The speech pathologist may help lead an aphasic patient from the trauma and despair of sudden loss of the ability to use or understand language. The speech pathologist may develop speech in the speechless laryngectomee or work with the psychologist to restore voice in a person suffering from hysterical aphonia (loss of voice as a result of psychological trauma). The evaluation of the audiologist may be critical in working with parents, pediatricians, psychologists, and speech pathologists in determining whether a child is mentally retarded, hearing-impaired, aphasic, or emotionally disturbed. Selection of a hearing aid and aural rehabilitation may permit a child and his or her teacher to achieve educational objectives or an adult to maintain his or her job and role in society.

The need for professionals to serve the communicatively impaired is a great one. Abnormal speech and hearing are frequently handicapping, sometimes devastating. As with other disabilities, this fact can be understood fully only by those so impaired. The communicatively handicapped require more than we presently can provide. The challenge to the communicative scientist and clinician and related professionals is a great one.

Glossary

Audiologist: A person who studies normal hearing and hearing disorders, evaluates people's hearing, and provides nonmedical rehabilitation.

Codification: The organization of a set of symbols arbitrarily used to represent words or concepts to convey meaning.

Communication: The transmission and exchange of information. Communication may be accomplished in many ways: biological systems, such as speech and hearing; machines; mass communication; and others.

Dyadic communication: Interaction that integrates two communication units into a single system. In speech and hearing, dyadic communication is a behavioral interaction.

Hearing: The sensory perception of sound, including the perception and comprehension of speech. Sounds are analyzed and encoded by the ear and decoded by the brain.

Language: In a general sense, language is any means—vocal or other—of expressing and understanding thoughts, ideas, or feelings.

Sensory feedback: Input to the body's sense organs, e.g., the auditory reception of one's own spoken language.

Servosystem: A self-regulating or self-controlling system. It may or may not be self-starting or stopping, but it controls its own operation.

Speech: The process of encoding a linguistic message by producing coded sound patterns which carry meaning.

Speech pathologist: A person who studies normal speech and language, evaluates speech and language disorders, and provides nonmedical rehabilitation.

Theory: In science, theory is a highly developed conceptual construct established through rigorous evaluation of facts, possible relationships among variables, and proof of many hypotheses. (A concept below the level of theory, a hypothesis is a conjecture put forth as a possible explanation of a certain phenomenon.)

Transduction: A process of changing from one form of energy to another, e.g., changing from acoustical to electrical energy.

Study Questions

1. What is communication and how is it accomplished?
2. What is the relationship between speech and language? Is speech a part of language, or is language a part of speech?
3. Explain how speech and hearing function as a servosystem and in particular how the ear functions as a component of the speaking system.
4. Speech and hearing can be described in physiological terms and also in behavioral terms. Distinguish between speech and hearing as a physiological system and as a behavioral system.
5. What concept does dyadic communication add to the traditional observation of two people talking to each other?
6. What are the implications of feedback in normal and disordered speech and language?
7. What are the normal processes that occur in speech production and auditory perception and comprehension of speech?
8. What are some problems that might be studied by the speech and hearing scientist in normal and disordered speech, language, and hearing?
9. What is the role of the audiologist? Distinguish that role from related professions.
10. What is the role of the speech pathologist? Distinguish that role from related professions.
11. What is the relationship among the basic scientist, applied scientist, and the clinician in speech and hearing?

Bibliography

CHERRY, C., *On Human Communication: A Review, a Survey, and a Criticism*, Cambridge, Mass.: M.I.T. Press, 1957.

CLEVENGER, T., AND J. MATTHEWS, *The Speech Communication Process*, Glenview, Ill.: Scott, Foresman, 1971.

CUTTING, J. E., AND J. F. KAVANAGH, "On the Relationship of Speech to Language," *ASHA* **17** (1975):500–506.

DENES, P. B., AND E. N. PINSON, *The Speech Chain,* New York: Bell Telephone Laboratories, 1968.

FAIRBANKS, G., "A Theory of the Speech Mechanism as a Servo-System," *J. Speech Hearing Dis.* **19** (1954):133–139.

MCDONALD, E. T., *Articulation Testing and Treatment: A Sensory-Motor Approach,* Pittsburgh: Stanwix House, 1964.

MYSAK, E. D., *Speech Pathology and Feedback Theory,* Springfield, Ill.: Charles C. Thomas, 1966.

NATIONAL ADVISORY NEUROLOGICAL DISEASE AND STROKE COUNCIL, *Human Communication and Its Disorders—An Overview,* Bethesda: National Institutes of Health, Public Health, 1969.

SMITH, A. G., *Communication and Culture,* New York: Holt, Rinehart and Winston, 1966.

VAN BERGEIJK, W. A., J. R. PIERCE, AND E. E. DAVID, *Waves and the Ear,* Garden City, N.Y.: Doubleday, 1960.

VAN RIPER, C., AND J. V. IRWIN, *Voice and Articulation,* Englewood Cliffs, N.J.: Prentice-Hall, 1958.

23

CHAPTER 2
Overview

Language is a primary means of communication. In this chapter we will look at language and how it functions. Speech sounds, word formation, sentence structure, and meaning will be considered. A particular perspective on language—linguistics—will be introduced. You will see that language is very complex—more so than you may have thought, perhaps—and also a highly organized system. Linguistics is a scientific discipline, although different linguists approach the study of language in different ways. A little background in linguistics will be helpful in considering language disorders later in the book; however, the study of language alone is not enough to understand communicative disorders. Language involves biological, psychological, and social processes, in addition to words, sounds, and sentences. With this information in hand, we will then focus on children's language acquisition. The stages that children go through as they develop skill in language will be outlined. We will note the importance of understanding as well as speaking and the interrelationship between intellectual development and language development. The chapter will conclude with a look at two environmental influences on language acquisition—the family and the peer group. Language is an aspect of being human that gives us striking advantages over other creatures. We invite you to a closer look at language and how it's acquired.

Robert D. Hubbell, Ph.D.
California State University, Sacramento

Language

Introduction

People communicate in many ways. Gesture, posture, facial expression, and the spoken voice are but a few of the ways we send and receive messages. In fact, all behavior has the potential of communicating some message. If I stand at a crosswalk and watch the oncoming traffic, an observer can "read" something about me just from this behavior: I want to cross the street, but I'm waiting until the cars have passed. With a closer look, one might be able to tell whether I'm in a hurry. Similarly, one can often tell much about other people by their clothes. Formal or casual clothes, recreational or work clothes can often be easily identified. Facial expression and posture also communicate a great deal to the observer. For example, they are often a source of information about whether one is happy or sad, eager or bored. A speaker's facial expression and tone of voice are used to help interpret the words being spoken. While I'm talking, my face is giving additional messages about such things as whether you should take me seriously, whether you should respond, and whether I'm pleased with what I'm saying.

Human **communication,** then, can be defined as exchange of information between people. This idea of information exchange embodies two further ideas. First, the information involved doesn't have to be correct or true. Any poker player knows that. Second, an individual will transmit information unintentionally, as well as intentionally. In fact, it can be said that it is impossible not to communicate. Even by refusing to communicate, one is communicating. The point is that one can't help but exude information simply by being alive and doing things. For further information on this view of communication, including a fascinating analysis of Albee's play *Who's Afraid of Virginia Woolf?*, see Watzlawick, Beavin, and Jackson (1967).

From this perspective, communication consists of many individual bits of behavior, usually with several occurring at once. In order to interpret this complex of information, some sort of organization is needed. A primary means of organization in human communication is **language.** Through language we have a set of symbols to represent the things we wish to communicate and a method for combining these symbols into coherent statements expressing what we have in mind.

If all behavior implies communication, language can be seen as a subset of all behavior that involves various vocal activities used for communication. Thus, for example, we can make many different sounds with the vocal mechanism, but only certain sounds are used to form words. These sounds are called vowels and consonants. Other sounds, such as coughing and humming, are still communicative, but they are not part of language per se. Not all experts define language in terms of behavior, though. Some see language as the system of rules underlying such behavior; in other words, language is a set of rules which governs our use of vocabulary, **syntax,** and other aspects of spoken communication.

There are many types of language: sign language, bee language, body language, even computer language. We will be concerned primarily with human verbal language, commonly defined as an arbitrary system of symbols. Let us look at each of the terms in this definition separately. A symbol is something that stands for something else. Thus the spoken word "tree" or the printed form of that word can be used to refer to one of those things with a trunk, branches, and leaves. The term "system" indicates that these symbols can be combined in regular ways to express more complicated ideas. The system of language is the set of rules for the construction of words and sentences. Finally, language is arbitrary. There is no inherent relation between a word and what it stands for. Words mean what they do by convention. In principle, for example, there is no reason why we couldn't call a tree a "glimp," but we don't. By common usage we agree on the term "tree."

In addition to providing a relatively efficient way of organizing communication, language provides a powerful tool for handling abstractions. Through language we can discuss beauty, truth, fiction, Babylonian civilization, Martians, and Tinkerbell. In a very real sense, language permits us to expand our horizons way beyond what we have personally experienced. Similarly, language is a primary means of dealing with concepts and problem solving. In short, although language and thinking are not the same, language is the most important tool in much of our intellectual activity.

If language behavior is a subset of communicative behavior in general, speech may be seen as a subset of language behavior. From this view, speech is defined as vocal-auditory language—language that is spoken and heard. In other words, speech is the spoken expression of meaning in a language system. The term "speech" is also sometimes used to refer to all the sounds made by the vocal mechanism. In particular, the vocal sounds made by babies before they've learned any real language are often called "infant speech."

Linguistics and Language

Linguistics is the scientific study of language. In general, linguists are interested in discovering the rules for the formation of words and sentences in any particular language. This set of rules is called the **grammar** of the language. Linguists use the term "grammar" to refer to descriptions of how people actually talk or to the rule system that underlies the production and comprehension of utterances. This is a different approach from the traditional grammar book, which is used to teach students how to talk "correctly." Linguists are descriptive, whereas traditional grammar books are prescriptive.

Linguists concentrate on spoken language, not the written form. This focus is necessary because most languages do not have a written form. There are perhaps three to five thousand languages alive in the world today. Considerably less than a thousand have been written down, many of these only by linguists. Further, in the history of language, the spoken form far antedates any written form. This is not to say that writing systems are ignored, only that they are a separate branch of study.

As you consider speech and language in this book, it will be helpful to keep in mind this distinction between the spoken and written language. Consider the following words:

> though
> bough
> through
> thought
> tough
> cough
> hiccough

Say each word out loud carefully. Each of these words contains the sequence "ough," but in each word the pronunciation of this sequence is different. This example illustrates the fact that often there is no obvious correspondence between spelling and pronunciation in English.

The study of language can be broken down into four areas: **phonology,** the study of speech sounds; **morphology,** the study of words and word forms; syntax, the study of phrases and sentences; and **semantics,** the study of meaning. Each of these areas will be discussed separately.

Phonology

Phonology is the study of phones, or the sounds we use in speaking. Consider this pair of words:

> bin
>
> pin

Each word is made up of three sounds. By changing the first sound, we change from one word to another. Thus /p/ and /b/ are distinctive sounds in English. They differentiate one word from another. Such sounds are called **phonemes.***

We use each speech sound many times a day as we talk. However, we do not produce the sound exactly the same way each time. Repeat each of the following words out loud, several times, quickly:

> tea
>
> butter

Most speakers of American English will pronounce the /t/ in these two words

---

*   Letters representing phonemes are placed between slashes to indicate that they refer to phonemes, not letters of the alphabet.

differently. In *tea* the /t/ includes an audible burst of air as the sound is produced. In *butter* it does not. In fact, most people pronounce the /t/ in *butter* as a lightly produced /d/. The point is that although the two productions do not sound the same, we recognize both of them as versions of the /t/ phoneme. (Don't let the two t's in *butter* confuse the issue. In the spoken form there's only one. In these two examples, consider only the spoken form. Forget that you know how to spell.)

Consider another example. Say the following phrase as an American waiter might say it: *Very good, sir*. Now say it as a British butler might say it in a "B" movie. You might come out with something like this: *Veddy good, suh*. Listen to the /r/ phoneme as you repeat these utterances. In the American waiter version, both productions of /r/ will sound much the same. In the British butler version, the first /r/ will sound something like a /d/ and the second something like an "uh." Neither will sound like the American waiter's /r/. Again, the point is that we recognize all three as belonging to the /r/ phoneme.

These examples help to illustrate what a phoneme is. A phoneme is a group of sounds considered the same for the purpose of distinguishing between words. To put it the other way around, the differences between versions of a particular phoneme are ignored. A phoneme then is an abstraction. It is a category which includes all variants of a particular sound. Thus both variations of /t/ are recognized as representing the /t/ phoneme, and all three variations of /r/ are recognized as representing the /r/ phone. Consequently, in our examples the /t/ phoneme consists of two **allophones,** the /r/ of three.

Which allophone you use in a specific instance depends partly on which speech sounds precede and follow the sound in question and partly on which particular **dialect** of English you are speaking. More specifically, some allophones are said to be in "free variation." That is, it doesn't matter which allophone is used in a particular occurrence of a phoneme. Thus I can say "bet" by ending the word when the airflow is stopped by the /t/, or I can end it with an audible burst as the /t/ is released. In other cases, allophones of a phoneme are said to be in "complimentary distribution." In these situations one allophone must occur in certain contexts and other allophones in other contexts. For example, speakers of English cannot use the allophone of /t/ that occurs in the word "butter" to begin the word "tea." In studying the sound system of a language and identifying its phonemes, a linguist must take all this variation into consideration.

There are 43 phonemes in American English. In order to represent all of these phonemes on paper, dictionaries provide pronunciation guides, which generally employ our standard 26-letter alphabet with many special markings (diacritics) above the letters. Linguists have attempted to devise phonetic alphabets which provide separate symbols for each sound without extensive use of diacritics. In addition, these alphabets are designed to handle the phonemes of many different languages. Most speech pathologists have adopted the International Phonetic Alphabet. This system is very helpful, particularly in the study of articulation disorders (see Chapter 8).

The phonemes in any language are classified according to how they are produced by the vocal mechanism and how they sound. The most general distinction is between vowels and consonants. In terms of production, the vocal tract is open to a greater degree for a vowel than for a consonant. The air flows freely through the vocal tract in a vowel, but the flow is constricted in a consonant.

There are two large classifications of consonants. If some point in the vocal tract is constricted so there is only a small opening, a sound will be generated as the air rushes past. In principle, this sound is similar to the noise you can make by holding a piece of paper very close to your lips and blowing on it. These consonants are called **fricatives.** Examples of English fricatives are /s/, /f/, and /sh/.

The second classification of consonants is the **stop.** A stop is produced by momentarily closing the vocal tract completely at some point, allowing no air flow at all. Examples of English stops are /p/, /t/, and /k/. In normal speech, stops are produced so rapidly that the speaker is often not aware that the air flow has been broken. Say a word with a stop in the middle, such as "upper," in slow motion. You can feel that the air flow is blocked by the lips just before the /p/ is released.

Most consonants are produced by the tongue, lips, teeth, and palate. However, the larynx also plays a part. Take a big breath and make a long /z/ out loud: /zzzzzz/. While you are producing this sound, feel your Adam's apple with your fingertips. You will feel a vibration coming from your larynx. The sound /z/ is a **voiced** sound because the vocal folds are vibrating. Now do the same with /ssssss/. There is no vibration, because /s/ is **unvoiced,** or "voiceless." The vocal folds do not vibrate. Thus we have not only stops and fricatives, but also voiced stops, voiceless stops, voiced fricatives, and voiceless fricatives. There are several other kinds of consonants as well. Further discussion of the production of speech sounds will be found in Chapter 3.

Morphology

Morphology is the study of the minimal meaningful units of language and the minimal grammatically pertinent units of language. Such a unit is called a **morpheme.** Every word contains one or more morphemes. The following words contain one morpheme each, because they cannot be divided into smaller units and retain meaning:

car
boy
purple

The following words contain two morphemes, because each word can be divided into two units, each of which retains a meaning of its own:

> cookbook
> baseball
> sailboat

The words cited so far are examples of **free morphemes,** that is, morphemes which can stand alone.

There are also **bound morphemes,** which can occur only in combination with other morphemes. For example, there is the *un-* in the following words:

> undo
> uncover
> unhappy

Note that the *un-* has the same meaning in each word—a negation of the rest of the word. In the same way, many words contain several morphemes:

> un-know-ing-ly
> help-less-ness
> cup-cake-s

Just as there are phonemes and allophones, so too there are morphemes and allomorphs. The standard example in English is the plural morpheme. Read the following words out loud:

> books
> tubs
> buses

In spoken form, all three words end differently: *books* with /s/, *tubs* with /z/, and *buses* with a short vowel something like "uh" and then /z/. All three endings mean the same: "more than one." Thus these words demonstrate three allomorphs of the plural morpheme. Which allomorph is used depends on what kind of consonant precedes it. The allomorph /s/ is voiceless and is used after voiceless consonants. The allomorph /z/ follows voiced phonemes. The word *buses* already ends with /s/, so adding the /s/ allomorph would not be heard. Therefore, a little "uh" is added to separate them, but since it is voiced, it is followed by /z/.

In summary, morphology is the study of the rules for the formation and combination of morphemes in various languages. The examples above merely illustrate a few of the principles involved. From the last example it can be seen that the study of morphology cannot be entirely separated from the study of phonology.

Syntax

As was said earlier, language is a means of organizing communication, a method for combining words into meaningful statements. This function operates at all levels of language: combining phonemes into morphemes, joining morphemes, combining morphemes into phrases and sentences, and combining phrases and sentences. A basic function of this organizational process is to show what is related to what in the sentence. Consider the utterance: *John Mary bit*. It is hard to tell just what this utterance means, though we may have some ideas about it. Rearranging the words according to the rules of English syntax, we could get: *Mary bit John*. Now, through the syntax, we know that Mary did the biting. The relationship between Mary and John is clear. (Well, as far as who bit whom, it is.)

The study of syntax is based on distributional evidence. The linguist attempts to discover which elements of the sentence can go in which positions in the sentence. To borrow a phrase from linguistics, the elements of a language are described according to their "privileges of occurrence." In English, for example, proper nouns can occur as subjects of sentences. In the example above, the subject came first in the sentence. Thus we have a class of words (proper nouns) and information about where this class can appear in a sentence (first position). In addition, we have information about the function of this class in that position. Proper nouns in first position function as subjects. By a similar analysis we see that proper nouns in final position function as objects. Although this analysis is incomplete (for example, "Detroit" is a proper noun, but it would hardly fit in our sample sentence), it will suffice for present purposes.

Note also that the form of the past tense of "bite" in our example is a morphological matter. Thus syntax cannot be separated entirely from morphology any more than morphology can from phonology. In general, it is not accurate to look at phonemes as the building blocks of morphology and morphemes as the building blocks of syntax. Rather, they form an interlocking hierarchy.

A description of the syntax of a language is based on an analysis of hundreds of sentences elicited from a native speaker of that language. These sentences are elicited in such a way as to reveal the patterns of the language as efficiently as possible. This collection of sentences is called a **corpus.** The same general technique is followed in studying phonology or morphology. Through analysis of this corpus, the linguist writes a grammar of the language under study. The grammar is usually written as a series of rules, stated in a form reminiscent of algebraic formulas. These rules start with the most abstract—a general statement of how a sentence is constructed—and become increasingly specific in spelling out details.

Let us consider a very simple example of how the syntax of a set of utterances might be analyzed. Supposing we collect the following corpus from a young child:

doll
that doll
my doll
book
that book
my book

If we arrange the items in this corpus so that recurring items are placed in the same columns, we have:

doll

that doll

my doll

book

that book

my book

We can now discuss privileges of occurrence. We note that there are two word positions and that there is no utterance in which the word order is reversed. The words in the first column occur only in first position and those in the second column only in second position. Thus we can say that there are two classes of words—those that occur in first position and those that occur in second position, or Class One (C_1) and Class Two (C_2), respectively. We can now write a rule that shows where these two word classes can occur in relation to each other:

$$S \to C_1 + C_2,$$

where "S" stands for "sentence." (Although these utterances may not be complete sentences by adult standards, they were complete utterances by the child, and we will label them as sentences.)

The analysis is not yet complete, however. Doubtless you have noted that whereas a Class Two word occurs in every utterance in the corpus, some utterances do not contain a Class One word. In technical terms, Class Two is obligatory, that is, it must always occur; and Class One is optional, that is, the speaker has the choice of whether or not to use a Class One word. We show the optional character of Class One by enclosing it in parentheses:

$$S \to (C_1) + C_2.$$

This process may seem very simple-minded, but remember that the sample corpus is very simple. The point is that a set of rules can be written that represents the structure of a set of utterances.

To make our set of rules complete, we need to specify what is included in Class One and in Class Two:

$$S \to (C_1) + C_2$$
$$C_1 \to that, my$$
$$C_2 \to doll, book.$$

We now have a set of rules that completely represents the original corpus. All the utterances in the corpus can be generated from this set of rules, but no additional utterances can.

The analysis so far has been based purely on describing the order in which the words occurred, without any reference to what the words mean or how they function in the utterances. Because these latter aspects are important in understanding the structure of the utterances in the corpus, most linguists would make an interpretation about the functions of the two classes based on the meanings of the words in each class. Thus we note that "doll" and "book" are both names of things. On this basis, we could call Class Two "Topic" (T), because it's a reasonable guess that "book" and "doll" are indeed the topics of the child's utterances. Similarly, we could call Class One "Modifier" (M), because these words appear to modify the topic words. More precision in these labels would not be prudent with this small sample. With these considerations in mind, we write our set of rules a final time:

$$S \rightarrow (M) + T$$
$$M \rightarrow \text{that, my}$$
$$T \rightarrow \text{doll, book.}$$

It should be emphasized that this corpus is much too short and much too simple to be of any use in a linguistic analysis. It is used here merely to illustrate the process of abstracting a set of syntactic rules from a corpus. The important points are as follows. (1) We have derived a set of rules specifying where each word can occur and which words are optional. (2) This set of rules also specifies the function of each word. Note that privileges of occurrence and optionality are determined by inspecting the data, but that function is determined by interpreting the data. (3) Finally, the entire analysis is based on the corpus, that is, what the child actually said, rather than on any ideas we may have about how to construct sentences. For a more extended, but still simplified, example of this type, see Hubbell (1972).

Schools of Thought in Linguistics

The matter of the interpretation of linguistic data has become an important aspect of linguistic theory. Linguists differ on how freely they should make interpretations beyond the observable data. The approach to linguistics described so far is usually called **structural linguistics.** Structuralists are relatively conservative in the interpretations they make. They emphasize an objective analysis of language, making as few assumptions as possible, sometimes with relatively little emphasis on meaning. Their focus is on actually observed utterances.

There are several other schools of thought in linguistics, of which the most well known is **generative grammar.** Generative grammar is more abstract and theoretical than structuralism. The whole approach of the generative grammarian is based on interpretation. Not restricted to the analysis of objective data, such as a corpus of utterances, the generative grammarian's analysis is extended to include an in-depth consideration of the meanings of those utterances and people's judgments of whether or not those utterances are grammatically acceptable. The focus is on the abstract structure of language rather than on the analysis of actual utterances.

Thus a generative grammarian may analyze a sentence in terms of the morphologic and syntactic relationships reflected in the strings of words actually uttered, called the **surface structure,** and in terms of the underlying structure of the sentence, called the **deep structure.** Similarly, generative grammarians make a distinction between what they call **competence,** that is, everything one knows about one's language, and **performance,** or what one actually does with language.

The two categories—competence and performance—are not the same. Consider a simple card game. Each player knows the rules of the game, the name of each of the 52 cards in the deck, and perhaps some strategies which can be used in an attempt to win. All of this information is part of the player's competence for that card game. During the game, though, the player may forget some of the cards that already have been played or may get confused about strategy. These problems are not in the player's knowledge of the game (competence), but in performance, that is, use of that knowledge. Thus performance is affected by psychological factors such as memory and motivation, whereas competence is the "pure" knowledge of the game and how to play it.

Generative grammarians apply this same distinction in studying language. For example, one may have the grammatical knowledge (competence) to understand a 1000-word sentence, but be unable to actually utter or comprehend such a sentence simply because of being unable to keep the whole thing in memory. It can be seen that the study of competence is ultimately based entirely on interpretation. That is, one can never study competence directly. It can be studied only by speculating on what knowledge lies behind various aspects of performance.

In summary, the generative grammarians' willingness to theorize and speculate has enabled them to make many insightful hypotheses concerning the nature of language. At the same time it has taken them farther and farther from the objective analysis of the structural linguists. There has been considerable debate about which approach is "better," but perhaps it would be more useful simply to consider them as representing two different approaches to the study of language and knowledge in general, the one more objective and the other more intuitive.

As you will discover in the chapters on clinical disorders and their management, clinicians and teachers are forced to operate primarily with objective data because they must deal directly with what their clients or students are actually doing. For a more thorough introduction to linguistics and the issues that have been raised above, you may wish to look at Bolinger (1975), Lyons (1968), Palmer (1971), or Langacker (1973).

Semantics

The last area of linguistics to be discussed is semantics, the study of meaning. If there were no meaning, no content, there would be no point in using language. Meaning is the bridge between the thoughts and ideas of individuals and the sequence of vocal sounds they produce to symbolize those thoughts and ideas. Words symbolize concepts, and concepts represent segments of reality.

In general, there are two kinds of meaning: denotative and connotative. The denotative meaning of a word refers to its referent in reality or in somebody's conceptual field representing reality. The denotative meaning of a word is analogous to its dictionary definition. The connotative meaning of a word refers to the emotional reactions and associations one has to that word. The denotative meaning of "fire," for example, might refer to the chemical process of combustion or to flames consuming a house; the connotative meaning of "fire" might be related to fear or fascination. The denotative meaning of "rose" might be a pink-petalled, perfumed flower; the connotative meaning might be "he loves me."

One problem in studying the meanings of words is that some words don't seem to have any meaning of their own, such as *the, if, some,* and *a.* Rather, they take on their meanings from the context in which they are used. Another problem is that sometimes a sentence means more than a combination of the meanings of the words it contains. The total is more than the sum of the parts. This phenomenon became a problem during attempts to develop machine translators from one language to another. The machine could translate the meaning of each word, but could not always translate the meaning of the sentence as a whole. Poetry is an obvious example of this situation.

The study of meaning is extremely complex. Research in this area is so varied that one is reminded of the story of the blind men and the elephant. A good part of the problem is that meaning exists in the mind, and so far our means for exploring the mind are limited. Nevertheless, meaning is at the very core of language. Meaning is the heart of all communication.

Psycholinguistics and Sociolinguistics

The study of the individual as a language user is called *psycholinguistics.* The term reflects an interdisciplinary effort to relate linguistic theory and psychological theory in the study of how the individual produces and comprehends language. One area of interest in psycholinguistics is the psychological reality of grammar. Linguists describe the grammar of a language in terms of various levels, such as phonology and syntax, and in terms of systems of rules, such as those for constructing a declarative sentence. Through such hierarchies of rules and levels, linguists impose a structure on language. That is, linguistic descriptions are not handed down on stone tablets. They are invented by linguists. Psycholinguists want to know if the linguists' systems for organizing language have any psychological reality. In other words, does the mind process language through such structures as phonemes, morphemes, and grammatical rules? Or does the mind process language in some other way, perhaps related to the sequence of words or their information load? Although these questions are not yet resolved, it appears that we do behave as if we know a set of grammatical rules, but it may be that we construct our sentences more on the basis of the meanings involved than on purely syntactic rules. For a good summary of psycholinguistic work in this area, see Fodor, Bever, and Garrett (1974).

Another important area in psycholinguistics is the study of specific psychological processes involved in using language. These processes, often called psycholinguistic skills, are related to how information is processed in the human nervous system. Of interest are questions about comprehension and expression, memory, and the relationships between various sensory modes. How, for example, do we distinguish among the various speech sounds we hear? How do the content and organization of a sentence affect our ability to comprehend or say it? How can we comprehend a sentence that is longer than we can remember? The answers to such questions have important implications for specialists working with language disorders. In fact, some teachers and speech pathologists base their work with language-disordered children and adults on a careful analysis of each client's psycholinguistic skills. A test for these skills will be described in Chapter 11. Psycholinguistic skills are also important in articulation and aphasia, as discussed in Chapters 8 and 12. For a view of psycholinguistic skills developed by educators, see Kirk and Kirk (1971), especially Chapter Two. For a general discussion of human information processing, see Lindsay and Norman (1972).

Children's language acquisition is another focus of attention in psycholinguistics. Here the emphasis is on not only describing the sequence of language development in the child, but also determining how language acquisition occurs. It has been argued, for example, that the principles of learning that have been well established over years of research in psychological laboratories are insufficient for explaining how children acquire language. Some psycholinguists have therefore proposed that children must be born with a predisposition for learning language or that the basic structures of language are somehow prewired in the brain. This proposal is a variant of the "nature/nurture" controversy in psychology. The problem here is that brain function changes as the child interacts with the environment. It follows that in considering child development, it is difficult to separate nature (the makeup of the child's body and brain, which would include any prewiring that might exist) from nurture (the influence of environment, which would include language-learning experiences). The two are continually affecting and changing each other. For some interesting theoretical views on how children acquire language, see Braine (1971), Slobin (1971), and Fodor, Bever, and Garrett (1974). The rapid development of psycholinguistics has provided a rich source of material for those who are interested in training children with language disorders. Some applications of this material will be discussed in Chapter 11.

The term "sociolinguistics" refers to a similar cooperative endeavor between sociology and linguistics. Sociolinguists study the interplay between social structure and language. They are interested in the many ways in which social status and group identification are reflected, complimented, and enhanced by differences in language usage. Of particular interest in the United States are the various dialects, or regional varieties of English, such as those used by black Americans. Another area of great interest is the study of bilingualism, or the use of more than one language by individuals and groups, such as American Indians and Mexican-Americans. Children who are not skilled in the standard English dialect because they speak some other dialect or language present a special challenge to speech pathologists and educators. In designing training programs for these children, we must decide which form of language to use—standard English or the dialect employed by a subgroup. There has been considerable debate about this matter.

Another area of sociolinguistics particularly relevant to speech pathology and education is the relationship between how one talks and the situation the person is in. It is clear that people do talk differently in various situations. This fact can be a problem for the professional who wants to evaluate a child's language skill, but sees the child in only one setting, usually a school or clinic. We will consider this topic in Chapter 11 when we discuss the evaluation of children's language skill. For interesting collections of papers in sociolinguistics, see Fishman (1968) and Labov (1972).

One sociolinguistic unit of particular interest in considering speech, hearing, and language disorders is the family. Children learn to talk in their families. Many people of all ages with problems of communicative disorders do much of their communicating in their families. The family functions as a source for learning language, a context in which much verbal and nonverbal communication takes place, and a place in which many attitudes about one's self as a communicator develop. We will return to the family later in this chapter and again in Chapter 11.

Linguistic description is but one of many ways in which language is studied. That is, although language can be thought of as an abstract system of and by itself, the use of language involves much more. In particular, anyone who uses language to communicate is involved in two overlapping sets of processes. The first is internal and includes memory, perception, and thought. It is the area of human information processing and psycholinguistics. The second set is external and involves social and interpersonal factors and the use of language to deal with other people. It is the area of interpersonal communication and sociolinguistics.

At the same time, these two sets of processes do not occur in isolation from each other. They are mutually interdependent. This fact is of prime importance in considering disorders of speech, hearing, and language. A hearing loss affects social behavior as well as language comprehension. An impairment of language affects learning and thought processes as well as interpersonal communication.

The mutual influence between internal processes and external processes is also important in studying how children normally acquire language. It is to the topic of children's language development that we now turn.

Children's Language Acquisition

Development During the First Year

Children begin communicating at a very early age. After a few weeks of life they may stop crying when picked up. After one month or so, many mothers can begin to tell from the cry what the baby is complaining about. Around the same time the baby begins to smile. The mother responds to these behaviors by picking the infant up, talking and playing with the baby, as well as feeding, changing, and generally caring for the baby. Of course, there is considerable variation in the ways mothers or caretakers respond to their babies, but because babies cannot take care of themselves, all babies get some response.

Thus interaction between parent and child begins to develop with the first feeding and changing. This early communication involves a great deal of physical contact. Physical communication is important primarily in the communication of affect—of feelings and emotions. Clearly this early communication by the baby is gross and unfocused. It seems safe to assume that much of it is not purposefully communicative. Its importance lies in the fact that there is two-way communication of some sort between mother and child even during infancy.

At one month or so, most babies begin to develop some sort of pleasure sounds in addition to their cries. These **cooing** sounds are vowellike in nature. Gradually over the next three or four months, these vocalizations become more frequent and varied as they develop into vocal play. At this stage, often called **babbling,** the child is using both vowellike and consonantlike sounds. At first these sounds cannot be called phonemes of any language, but gradually they get closer to the phonemes of the language spoken in the child's environment. Vocal play continues throughout childhood and remains in adulthood in such forms as singing in the shower, puns, and nonsense songs.

At about six months many children begin to repeat syllables, that is, to imitate their own babbling. This behavior implies that babies are aware of their own utterances, at least in some form. (More will be said about perception in a later section.) Some people have interpreted this imitation, called **lalling,** to mean that some sort of feedback system is now operating in the baby. The reasoning is that in order to repeat an utterance two or three times, a child has to be aware of what she or he said the first time. This is an important development, because there is little doubt that feedback plays a role in the control of mature speech.

Between six and nine months, many babies begin to imitate utterances from other people in the environment. This process, called **echolalia,** is clear evidence that children can now differentiate at least some remarks made to them and have sufficient control of their vocal mechanisms to imitate those remarks, at least in gross fashion. This imitation is accompanied by and probably preceded by imitation of the children by the parents. It's not hard to imagine a situation in which a child makes an utterance which the mother hears as "mama." The mother then repeats "mama, mama" back to the child, perhaps along with a cry of "Hey, Harry, Sally said her first word!" to her husband. In any case, it seems probable that through the mechanism of echolalia, the child might begin to direct vocal play more toward the sounds of the language spoken by the parents. The speech of some communicatively handicapped individuals may consist primarily of echolalia. These individuals usually do not appear to comprehend what they are saying, but they may imitate rather long sentences quite precisely.

Some children use an interesting type of vocal play called **jargon.** In young children, this stage may be described as "pretend conversation." The child will use "sentences," with inflectional patterns clearly representing statements, commands, and questions, but made up entirely of nonsense syllables. It is as if the child role plays, using language. Occasionally such a child will engage someone in a "conversation" and wait for a reply! Jargon is also seen in certain pathological cases in which the person attempts to talk but cannot produce intelligible, meaningful speech.

Babies seem to seek stimulation. As their motor skills begin to develop, they will watch, touch, mouth, listen to, and otherwise explore increasingly complex stimuli. At first the baby seeks stimulation indiscriminately, anywhere in the environment. Slowly attaching more and more attention on other human beings, the baby finally focuses on the mother or caretaker. This attachment on the mother develops at about the same time that echolalia appears. Thus after nine or ten months, parent and child are participating in a rather rich social exchange.

Many children utter their first words at approximately one year of age. Of course, the first word may not be a word in the adult sense, but it will be a recognizable utterance, used consistently with some referent. My son's first word was "eeee," which referred to anything to do with eating. After the first word, children's vocabularies begin to grow, slowly for the next half year or year and then more rapidly.

It is worth emphasizing that there is no hard-and-fast time schedule for the development of speech and language in children. Not all children exhibit all the stages of development that I have described. Some children do not utter their first words until after two years of age and develop normal speech. The age levels I have described reflect very general trends and are intended merely to add additional perspective. They should not be applied literally to measure a particular child's development.

Words and Concepts

As was mentioned earlier, words represent concepts or ideas. We do not know whether or not a child has to know a concept before learning the word for it. Nelson (1975) has argued convincingly that children can indeed form concepts they do not have words for and then later acquire the word; Werner and Kaplan (1964), by contrast, have argued that learning the word is a primary component of learning the concept.

Underlying this disagreement is the question of how children acquire concepts in the first place. Some experts feel that children develop concepts primarily through their own activity in manipulating and interacting with the environment. One can easily imagine concepts developing in this fashion without accompanying words. Others feel that concept acquisition is more of a perceptual process than a motor process. In either case, the provision of an appropriate word might highlight the important aspects of the concept for the child and thus provide a focus for organizing that concept.

The situation is further complicated by the fact that young children's concepts may be directly related to dealing with their environment and the people in it, but older children and adults have many concepts which have no basis beyond words, and they learn many concepts through language rather than through direct experience with the environment. However these matters get resolved, there is no doubt that the acquisition of words and the acquisition of concepts are interrelated in very complex ways.

Grammatical Development

Between one and a half and two years of age, most children begin combining words into longer utterances. That is, they begin developing a grammar, a set of rules for constructing sentences. Research in children's grammar has developed rapidly in the last 15 years. Recent studies in this area differ in a fundamental way from previous studies. In the earlier approach, the adult grammar was taken as the model, and children's language was studied from that viewpoint; children's utterances were compared with the adult grammar, and differences and developmental trends were noted. The current approach is to study children's utterances as if they were a foreign language, without reference to adult grammar. The linguist gathers a corpus, just as in studying any other language. With an adult informant the linguist can work efficiently, eliciting various types of constructions. Two-year-olds, however, do not respond as adults do. Therefore, the linguist must gather the corpus by following the child around and recording everything said. Even with this method, and the fact that it is difficult to get a large enough corpus, considerable strides have been made in describing young children's grammar.

Children's early sentences have been described as **telegraphic speech**, because they have much the same form a telegram has. In comparison with adult speech, important content words are retained and other words are dropped. It appears that children rarely combine words by chance in these utterances. The sentences they produce follow regular rules. However, they are the rules of the child's grammar, not the grammar of mature speakers.

Some students of children's grammar have proposed that children's two-word combinations are based on two classes of words: a topic class and a modifier class. (Sometimes these classes have been called "open" and "pivot," respectively.) As their names imply, the topic word names or identifies something, and the modifier says something about it: *my daddy; milk allgone*. The two classes can come in either order. You will recall that the topic-modifier construction was used earlier in this chapter to illustrate how grammatical rules are derived from a corpus. It is worth emphasizing once more that this construction is based on analysis and interpretation of what the child actually says, rather than on reference to adult ways of talking. There is always the possibility of error in such analysis, because one cannot ask the child if the interpretation is correct, as one can with an adult informant.

In increasing utterance length, the child sometimes takes a topic and modifier, treats them as a single unit, and says something about this unit with another modifier: *my daddy byebye; see milk allgone*. Thus the child is developing phrases within sentences. In similar fashion, the child continues to elaborate the grammar. In a relatively short time, say by age three and a half, the child is making rather complex utterances.

A surprising degree of uniformity in grammatical structure has been found in the descriptions of utterances from a number of children, some of them speaking languages other than English. However, it does not appear that these descriptions of utterances are equivalent to describing the child's grammar. The child is capable of more varied grammatical structures than may be demonstrated in expressive language. For example: *look mama* could be analyzed simply as modifier-topic. However, if observations are made of the child's behavior while this utterance is being produced, one can infer more about the grammar. Suppose the child says the remark above twice, in different circumstances: *look mama* (pointing at mother as she comes up the walk) and *look mama* (pulling at mother's sleeve and pointing at something else). The first is a declarative sentence in which the child remarks on seeing mother; the second is an imperative in which the child tells mother to look at something. Thus the topic-modifier analysis may oversimplify what the child knows about how to use language. Further, some children do not seem to use topic-modifier constructions at all. For further discussion of these matters, see Bloom (1970) and Braine (1971). The most extensive study of grammatical development is in Brown (1973).

We have seen in the example above that children can be given credit for knowing more elaborate grammars than their utterances directly demonstrate.

The key to this type of analysis is that the focus is not only on the utterances themselves, but also on the context in which each utterance occurs. Including the context in the analysis allows the linguist to guess at the child's intentions and therefore to interpret utterances as representing different sentence types, as in the example above. More broadly, this technique represents an attempt to study how meaning relates to children's sentence structures. Many experts now believe that the child's early sentences are constructed around the meaning the child wants to express, rather than on strictly grammatical categories. This idea makes sense intuitively, because we know that meaning is the heart of language. However, it puts us right back in the dilemma concerning how much interpretation is appropriate in linguistic analysis. If we restrict ourselves to describing what children say, we may miss some of the richness and meaning of their utterances. If we interpret children's utterances in terms of their meanings, we surely run a greater risk of making errors. Perhaps a combination of both approaches will prove most useful in the long run. In addition, studies of comprehension can provide a different type of information on how children deal with meaning.

Comprehension

So far, the discussion has focused on expression, the utterances that babies and children actually produce. However, the child has been developing comprehension skills at the same time. Researchers have found that babies as young as one month old have the auditory skill to differentiate between different phonemes. It is not known how much or in what ways the baby uses this skill. It is not until around ten months or so that babies begin to clearly demonstrate the rudiments of comprehension. Children at this age may respond to a few words, such as their name, "no," and perhaps a word for food. It is highly probable that they read the total situation rather than only the words spoken to them. A classic example is the parent's stern "no, no!" said while bending over the child, frowning, and shaking a finger. Still, comprehension does begin before the child starts to utter verbal expressions. In some ways comprehension remains ahead of expression throughout life. Adults' recognition vocabularies are always larger than their expressive vocabularies.

Studying comprehension has a singular advantage. We can limit the language stimuli to the area we are interested in. Instead of waiting for the child to say things and hoping that those utterances will be appropriate for our purposes, we can select the words and sentences the child will hear. Studying comprehension also has a singular disadvantage. We can never know if something is comprehended exactly as we intended it. We can only infer comprehension. We may interpret a child's behavior as showing comprehension of what was said, such as complying with a request or saying "I gotcha," or words to that effect.

We are back to interpretation again. Nevertheless, comprehension can be measured to a certain extent. This matter will be discussed further in Chapter 11.

In summary, we have seen that in the abstract, there is one unitary phenomenon: language. In actual use, however, there are two processes: comprehension and expression. The relationship between these two is not well understood. It is usually assumed that children's comprehension exceeds their expressive functioning. As was just mentioned, however, it is very difficult to test just what a small child does comprehend. The younger the child, the truer this is. Further, in order to comprehend a sentence, a child must have some knowledge of its elements and structure. In this case, why shouldn't the child be able to express that sentence as well as comprehend it? Perhaps comprehension requires only enough knowledge for recognition, whereas expression requires much more detailed knowledge.

The relationship between comprehension and expression is important to teachers and clinicians working with adult aphasics and with children who are having difficulty learning language. One must decide whether training should focus on comprehension or expression or on both together. We will return to this matter in Chapters 11 and 12. Various points of view on the relationship between comprehension and expression will be found in Braine (1971), Olson (1970), and Schiefelbusch and Lloyd (1974, especially Section IV).

Articulation

Articulation refers to the production of speech sounds. The study of articulation involves concepts of phonology such as those presented earlier, especially the psychological and motor skills of sound production. There has been considerable research on the order in which children acquire the sounds of English. Most investigators have begun developmental studies with three-year-olds, because there is so much variation in the articulation of younger children. At around age three, most children can articulate the vowels of English adequately. They can also produce some consonants, mostly sounds made with the lips, such as /m/, /p/, /b/, and /w/. It may be that these sounds are easier to make because they are "visible," that is, the child can see as well as hear how other people articulate them.

An interesting aspect of articulation development is that the child has probably made these same sounds or similar ones many times during vocal play, but they are not used consistently in spoken words until age three. Stated more formally, many of these sounds may be in the one- or two-year-old's repertoire, but are not used as members of phonemes until the child reaches a later age. The child continues to articulate more sounds correctly each year, but it is not until age seven or eight that most children are using all the phonemes of English correctly. Many children develop standard articulation before that age. Some of the last sounds to develop are /r/, /s/, and /z/. Children with deviant articulation are discussed in Chapter 8, which also contains additional information on normal articulatory development.

Environmental Influences in Language Acquisition

It is obvious that certain environmental factors are necessary for general growth and development as well as language acquisition: adequate food, shelter, warmth, and human contact. For example, malnutrition in the infant or young child seems to permanently limit the development of the brain and intellectual functioning. This chapter will close with reference to two aspects of the child's environment that have particular relevance to language acquisition: the family and the peer group.

I have already emphasized the importance of the interaction between mother and child during the first year of life. In more general terms, language acquisition is an interactive process, involving both child and parents. The child learns to communicate by participating in the communication system the family has already developed. The family's system, in turn, reflects cultural patterns. This situation applies to language and also to the many other communicative behaviors that the family engages in, such as facial expression, gesture, body movement, and posture. Behavior of this type is often thought to be "natural," but in fact much of it is learned and varies from culture to culture. Very little is known about how this learning takes place.

Generally, family members adjust their level of language to accommodate a young child. This is an important point, because it means that not only does the family influence the child, but also the child influences the family. Parent-child communication cannot be thought of in terms of the parent stimulating and the child responding. It is a two-way street, with both participants initiating and both responding. Typically this process works out to the benefit of all concerned. The child and parents work out a balance in their communicative behavior which produces relatively effective communication and at the same time, almost as a side effect, provides the child with an appropriate model and encouragement to further develop communication skills. As the child develops further, the family changes to take advantage of the youngster's new skills, at the same time encouraging the child to progress a little more. Broen (1972) presents some interesting examples of how mothers adapt the level of their language usage according to whether they are talking to a preschooler, a school-age child, or another adult.

It is not yet clear precisely what types of home experiences will enhance the child's language development. The single most important factor seems to be responsivity in the parents. Parents who are responsive to their children are able to provide appropriate language as input and useful feedback following the child's utterances. Such parents are able to recognize growth in their children and encourage continued development without pushing. Usually parents don't engage in such activities with any special teaching purposes in mind, but rather just in the normal course of events. It is an open question whether the amount of interaction with parents is as important as the quality of that interaction for the child's language development. In any case, the child must hear a sample of language that can be related to directly, have sufficient opportunity for self-expression, and receive some feedback for communicative efforts. Stimulation alone is not the answer; children don't learn much language by watching television. Rather, human interaction is the key to language development.

Clearly, the parents and older siblings provide the model of language the child will learn, as well as other communicative behaviors. The child learns the basic structure of language by following the parents' model. However, the details of how the child speaks will be increasingly determined by the peer group. It has been shown that the way one talks is closely related to peer identification and social status. Thus no matter how the parents talk, if the family lives in New York the child will grow up speaking like a New Yorker. Indeed, the child will be a New Yorker, and language patterns will reflect this identification. The same principle will apply no matter where the child grows up.

Conclusion

This chapter has presented brief discussions of language and linguistics and language acquisition in children. Speech may be considered the auditory-vocal form of language. Linguistics is helpful in developing a more precise understanding of what language is and how it operates. Linguistics is also helpful in studying language acquisition, but it is clear that much more than linguistics is needed to understand the process of acquisition. This process also involves **cognition**, nonverbal communication, interpersonal relations, group behavior, and other factors. The information in this chapter will provide background for Chapters 3 and 4 on speech production, and on Chapters 8, 11, and 12 on articulation and language disorders.

Glossary

Allophone: A systematic variation of a phoneme; a variant of a phoneme whose use is governed by the rules of pronunciation for that language.

Babbling: Stage in the baby's vocal development involving nonmeaningful combinations of consonants and vowels into syllables; includes much variation in the sounds and combinations of sounds produced.

Bound morpheme: A morpheme that cannot stand alone, such as a word ending.

Cognition: Thinking and thought processes, including concept formation and problem solving.

Communication: Transfer of information between individuals by any means. The information does not have to be true or complete.

Competence: In linguistics, everything one knows about one's language; includes more than those aspects of language that a person can actually express. (Compare with Performance.)

Cooing: Stage in the infant's vocal development involving pleasure sounds consisting of imprecisely formed vowel sounds.

Corpus: A collection of utterances used by a linguist to analyze part of a language.

Deep structure: In linguistics, the abstract structure of a sentence from which an actual utterance is ultimately derived. (Compare with Surface structure.)

Dialect: A local variation of a language. The locality may be small or large. The variation usually includes pronunciation, vocabulary, and grammar as well as the tonal or melodic contours of different sentences.

Echolalia: Stage in vocal development in which the baby repeats utterances of others, although not always precisely; also refers to pathological cases in which the individual repeats what is said, but apparently without comprehension.

Free morpheme: A morpheme that can stand alone; a morpheme that can function as a word.

Fricative: A consonant produced by forcing the air stream through a small opening so that turbulence is produced, as in /th/ or /z/.

Generative grammar: A school of thought in linguistics that bases grammatical analysis on the study of the abstract structure of language; the emphasis is on theoretical constructs. (Compare with Structural linguistics.)

Grammar: Term in linguistics which refers to the set of rules for producing utterances in a particular language; sometimes used to refer primarily to the rules of morphology and syntax combined for a particular language; also used to refer to the rules of all four levels of linguistics combined for a particular language.

Jargon: Type of vocal play in babies in which they pretend to talk or enter into conversation, but their utterances consist of meaningless babble; also refers to pathological cases in which the individual attempts to speak meaningfully, but the utterances do not consist of legitimate words.

Lalling: Stage in vocal development in which the baby repeats some of his or her own syllables (more than once) consecutively.

Language: An arbitrary system of symbols used for human communication.

Linguistics: The scientific study of language; includes four levels: phonology, morphology, syntax, and semantics.

Morpheme: A minimal unit of meaning or grammatical pertinence in a language.

Morphology: The level of linguistics concerned with words and word formulation and with word inflections, such as past tense and plural.

Performance: In linguistics, what one actually does with language, the process involved in the comprehension and production of language; is limited by psychological factors that do not affect one's knowledge of language in the abstract. (Compare with Competence.)

Phoneme: An abstract category representing a group of sounds that are considered the same for purposes of distinguishing between words in a language.

Phonology: The level of linguistics concerned with speech sounds, their production, and how they function in the language system.

Semantics: The level of linguistics concerned with the relationships between meaning and the language system.

Stop: A consonant produced by stopping the air stream momentarily; also called a plosive or stop-plosive.

Structural linguistics: A school of thought in linguistics that bases grammatical analysis of language on objective analysis of utterances; the emphasis is on the study of observable data. (Compare with Generative grammar.)

Surface structure: In generative grammar, the actual string of words used in a sentence, along with the morphologic and syntactic relations reflected by this string of words. (Compare with Deep structure.)

Syntax: The level of linguistics concerned with phrase, clause, and sentence structure.

Telegraphic speech: A type of child language in which content words are used but function words are omitted.

Unvoiced sound: A sound that does not include vibration of the vocal folds.

Voiced sound: A sound whose production includes vibration of the vocal folds.

Study Questions

1. List at least seven ways of communicating, other than spoken or written forms of language, that you have used in the past 24 hours. Be specific.

2. Give the total number of phonemes in each of the following words. Remember to say each word out loud and to ignore its spelling.

done	lunch	dumb
trust	enough	bloom
honest	blessing	trainer
golf	shoe	chew

3. List five morphemes that can stand alone. List five morphemes that cannot stand alone.

4. Divide each of the following sentences into morphemes and give the total number of morphemes in each sentence.

   His honesty is undoubtable.
   Bill's donkey is going nowhere fast.
   Mother cooked cupcakes for the workers.

5. Define "phoneme" and "morpheme" in your own words. What is the difference between the two? How does each relate to meaning?

6. We mentioned that the amount of interpretation involved in a linguistic analysis is one of the major differences between the structural and generative approaches to linguistics. Consider the following two sentences:

   John built the barn.
   The barn was built by John.

   Describe these two sentences in terms of sentence structure. Are they different? Now describe them in terms of meaning. Are they different? How does your interpretation of the meaning of these two sentences affect your descriptions of them?

7. Make up a list of 12 unrelated words, so that the whole list doesn't make any particular sense. Study the list until you can say the words in order without looking. Now make up a sentence containing 12 different words and do the same thing. Does grammatical structure help us process language?

8. Suppose that you wanted to teach a child an unfamiliar word. You could have the child say the word while you pointed to objects which that word symbolizes, or you could say the word and have the child point to the objects. Analyze the problems involved in each approach and how they might be solved. Is language learned primarily through comprehension or expression?

9. List three social situations which might influence the way you talk in terms of choices of vocabulary items and grammatical structures. Now analyze each of the three situations carefully to determine just what factors within each situation influence your use of language.

10. A deaf baby's babbling is very similar to that of a hearing baby. How would you explain this fact? At which stage in prespeech development should the baby begin to behave in ways that might suggest the presence of hearing loss?

Bibliography

BLOOM, L., *Language Development: Form and Function Emerging Grammars*, Cambridge, Mass.: M.I.T. Press, 1970.

BOLINGER, D., *Aspects of Language*, 2d ed., New York: Harcourt Brace Jovanovich, 1975.

BRAINE, M., "The Acquisition of Language in Infant and Child," in C. Reed, ed., *The Learning of Language*, New York: Appleton-Century-Crofts, 1971.

BROEN, P. A., "The Verbal Environment of the Language-Learning Child," *ASHA Monograph*, No. 17, Washington, D.C.: American Speech and Hearing Association, 1972.

BROWN, R., *A First Language: The Early Stages*, Cambridge, Mass.: Harvard University Press, 1973.

FISHMAN, J. A., ed., *Readings in the Sociology of Language*, The Netherlands: Mouton, 1968.

FODOR, J. A., T. G. BEVER, AND M. F. GARRETT, *The Psychology of Language*, New York: McGraw-Hill, 1974.

HUBBELL, R., "Children's Language," in A. Weston, ed., *Communicative Disorders*, Springfield, Ill.: Charles C. Thomas, 1972.

KIRK, S. A., AND W. D. KIRK, *Psycholinguistic Learning Disabilities: Diagnosis and Remediation*, Urbana: University of Illinois Press, 1971.

LABOV, W., *Sociolinguistic Patterns*, Philadelphia: University of Pennsylvania Press, 1972.

LANGACKER, R. W., *Language and Its Structure*, New York: Harcourt Brace Jovanovich, 1973.

LINDSAY, P. H., AND D. A. NORMAN, *Human Information Processing*, New York: Academic Press, 1972.

LYONS, J., *Introduction to Theoretical Linguistics*, Cambridge, England: Cambridge University Press, 1968.

NELSON, K., "Concept, Word, and Sentence: Interrelations in Acquisition and Development," *Psychological Rev.* **81** (1975):267–285.

OLSON, D. R., *Cognitive Development: The Child's Acquisition of Diagonality*, New York: Academic Press, 1970.

PALMER, F., *Grammar*, Baltimore: Penguin Books, 1971.

SCHIEFELBUSCH, R. L., AND L. L. LLOYD, eds., *Language Perspectives: Acquisition, Retardation, and Intervention*, Baltimore: University Park Press, 1974.

SLOBIN, D. I., ed., *The Ontogenesis of Grammar: A Theoretical Symposium*, New York: Academic Press, 1971.

WATZLAWICK, P., J. H. BEAVIN, AND D. D. JACKSON, *Pragmatics of Human Communication*, New York: Norton, 1967.

WERNER, H., AND B. KAPLAN, *Symbol Formation*, New York: Wiley, 1964.

CHAPTER 3
Overview

The production of speech is dependent on the respiratory system, larynx, articulators, and nervous system. Voice is produced by exhaled air placed into audible vibration as it passes between the approximated vocal folds of the larynx. Speech sounds are produced by positioning the articulators, which include the tongue, soft palate, teeth, and lips, in the way of the breath stream. Passage of air through a narrow orifice created by two articulators causes an audible friction, and the stoppage and quick release of air by articulators cause a burst of sound. The use of voice, friction, and plosion in the production of speech is described in this chapter.

The speech-production process requires precise coordination of the articulators mentioned, and that coordination is provided by the nervous system. Attention is given both to the transmission of motor commands from the cortex of the brain to the muscles that move the speech mechanism and to feedback of information from the speech mechanism to the brain in the control of the production process. Although the structures used in speech also serve such life-support functions as breathing and eating, portions of the central nervous system are devoted exclusively to communication processes. The chapter ends with a brief consideration of theoretical viewpoints that have been developed to help understand the complex matter of neural control of speech.

Ralph L. Shelton, Ph.D.
University of Arizona
Clifford A. Wood, Ph.D.
Department of Defense

Speech Mechanisms and Production

Introduction

In Chapter 2, speech was defined as language that is spoken and heard, and the term was used to refer to the sounds made by the vocal mechanism. The generation of sounds of any kind is dependent on certain mechanical factors. In speech production, those factors are provided by physiological functions of anatomical structures. This chapter describes the anatomy and physiology of key components of speech production: (1) respiration, which provides an energy source for speech; (2) phonation, or the production of voice; (3) articulation, or the production of speech sounds; and (4) nervous system control of the speech-production process. The acoustics of speech production are presented in the next chapter.

Respiration

The energy necessary for speech is produced by the movement and pressure of air from the lungs, which along with the heart almost fill the thoracic cavity (chest). The lungs are of a porous, spongy texture and have elasticity, which is important in exhalation. However, the lungs do not have muscles, and their expansion in inhalation is dependent on movements of the rib cage and diaphragm (see Fig. 3.1). For detailed presentations, see Zemlin (1968, Chapter 2) and Hixon (1973).

The thoracic cavity is bounded by the thoracic vertebrae of the spinal column* (backbone), the sternum (breastbone), the 12 ribs on each side, and the diaphragm muscle. Inspiration for speech involves the elevation and expansion of the rib cage, which is accomplished by muscles that connect the rib cage to the neck, shoulders, and arms and that join the ribs to one another and to the thoracic vertebrae. Inspiration also involves contraction of the diaphragm, a thin, arched muscle that separates the thoracic cavity from the abdominal cavity.

The diaphragm forms the floor of the chest and attaches to the bottom of the sternum, the lower ribs, and the lower thoracic vertebrae. When the diaphragm muscle contracts, it flattens and thus contributes to an increase in the volume of the thoracic cavity. The largest change in chest volume is caused by diaphragm movement, but as we indicated above, elevation and expansion of the rib cage also increase the volume. Most people use both kinds of movement in respira-

---

* The entire vertebral column extends from the base of the skull to the pelvis. From the top, the first seven vertebrae are termed "cervical vertebrae." They are located in the neck above the rib cage, and the first two of these vertebrae are arranged to support the skull and facilitate its rotation. Change in cervical vertebrae posture changes the diameter of the airway in the pharynx, which is adjacent to it and involved in speech.

54

Figure 3.1

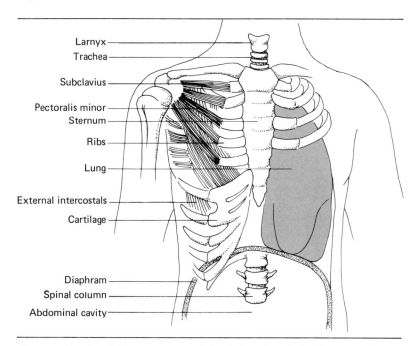

Larnyx
Trachea
Subclavius
Pectoralis minor
Sternum
Ribs
Lung
External intercostals
Cartilage
Diaphram
Spinal column
Abdominal cavity

Organs involved in respiration. The left side of the drawing depicts the rib cage and some of the muscles that elevate it in respiration. The rib cage is partially removed on the right side to show a lung. The diaphragm, which is important to respiration, is also shown.

tion. The changes in chest volume that occur in inspiration and expiration are shown in Fig. 3.2.

As the ribs lift and expand and the diaphragm contracts and lowers, the airtight, fluid-covered *pleural membrane* enclosing each lung is pulled out with the chest walls. The pleural membrane pulls on the lungs, and the lungs increase in volume. Atmospheric air rushes through the upper respiratory tract into the lungs and balances the drop in lung pressure resulting from the expansion of the thoracic cavity.

The pressure and flow of air required for speech production are provided through expiration, which has both passive and active components which reduce the volume of the thoracic cavity (Hixon, 1973). The passive component includes gravitational pull on the elevated rib cage, elastic recoil of the lungs, and a pushing up on the relaxing diaphragm by the compressed abdominal organs. The active component of expiration includes muscular pull downward on the

Figure 3.2

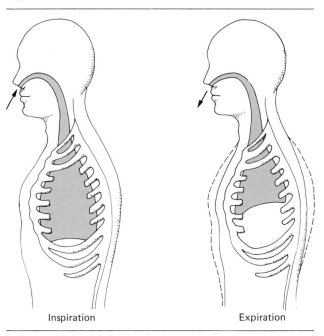

Inspiration   Expiration

*During inhalation, the ribs are lifted up and outward,
and the diaphragm contracts and lowers. These actions are reversed in exhalation.*

rib cage and contraction of abdominal muscles which raise abdominal pressure,
thus helping to force the diaphragm upward. The air pressure in the lungs is
increased by these expiratory forces, and as it exceeds atmospheric pressure, air
is expelled from the lungs. This positive lung-air pressure is what furnishes the
energy necessary for speech production.

During quiet breathing for life support (i.e., carrying oxygen to body tissues
and carbon dioxide from them), expiratory air merely returns to the atmospheric
air through the respiratory tract. This type of breathing is a semiautomatic body
function that is peformed about 14 to 18 times every minute of our lives. Rate
varies with maturity and activity. About half of the respiratory cycle is devoted
to inspiration and half to expiration; however, this pattern changes during
speech production. The human being has learned to inhale quickly just a little
more air than is necessary for a spoken phrase and to sustain exhalation. The
exhalation is controlled and checked by muscles to sustain expiratory air pressure for the relatively long period necessary for speech production. Skillful execution of voluntary respiration for speech is carefully developed and maintained
by singers, public speakers, and other performers. Indeed, the semiautomatic

performances of respiration, phonation, chewing, and swallowing all involve voluntary muscles that can be influenced by training. Many of the same muscles are used in speech, but their speech coordination requires a special neural integration, which is described in a later section.

Phonation

As shown in Fig. 3.3, the passageway from the lungs to the pharynx consists of bronchi, which leave each lung and join in midline to form the trachea, or windpipe. The larynx (Fig. 3.4), which is continuous with the top of the trachea, is

Figure 3.3

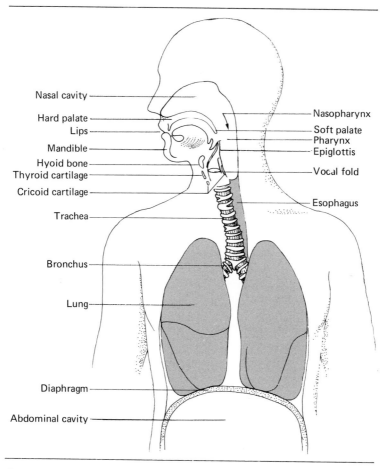

Organs involved in speech.

Figure 3.4

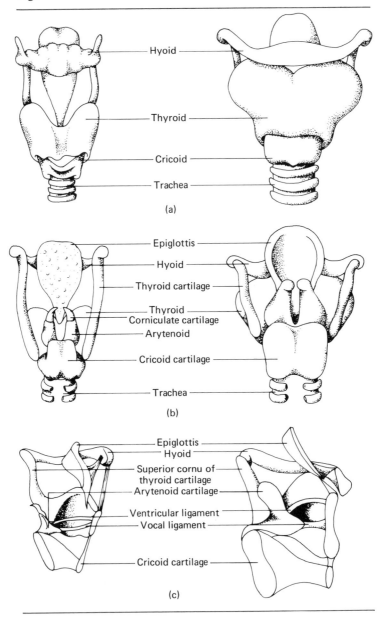

Hyoid

Thyroid

Cricoid

Trachea

(a)

Epiglottis

Hyoid

Thyroid cartilage

Thyroid
Corniculate cartilage

Arytenoid

Cricoid cartilage

Trachea

(b)

Epiglottis
Hyoid

Superior cornu of
thyroid cartilage

Arytenoid cartilage

Ventricular ligament
Vocal ligament

Cricoid cartilage

(c)

◀ *The adult (left) and infant (right) larynx. With growth and maturation, the speech mechanism changes in both size and form, and relationships among structures are altered. These age-related changes in the speech mechanism are studied for understanding of both normal and pathological functions. (a) The larynx from the front; (b) from the back; (c) to the side of the larynx from midline, showing the vocal ligaments that support the muscles of the vocal folds, which place air into vibration. (J. F. Bosma, "Anatomic and Physiologic Development of the Speech Apparatus," in D. B. Tower (Editor-in-Chief),* The Nervous System, *Vol. 3, ("Human Communication and Its Disorders," ed. E. L. Eagles, New York: Raven Press, 1975. Reprinted by permission.)*

the organ of phonation, or voice production. Through its several closing, or valving, mechanisms, the larynx also defends the trachea and lungs from the intrusion of material taken into the mouth. Failure of this defense mechanism results in the death of persons who inhale chunks of food, and a first-aid procedure, the Heimlich maneuver, has been devised to pop food from the larynx by compressing air in the lungs (American National Red Cross, undated).* We once participated in the evaluation of a young child who was undergoing tests in a teaching hospital because of respiratory deficit and associated disordered phonation. The child was found to have a penny lodged in the vestibule of the larynx, partially obstructing the airway.

Laryngeal Functioning

Sound generation requires that air be set into vibration (Chapter 4), and for voice this is accomplished in the larynx (voice box) by movement of the *vocal folds*, which disrupt the flow of expiratory air. The process of phonation is described below. First, however, let us consider the structure of the larynx. What supports the vocal folds, and how are they brought together?

The framework of the larynx is provided by its nine cartilages. The largest and most prominent is the thyroid cartilage, or Adam's apple (see Fig. 3.4). The thyroid is attached to and pivots on the ring-shaped cricoid cartilage, which attaches to the first ring of the trachea. At the back (Fig. 3.4b), the cricoid is enlarged something like the signet of a ring, and attached to the top of this signet

---

* Malfunction of the upper respiratory apparatus may threaten life in many ways. A conference report (Bosma and Showacre, 1975) relates basic information about the airway to sudden death of unknown etiology that occurs in some infants (so-called "crib death").

are two pyramidal-shaped cartilages, called the arytenoids. Extending from the arytenoids to the inside of the front portion of the thyroid cartilage (Fig. 3.4c), across the airway from the lungs, are shelves of muscle called the *true vocal folds* (see Fig. 9.1). The air passage between the left and right true folds is called the *glottis*. The movements of the arytenoids from side to middle and the pivoting of the thyroid on the cricoid, which are accomplished by muscles within the larynx, help to open and close the glottis and to stretch the vocal folds.

Several parts of the larynx are not as directly involved in vocal-fold vibration as are those just discussed. Above the true vocal folds are the *false vocal folds,* which attach to the thyroid cartilage just above the true folds and to the upper front surfaces of the arytenoids. There are few muscle fibers in the false folds, and many voice scientists believe that they seldom vibrate and that they have little or no function during normal phonation.

Another laryngeal cartilage is the leaflike *epiglottis* (Fig. 3.4b) that partially hangs over the folds. This cartilage and the tissue that covers it are thought to fold during swallowing, thus closing the vestibule to the larynx and protecting the airway.

Another structure that functions with the larynx is the horseshoe-shaped *hyoid bone,* located above and to the front of the thyroid cartilage. The hyoid bone, the only bone that does not connect directly to another bone, seems to be used primarily as a connection point for several groups of muscles. It serves a support function for the larynx, tongue, and **mandible** (jaw), and through muscular attachments it contributes to the posture of the head and neck.

The position of the vocal folds across the breath stream allows them to act as a valve to control air flow. If the glottis is closed during exhalation (expiration), air from the lungs builds pressure below the tensed true vocal folds until it reaches a level sufficient to blow them open. Once a puff of air has passed through the glottis, the subglottal air pressure will drop slightly, and the tensed elasticity of the folds will return them to their closed position.* The subglottal air pressure will rebuild until it has sufficient force to overcome the folds' tensed elasticity, and the cycle is repeated (Fig. 3.5).

The movement of the folds from closed to open and back to closed releases one puff of air. When this action is repeated about 125 times per second, a tone is generated that has the fundamental frequency of the average adult male voice. For the average adult female, the puffs are produced at a rate of about 250 per second. Fundamental frequency and the acoustics of voice production are considered in the next chapter.

---

* Passage of air through the partially closed glottis causes negative pressure, or suction, which contributes to closure of the vocal folds. This phenomenon is known as the Bernoulli effect.

Figure 3.5

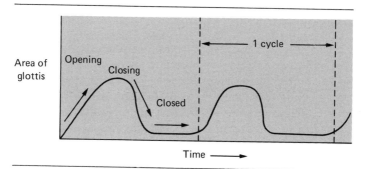

Schematic representation of changes in glottal opening
during each phonation cycle. (*Adapted from F. D. Minifie,
"Speech Acoustics," in F. D. Minifie, T. J. Hixon, and
F. Williams, eds.,* Normal Aspects of Speech, Hearing, and
Language, *Englewood Cliffs, N.J.: Prentice-Hall, 1973.*)

Vocal Pitch and Loudness

When muscular action pivots the thyroid cartilage forward on the cricoid, the
result is a rise in vocal **pitch.** This action increases the distance between the thyroid and the arytenoids, which are attached to the cricoid. While this action
lengthens the vocal folds, which serves to lower pitch, simultaneous contraction
of the vocal-fold muscle increases vocal-fold tension. The combined effects of
thyroid rotation and vocal-fold muscle contraction thin the folds somewhat, allowing them to move faster (releasing more puffs of air in a given period of
time) and thus increasing the **frequency** and pitch of the tone produced. In other
words, the pitch of the human voice changes in concert with changes in the mass,
tension, and length of the vocal folds. Men's voices are lower-pitched than
women's because the male larynx, which undergoes a growth change at puberty
that is related to sexual maturation, is larger and has longer folds than the female larynx.

The intensity of the voice is changed by adjustment of subglottal air pressure; that is, the greater the subglottal air pressure, the more intense the voice.
Pitch is primarily a function of the laryngeal mechanism, and **loudness,** which is
related to intensity, is primarily a function of the respiratory system. However,
these two systems do not work independently of each other, and to maintain
good voice control, the speaker must use the larynx and the air stream in skillful
balance. This coordination requires the participation of many components of the
nervous system.

Sound produced by laryngeal vibration resembles a low-pitched buzz. Speech,
of course, differs from a buzz that changes only in pitch and loudness. What
happens to modify and add information to the laryngeal source signal?

61

Articulation

Articulatory Structures and Their Function

The larynx opens into a passageway called the **pharynx,** which in turn opens into two more tubelike cavities—the nose and the mouth. The walls of the pharynx and also the soft palate (velum), tongue, mandible, and lips are somewhat free to move and thus to change the configuration of the pharyngeal and oral airways or tubes. These structures (see Fig. 3.3) are called *articulators* because they are involved in the production of speech sounds—articulation.

Pharynx   The pharynx is a muscular tube that extends from the **esophagus** and larynx to the base of the skull. It is convenient to discuss the pharynx as having three regions, which are named in terms of either adjacent structures or location. Starting from the bottom, these regions are the laryngopharynx (also called the hypopharynx), the oropharynx (also termed mesopharynx), and the nasopharynx (epipharynx). The pharyngeal tube is composed primarily of three overlapping constrictor muscles and connections to other parts of the speech mechanism. The pharynx serves two primary life-support functions: (1) to aid in pushing the bolus of food from the mouth to the esophagus (Fig. 3.3), which is a tube for the passage of food; and (2) to allow the passage of air from nose or mouth to the larynx. Because the pharynx is quite flexible, it can serve to help modify sound from the larynx as it passes on its way to the oral-cavity articulators.

Oral cavity   The floor of the nasal cavity and the roof of the oral cavity, which are essentially one and the same, are formed by the soft palate, or velum, and the hard palate. The hard palate is composed primarily of bone and its mucous-membrane covering, and it begins just behind the upper teeth with the **alveolar ridge** and continues as a vaulted structure backward for about three-quarters of the length of the oral cavity. The hard palate, as we have described it, consists of both palatine bone and some of the **maxilla,** or upper jaw.

The soft palate is a muscular continuation of the hard palate. It is very mobile and can move rapidly to close or open the pharyngeal airway between the oral and nasal cavities. (Movement of the pharyngeal walls toward the palate often contributes to the closure.) This closing is called, logically, *velopharyngeal closure.* During breathing, the soft palate is down, allowing air to travel between the nasal passages and the larynx (see Fig. 8.3). During swallowing, however, the soft palate rises, thus closing the velopharyngeal passage and preventing leakage of the material swallowed into the nasal passages. One cannot breathe and swallow simultaneously.

The velopharyngeal port is usually closed during speech, except during production of the nasal consonants /m/, /n/, and /ŋ/. During sounding of these three consonants, the port is open, allowing sound from the larynx to be modified by the nasal cavities as well as by other articulators. Opening of the velopharyngeal port at an inappropriate time during speech results in an unwanted nasal voice quality and sometimes in audible escape of air through the nose. Oral pressure required for the production of certain consonants may be inadequate because of the escape of air through the nose.

The nasopharynx opens into the nasal cavities, which are made up of bone, cartilage, and mucous-membrane covering. These structures move little, if at all. In life support, the nose allows passage of air and also contributes to the sense of smell, or olfaction. The nasal cavities do not contribute to articulation, in that they do not move, but they influence voice through a process of resonance, described in the next chapter.

Tongue　The oral cavity is anterior to the mesopharynx and houses the most important and mobile articulator—the tongue. The tongue helps position food for chewing and for transporting the bolus of food into the pharynx as a part of the swallow act (deglutition). It also contributes to the sense of taste.

The tongue is composed primarily of two sets of muscles. The intrinsic muscles (Fig. 3.6a), which begin and end within the tongue, allow the tongue to assume a wide gradation of shapes. The extrinsic muscles (Fig. 3.6b) connect the tongue to the mandible, hyoid bone, and skull, position the tongue within the oral cavity, and allow the tongue to be protruded from the mouth.

The sensitivity of the tongue to touch-pressure contacts contributes to the coordination of tongue movements in speech. For the production of many consonant sounds, the tongue either constricts the flow of expired air, thus creating audible turbulence or a hisslike sound, or stops and then quickly releases the flow of air, thus generating a burst of sound. These *frictional* and *stop* sounds involve positioning a portion of the tongue near or against the hard palate, alveolar ridge, or teeth. Vowels and consonants that resemble vowels are also dependent on tongue position. Although different tongue positions result in different vowels, Kent (1972) observed from a study of motion picture X-rays that the shape of the tongue is similar for different vowels. For vowels, the flow of air must not be so restricted that audible friction results.

The production of different sounds is considered further in the next section, which is concerned with the classification of speech sounds. However, it should be evident at this point that although voice is produced at the larynx, speech sounds are also produced by air turbulence higher in the vocal tract. Fricatives and stops may be formed by the lips or lips and teeth as well as by the tongue working with other structures. If these **turbulent** sounds occur while the larynx is producing voice, voiced consonants result. If they are produced in the absence of voice, voiceless consonants result.

Figure 3.6

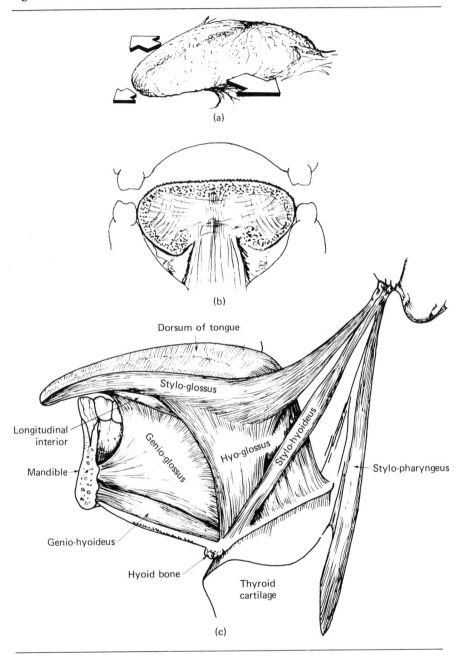

(a)

(b)

Dorsum of tongue

Stylo-glossus

Longitudinal
interior

Genio-glossus

Mandible

Hyo-glossus

Stylo-hyoideus

Stylo-pharyngeus

Genio-hyoideus

Hyoid bone

Thyroid
cartilage

(c)

Other articulators   Anterior to the tongue are the central teeth, which contribute to articulation as they are approximated by tongue or lips as just described. The lips are important articulators, and of course they contribute to life support through their role in sucking and eating. The facial muscles can cause the lips to purse, round, elongate, or close—actions that are involved in the production of both vowels and consonants. That is, the lips supplement the tongue in shaping the vocal tract for the production of vowel sounds. The facial muscles also contribute to nonverbal communication as the individual smiles, frowns, or projects other facial expressions. The lip (labial) sounds are among the first speech sounds that a baby acquires, and these sounds can be found in all oral languages.

We have not mentioned the mandible except to say that it helps support the tongue. Its movements do influence the position and movement of both the tongue and the lower lip, and consequently the lower jaw is an articulator. It also contributes to chewing and swallowing.

Classification of Speech Sounds

To complete our consideration of articulation, it is appropriate to introduce the sounds of speech in terms of the articulators and movements that produce them. The section on phonology in Chapter 2 introduced the concept of phonemes and described a few of the approximately 46 phonemes in American English. Sounds belonging to different phonemes will now be classified according to the movements and positions of the articulators that produce them.

It is convenient to divide speech sounds into consonants and vowels. Consonants involve use of air turbulence produced by an articulatory constriction of the vocal tract, whereas vowels involve a more open vocal tract and **laminar**

◄ *The muscles of the tongue. The drawings of the tongue dorsum (a) and of the tongue in cross-section in relationship to the mandible and maxilla (b) schematize the intrinsic muscles of the tongue. These muscles are contained within the tongue and permit change in tongue shape. The intrinsic muscles run in all directions but primarily laterally, vertically, and longitudinally; and they may flatten, narrow, elongate, or shorten the tongue, and they may curl the tongue tip upward or pull it down. The extrinsic muscles of the tongue (c) originate on the skull, mandible, or hyoid bone and insert into the tongue or influence the tongue by action on the larynx or hyoid bone, which provide support to the tongue. The extrinsic tongue muscles serve primarily to position the tongue. The longitudinal inferior muscle is an intrinsic tongue muscle. (The bottom drawing was adapted by permission from H. Gray,* Anatomy of the Human Body, *29th ed., ed. C. M. Goss, Philadelphia: Lea and Febiger, Copyright 1973).*

(quiet) air flow. Table 3.1 presents two charts that classify the phonemes of American English according to the International Phonetic Alphabet. The top chart pertains to consonants; the bottom one to vowels.

Consonants Consonants are differentiated by place of constriction (horizontal axis of the consonant chart), manner of constriction (vertical axis), or the presence or absence of voicing or laryngeal tone. Any two consonants will differ from each other in terms of one or more of these three features.

Place of articulation encompasses the structures from the front to the back of the mouth, and two articulators are necessary to establish a place of constric-

Table 3.1 Charts of the phonemes of American English.

CONSONANTS

Manner of Articulation	Voicing*	Bilabial	Labio- dental	Inter- dental	Apico- alveolar	Fronto- palatal	Dorso- velar	Glottal
Stop (plosive)	VL	p (pit)			t (tip)		k (kit)	
	V	b (bit)			d (dip)		g (get)	
Affricate	VL				tʃ (chip)			
	V				dჳ (jet)			
Fricative	VL	wh (why)	f (fit)	θ (thin)	s (sit)	ʃ (ship)		
	V		v (vex)	ð (that)	z (zip)	ჳ (azure)		h (hit)
Nasal	V	m (moon)			n (noon)		ŋ (ring)	
Lateral (Glide)	V				l (loom)			
Semi-vowel (Glide)	V	w (wad)			r (bar)	j (yet)		

Position of Articulation

*   VL represents voiceless; V, voiced.

VOWELS

Tongue Position							Sample Diphthongs
high	i I	eat it	ɝ mother	suit book	u U		aI (sigh) ɔI (boy) aʋ (cow)
mid	e ɛ	vacation ever	ə sofa ʌ up	obey law	o ɔ		
low	æ a	at class		not father	ɒ ɑ		
		front	center	back			

TONGUE POSITION

tion. For example, the term "bilabial" describes sounds produced by closure of the lips (/p, b, m/). Constrictions produced by lips and teeth result in "labio-dental" sounds (/f, v/). "Interdental" sounds involve placement of the tongue just behind or between the upper and lower central teeth. (See the first chart in Table 3.1 for a listing of the interdental sounds and for sounds in the classes presented next.) The term "apicoalveolar" indicates that the tip ("apico") of the tongue is near or touching the alveolar ridge. In "frontopalatal" sounds, the tongue and hard palate form a constriction; in "dorsovelar" sounds, the back (dorsum) of the tongue is raised toward the velum. "Glottal" refers to sounds produced by friction as air passes between the true vocal folds. The folds are partially closed—enough to cause turbulence and sound, but not enough to produce voice.

The vertical axis of the consonant chart indicates *manner of production*, or the different categories of constriction used in the production of consonant sounds. In the stop manner of production, articulators momentarily occlude, or stop, the oral air passage, and air pressure is built up behind the occlusion. Release of the constriction results in a burst of air turbulence that produces a stop, or plosive, sound, such as /p/, /b/, /t/, and /d/. The affricates are much like the stops, except that the pulse of air is sustained a bit longer. Fricatives are caused by the approximation of two articulators, thus directing exhaled air through a narrow opening and causing a relatively continuous stream of noise. The nasals were discussed earlier as sounds that are made by lowering the velum, thus directing the sound stream through the nose rather than the mouth. The lateral and semi-vowel glide categories are a bit more arbitrary. There is only one lateral glide in English, the /l/. The term "lateral" refers to the flow of air around the sides of the tongue as it is pressed against the anterior portion of the palate. The semi-vowel glides (/w, r, j/) are made with more constriction than vowels, but not enough to cause turbulent air flow. These semivowels are viewed differently by different authors, and you may find them located differently in other phonetic charts.

The third type of consonant differentiation is the presence or absence of *voice;* some consonants are voiceless (VL) and some are voiced (V). The onset of vocal-fold vibration occurs earlier in voiced than in voiceless consonants. That is, vocal-fold vibration is present during portions of consonants that are perceived as voiceless.

Knowledge of place, manner, and voicing allows specification of each consonant. That is, only one sound is represented in each place, manner, and voice cell in the chart.

Vowels   A different system is required for the classification of vowels. All vowels have the same manner of production, and all are voiced. Differences among vowels are determined primarily by position of the tongue, although lip configuration is also important. The tongue includes the tongue tip, tongue edges, and tongue body. Denes and Pinson (1973) classify vowels in terms of the position of the highest part of the tongue body. For example, they state that when the tongue body is positioned as high and as far forward as possible without causing a constriction sufficiently narrow to create turbulence and when the lips are spread and voicing is produced, the vowel /i/ (as in "eat") results.

The vowel chart in Table 3.1 classifies vowels as front, center, and back and as high, middle, and low relative to position of the tongue body in the oral cavity. The chart indicates the approximate positions of American English vowels relative to one another. But the vowel positions given in the table are ideal positions, reflecting isolated sound production, and these ideal positions are rarely reached during running speech. A shift in tongue location from that associated with one vowel to that of another vowel results in a sound termed a *diphthong*. Diphthongs, like consonants and vowels, contribute to the expression of meaning by a speaker. Acoustic differences among vowels are described in Chapter 4.

Because speech is produced with structures that also serve life-support functions, speech is sometimes said to be an overlaid function. Nevertheless, speech production is a motor act distinct from the life-support functions, and it has its own neural control.

The Nervous System

Evolution of the human brain involved development of the cerebral **cortex,** which in turn supported the organization of speech and language into a tool that has allowed humans to dominate the animal world. An overview of the nervous system will aid in our appreciation of the brain and its place as originator of speech, language, and hearing.

The brain is part of a vast network of neurons termed the nervous system. The nerve cell, or neuron (see Fig. 5.8) is the smallest unit of the nervous system. Each neuron consists of a cell body, one axon (an extension, or arm, that carries impulses away from the cell body), and one or more dendrites (arms that carry impulses toward the cell body). The dendrites are receptive to impulses from surrounding neurons and may approximate many axons from many other neurons. These connections, or synapses, allow the flow of neural information to be passed from one neuron to another or coordinated among a group of neurons. A "nerve" is a bundle of nerve fibers which are the axonic and dendritic processes of many neurons.

Two principal divisions of the nervous system are the central nervous system (CNS) and the peripheral nervous system (PNS). The CNS is composed of the brain and spinal cord; the PNS, of cranial and spinal nerves and a portion of the autonomic nervous system.* The PNS connects various parts of the body to the spinal column and brain. Both the CNS and the PNS are essential to speech production.

---

* The autonomic nervous system innervates visceral organs and other structures that presumably function involuntarily.

Figure 3.7

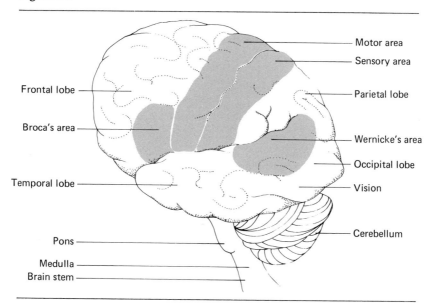

Lateral view of the cortex, showing areas important to speech production. Portions of the peripheral nervous system important to speech begin in the pons and medulla, which are also shown. (Adapted from A. T. Rasmussen, Outlines of Neuro-Anatomy, *3rd ed., Dubuque, Iowa: William C. Brown, 1943; and E. B. Steen and A. Montagu,* Anatomy and Physiology, *Vol. 2, New York: Barnes and Noble, 1959.)*

Central Nervous System

A portion of the CNS with special significance for speech and language is the cortex, or surface layer of the brain (Figs. 3.7 and 3.8). The cortex of each half, or hemisphere, of the brain is divided into four lobes. Those lobes and cortical regions important to speech, language, and hearing are shown in Fig. 3.7.

The motor area of the cortex controls bodily movements, including those involved in phonation and articulation. Impulses from the motor centers in each hemisphere are sent to lower coordinating centers and hence to the muscles. A large percentage of the neurons originating in the motor area of one cerebral hemisphere connects with PNS structures that control the opposite side of the body. For example, the left hemisphere controls the right arm. Midline structures of the body, such as the larynx and the articulators, require well-synchronized impulses from each hemisphere for skilled movement.

Just as the motor area of the cortex sends commands to muscles, the sensory area of the cortex receives information from muscles and other structures in-

Figure 3.8

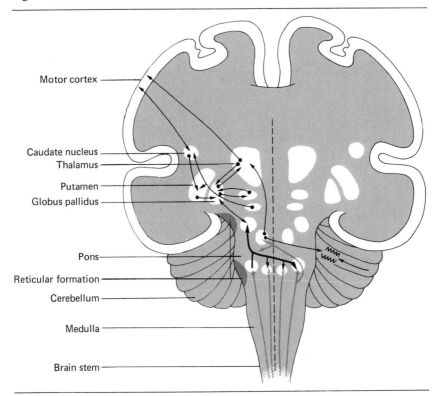

Frontal view of the brain, showing the two cerebral hemispheres and tracts from the cortex to the pons and medulla. (Adapted by permission from E. Gardner, Fundamentals of Neurology, *2d ed., Philadelphia: Saunders, 1975; and F. L. Darley, A. E. Aronson, and J. R. Brown,* Motor Speech Disorders, *Philadelphia: William C. Brown, 1975.)*

volved in speech and other bodily movements. Signals from muscles and joints may reach consciousness when they arrive at the sensory cortex, and this information helps to guide the production of normal speech and may be used in the correction of disordered speech.

For many communication functions, the left cerebral hemisphere is more important than the right. Anterior to the motor area of the left hemisphere is Broca's area, which programs speech production by coordinating neural signals which then travel to the motor area and hence to the articulators. Damage to Broca's area results in **apraxia**, the inability to make voluntary speech movements (see Chapters 8 and 12). The left side of the brain is also dominant for language (Penfield and Roberts, 1959; Sussman and MacNeilage, 1975) and brain damage involving the left hemisphere is much more likely to result in **aphasia** (see Chapter 12) than is similar damage to the right hemisphere. Wernicke's area in the left hemisphere controls the ability to understand spoken language; however, music and other sounds not involving speech are processed in the right hemisphere.

In order for speech or other movements to occur, neural information originating in the cortex must travel to the PNS and hence to the muscles. Two pathways starting in the motor cortex carry signals to synapse (connect) with the PNS. The pyramidal pathway is direct and involves no intermediate synapses. The extrapyramidal pathway from the motor area of the cortex to the PNS involves multiple synapses in portions of the brain beneath the cortex. Some of the **nuclei** (bundles of neuron cell bodies) along the indirect route are labeled in Fig. 3.8. Neurons in each pathway are termed *upper motor neurons,* and damage to either pathway can cause a disruption in speech production called **dysarthria** (see Chapters 8 and 12). **Lesions** involving upper motor neurons do not necessarily completely paralyze muscles, because some impulses may still reach muscles via alternative pathways. The nature of the dysarthria will depend on the location of the lesion, but the pattern of motor activity will be disrupted, and muscles may be spastic or malfunction in other ways.

Peripheral Nervous System

Neural signals traveling the upper motor neurons to the larynx or articulators make synapse with cranial nerves, whose nuclei are in the **pons** or **medulla** of the **brain stem** (see Figs. 3.7 and 3.8). Signals going to the respiratory apparatus, however, travel via spinal nerves. There are 12 cranial nerves, several of which are important for speech and hearing. The numbers, names, and functions of cranial nerves concerned with speech or hearing are as follows:

V. Trigeminal—controls the muscles of mastication which move the mandible.

VII. Facial—controls the facial muscles, including the lips.

VIII. Auditory—serves the sense of hearing.

IX. Glossopharyngeal—contributes to pharyngeal movement.

X. Vagus—contributes to movements of the pharynx and larynx and serves a sensory function for pharynx, larynx, trachea, bronchi, and lungs.

XI. Spinal accessory—controls movements of muscles of the neck, thus indirectly influencing the position of the larynx.

XII. Hypoglossal—controls tongue movements.

Figure 3.9 shows divisions of the trigeminal nerve, which mediates sensation from the oral and facial regions and innervates the muscles of mastication (chewing) which control the mandible.

The nuclei and axons of the cranial and spinal nerves are termed *lower motor neurons,* or the final common pathway. If they are destroyed, the muscles they serve will be totally paralyzed and **flaccid** because no neural impulses can reach it. If this flaccidity involves the speech mechanism, a form of dysarthria results.

We mentioned earlier that coordination of speech production requires that information from the speech mechanism be sent into the brain. This serves a feedback function (see Chapter 1) that allows the brain to guide motor performance and to correct errors when they occur. Signals picked up by receptors in muscles and joints are sent through the PNS and into the CNS. One receptor is the muscle spindle, which is found in some of the muscles of the speech mechanism (Bowman, 1971). As muscles contract and relax, information from the spindles is sent into the nervous system. Some of these signals may reach the cortical areas that contribute to conscious awareness, whereas others travel to subcortical centers which serve unconscious coordinating functions. Auditory signals about one's own speech also contribute to the guidance of speech production.

Figure 3.9

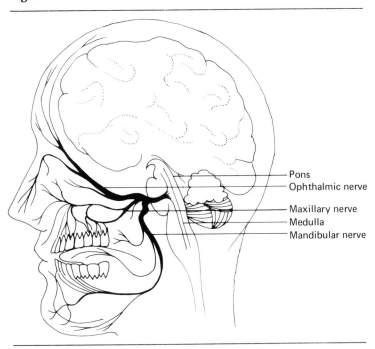

Pons
Ophthalmic nerve
Maxillary nerve
Medulla
Mandibular nerve

The nuclei and three branches of the trigeminal cranial nerve. (Adapted by permission from J. G. Chusid, Correlative Neuroanatomy and Functional Neurology, *16th ed., Los Altos, Calif.: Lange Medical Publications, 1976.)*

Speech-Production Theory

We have sketched a simplified picture of how the CNS controls speech production by sending commands to the muscles and receiving information back from the muscles as they respond to the commands. We have also pointed out that certain cortical regions serve language and hearing functions. Other areas of the brain are also involved in associations and other processes necessary for the production and perception of speech. The life-support functions that have been mentioned in this chapter are organized in lower brain areas and are semiautomatic, whereas speech, hearing, and language require a great deal of cortical involvement. Attempts to understand and explain speech production and the neural and physiological processes underlying it are in their infancy. Although the vigorous research being conducted on this topic promises new developments with explanatory and applied significance, many important questions are unanswered. For example, the brain does not instruct the muscles to produce strings of individual sounds, much like a typewriter, but we don't know what larger units, perhaps of syllable, word, or phrase size, are ordered by the nervous system. If scientists from various fields that are concerned with speech can use the same speech units in their research, correspondence can be sought in work being done in those fields. The matter of nervous-system organization of speech is of concern to speech pathologists, because they would use units in remedial work that are compatible with natural function. Persons studying reading disabilities wonder if reading training based on sound-sized units is incompatible with nervous-system processing of language (Rozin, Poritsky, and Spotsky, 1971; Kavanagh and Mattingly, 1972). So far no one has identified a unit for use in reading instruction that is relatively easy for all learners to use.

MacNeilage (1970) pointed out that many theorists attempting to explain speech production have used units the size of **phones,** or speech sounds (consonants or vowels), because those units have a psychological reality, and many components of the sound patterns of different languages can be described in terms of combinations of sound-sized units. However, our perception of sounds in speech lacks close correspondence with physiological measures of speech production (such as measurements from X-ray motion pictures) or acoustical analyses of the sounds produced (Curtis, 1970). That is, spectrographic tracings of repetitions of the same sound in various contexts are not identical. Consequently, speech-production theory based on the phoneme* concept has been modified to explain this lack of correspondence among speech perception, the physiology of production, and the acoustics of speech. Some investigators have theorized that the nervous system sends invariant commands corresponding to sound-sized

---

* *Phoneme* is used here to refer to a class of phones or sounds, but not to a given phone that is articulated. Elsewhere in this book, *phoneme, phone,* and *speech sound* may be used interchangeably.

units to the muscles, but that similar commands give different movements and acoustical results because of variability in the timing of the commands, mechanical limitations that influence the response of peripheral structures to the commands, or other reasons. An alternative explanation is that the nervous system directs the articulators to idealized target positions corresponding to phone-size units. The commands may differ, depending on the starting position of the articulators, and even so the ideal positions may not be realized for reasons similar to those mentioned in connection with the invariant motor-command viewpoint.

A phenomenon known as **coarticulation** is used as a tool in research directed to the identification of speech-production units. Speech specialists have long known that sounds represented by sequences of letters in written words actually involve movements that overlap in time as the words are spoken. Thus in the word *pod*, for example, the mandible may be dropping for the /ɑ/ before the lips have released the /p/. As a related matter, the place of articulation of a given sound may be influenced by neighboring sounds. Thus the contact of the tongue with the palate for a /k/ may be relatively forward in the mouth if adjacent sounds are forward in the mouth. For example, the tongue-palate contact for the /k/ in /ki/ (key) is more anterior than is the contact for /ku/ (coo).

Coarticulation may involve several articulators and can be more complex than it is in our example. The existence of coarticulation suggests that speech production is organized in units larger than single phones, and research findings which show coarticulatory effects across syllable and word boundaries suggest that at least some motor commands involve units larger than syllables and words.

Coarticulation has been studied and demonstrated by various instruments, including motion picture X-ray (cinefluorography), spectrographic displays of the speech signal, study of electrical signals associated with muscle activation (electromyography), and other means. Hopefully, its further investigation will enhance our understanding of how the nervous system controls speech production. Here we have tried to demonstrate that understanding of nervous-system control of speech production requires theory as well as data based on research.

Conclusion

We have described various components of the speech mechanism and their functions separately. However, we hope it is evident that no one part functions independently of the others. Speech-production structures also support life in different ways. The lungs and chest serve respiration, the larynx defends the airway, and the articulators are involved in respiration, eating, chewing, and swallowing. For this reason, speech is sometimes said to be an overlaid function. That is, it appears to have been added to the duties of structures that serve more essential purposes.

When the peripheral speech mechanism is viewed in connection with the roles of the CNS and PNS in the formulation, perception, and production of speech, it is evident that a complex neuroanatomical network devoted to speech and other aspects of communication does exist and that its function is of major importance to the distinction that is drawn between animal and human life. This speech-production system has been the object of a great deal of research that may be pursued in more advanced readings and courses. We hope that you have gained some appreciation for the complexities and order involved in the anatomy and physiology of speech production.

Glossary

Alveolar ridge: The bony ridge posterior to the portion of the maxilla that houses the teeth.

Aphasia: Loss of language function because of brain damage (see Chapter 12).

Apraxia: Inability to make voluntary speech movements even though involuntary movements of the articulators may be made normally. The disorder reflects neurological impairment even though neither muscle weakness nor spasticity is involved.

Brain stem: The portion of the brain beneath the cerebral hemispheres and excluding the cerebellum.

Coarticulation: The phenomenon whereby the speech mechanism moves simultaneously in the production of speech sounds that are perceived sequentially (see Chapter 8).

Cornu: A horn-shaped process. The thyroid cartilage of the larynx and the hyoid bone have two segments termed cornua (plural).

Cortex: The outer, or surface, layer of the brain.

Dysarthria: Neurologically based impairment of articulation and perhaps phonation, prosody, and respiration as well. Both voluntary and involuntary movements are consistently impaired.

Esophagus: A muscular tube used to convey food from the pharynx to the stomach. It is continuous with the pharynx and located behind the trachea.

Flaccid: Flabby, or lacking muscle tone.

Frequency: The number of sound cycles that recur within a period of time.

Laminar: Smooth, streamlined. Laminar airflow is likely to be quiet.

Lesion: An alteration of structure or function because of injury or disease.

Loudness: A perception of sound related to the intensity or energy of that sound.

Mandible: The lower jawbone.

Maxilla: The upper jawbone.

Medulla (medulla oblongata): A portion of the brain stem containing nuclei for some of the cranial nerves.

Nucleus (nuclei): A localized group of nerve cell bodies whose axons form nerves.

Pharynx: A tube of muscle and mucous membrane situated behind the nose, mouth, and larynx. It allows passageway for air into the larynx and food into the esophagus, and it serves as a resonating chamber for voice produced at the larynx.

Phone: A speech sound.

Pitch: A perception of sound related to the frequency of that sound.

Pons: An eminence at the base of the brain. The pons contains nuclei for some of the cranial nerves.

Turbulent: Agitated, disturbed. Turbulent airflow will create noise.

Study Questions

1. How is air taken into the lungs during inspiration?
2. How does expiration for speech differ from expiration in quiet breathing?
3. How does the larynx function in the production of voice?
4. What function does the larynx serve in addition to voice production?
5. What is the difference between the true and the false vocal folds?
6. How should a speaker go about increasing the intensity of his or her voice?
7. Describe the production of fricative and plosive sounds.
8. How may the passageway between the oropharynx and the nasopharynx be closed during speech?
9. Explain the classification of consonants in terms of voicing and place and manner of production.
10. How are vowel sounds produced?
11. Differentiate between the central nervous system and the peripheral nervous system.
12. Where in the nervous system do motor commands to the speech muscles originate?
13. How do cranial nerves contribute to speech production?
14. Why is it important that information about the performance of the speech mechanism be fed back into the central nervous system?
15. Why is theory needed to help understand the speech-production process?

Bibliography

AMERICAN NATIONAL RED CROSS, *First Aid for Foreign Body Obstruction of the Airway* (undated).

BOSMA, J. F., "Anatomic and Physiologic Development of the Speech Apparatus," in D. B. Tower (Editor-in-Chief), *The Nervous System*, Vol. 3, ed. E. L. Eagles, "Human Communication and Its Disorders," New York: Raven Press, 1975.

BOSMA, J. F., AND J. SHOWACRE, eds., *Development of Upper Respiratory Anatomy and Function*, Washington, D.C.: U.S. Government Printing Office, 1975.

BOWMAN, J. P., JR., *The Muscle Spindle and Neural Control of the Tongue: Implications for Speech*, Springfield, Ill.: Charles C Thomas, 1971.

CHUSID, J. G., AND J. J. MCDONALD, *Correlative Neuroanatomy and Functional Neurology*, 7th ed., Los Altos, Calif.: Lange Medical Publications, 1954.

CURTIS, J. F., "Segmenting the Speech Stream," in J. Griffith, and L. E. Miner, eds., *The First Lincolnland Conference on Dialectology*, University: University of Alabama Press, 1970.

DARLEY, F. L., A. E. ARONSON, AND J. R. BROWN, *Motor Speech Disorders*, Philadelphia: Saunders, 1975.

DENES, P. B., AND E. N. PINSON, *The Speech Chain*, Garden City, N.Y.: Bell Telephone Laboratories, Anchor/Doubleday, 1973.

GARDNER, E., *Fundamentals of Neurology*, 2d ed., Philadelphia: Saunders, 1952.

GRAY, H., *Anatomy of the Human Body*, 26th ed., ed. C. M. Goss, Philadelphia: Lea and Febiger, 1954.

HIXON, T. J., "Respiratory Function in Speech," in F. D. Minifie, T. J. Hixon, and F. Williams, eds., *Normal Aspects of Speech, Hearing, and Language*, Englewood Cliffs, N.J.: Prentice-Hall, 1973.

KAVANAGH, J. F., AND I. G. MATTINGLY, eds., *The Relationships Between Speech and Reading*, Cambridge, Mass.: M.I.T. Press, 1972.

KENT, R. D., "Some Considerations in the Cinefluorographic Analysis of Tongue Movements during Speech," *Phonetica* **26** (1972):16–32.

MACNEILAGE, P. F., "Motor Control of Serial Ordering of Speech," *Psychological Rev.* **77** (1970):182–196.

MATZKE, H. A., AND F. M. FOLTZ, *Synopsis of Neuroanatomy*, New York: Oxford University Press, 1967.

MINIFIE, F. H., "Speech Acoustics," in F. D. Minifie, T. J. Hixon, and F. Williams, eds., *Normal Aspects of Speech, Hearing, and Language*, Englewood Cliffs, N.J.: Prentice-Hall, 1973.

PENFIELD, W., AND L. ROBERTS, *Speech and Brain Mechanisms*, Princeton, N.J.: Princeton University Press, 1959.

RASMUSSEN, A. T., *Outlines of Neuro-Anatomy*, 3rd ed., Dubuque, Iowa: William C. Brown, 1943.

ROZIN, P., S. PORITSKY, AND R. SPOTSKY, "American Children with Reading Problems Can Easily Learn to Read English Represented by Chinese Characters," *Science* **171** (1971): 1264–1267.

STEEN, E. B., AND A. MONTAGU, *Anatomy and Physiology*, Vol. 2, New York: Barnes and Noble, 1959.

SUSSMAN, H. M., AND P. F. MACNEILAGE, "Studies of Hemispheric Specialization for Speech Production," *Brain and Language* **2** (1975):131–151.

ZEMLIN, W. R., *Speech and Hearing Science*, Englewood Cliffs, N.J.: Prentice-Hall, 1968.

77

**CHAPTER 4
Overview**

The production and perception of spoken language are taken for granted by many of us, yet these activities profoundly affect our daily lives. These activities, of course, encompass the study of speech and hearing in communication and communicative disorders.

Moreover, scientific developments in the study of speech production and acoustics and speech perception may lead to advances which may change our future communication remarkably. The use of "voice prints" (visual displays of speech), although controversial, now occurs in law enforcement in an effort to identify criminals. Machines have been developed which can produce, and with limited capacity recognize, spoken messages. Imagine "talking to a typewriter" and having it type the message you speak or talking through a "translator machine" to persons who speak another language. In fact, voice-controlled machines with computers are in common use.

This chapter obviously will not reveal the scientific principles to achieve these aspirations. It will

Speech Acoustics and Perception

introduce you, however, to many principles and problems that underlie the acoustics of speech and speech perception. The basic principles of acoustics are presented and applied to speech to give you an understanding of speech as an acoustical phenomenon. The significance of the acoustics of speech in speech perception is analyzed. Also, nonacoustic factors are analyzed in speech perception. Since speech is a linguistic, as well as an acoustic, phenomenon, knowledge of the language used, of course, is fundamental for the perception of speech.

Paul H. Skinner, Ph.D.
University of Arizona

Introduction

The mechanism and production of speech were discussed in the previous chapter, and that discussion provides appropriate background for the study of speech acoustics and perception. The mechanism and production of speech determine its acoustical characteristics, and in turn the acoustics of speech provide the basis for speech perception.

Speech was carefully defined in Chapter 1 and thus will be simply described here as coded sound patterns which vary over time and carry linguistic information. This description reveals the fundamental characteristics of speech which will be considered in this chapter. What is the acoustical basis of these coded sound patterns, and how are these coded sound patterns perceived?

Speech Acoustics

In order to understand the production and transmission of speech, we must acquire at least an understanding of certain principles of acoustics. Indeed, speech is an acoustical phenomenon. Thus speech is a special case of sound production. Although we might continue the classical debate that vibration is not sound unless it is heard, let us for convenience postpone that ponderous problem and accept simply that sound occurs as a result of vibration.

Sound Generation

For **sound generation** we need merely to set a vibrator in motion, and to do so we need a source of energy or an applied force. In the production of speech, described in Chapter 3, we may consider exhalation of air from the lungs to be the source of energy and the vocal folds to be the vibrator. The air in the cavities of the throat and mouth provides the elastic medium for the transmission of these vibrations, or speech sounds, to the ear of a listener. We may assume that the vibration of the vocal folds causes a series of **compression** waves or pressure changes in the surrounding air. We must give special attention to the mode of sound transmission in air, since reception of speech by the ear depends on air conduction.

Sound Propagation

Billions of molecules exist in each cubic centimeter of air, and these molecules normally are in continuous, random motion. Nevertheless, each molecule typically remains within a certain space—a position of "rest," or equilibrium—which is determined by the presence of neighboring molecules. Pressure waves are developed when molecules are displaced to and from their position of equilibrium.

Since air is an **elastic medium,** molecules tend to retain their position, or equilibrium, and thus when displaced will return to their original position. When force is applied to air molecules, the molecules become bunched together, or compressed, in the direction of the applied force. If the pressure is released or exerted in the opposite direction, the molecules become spread apart, or rarefied, in the opposite direction from their position of equilibrium. These alternating compression and **rarefaction** molecular displacements result in **sound propagation** and are shown schematically in Fig. 4.1.

When molecules are set into vibration, they collide with their immediate neighbors and set up a chain reaction. Hearing occurs as a result of such a chain reaction when molecules are displaced in the vicinity of the ear drum and set this delicate membrane into the same pattern of vibration as the original source of vibration. In this way, information may be transmitted by sound waves.

Thus sound waves travel as a result of the patterns of molecular displacement in the same direction as the applied force. Since the molecular movement in air is horizontal, or parallel to the driving force, sound waves in air are described as longitudinal waves.

It should be apparent, then, that sound cannot travel in a vacuum, that is, in an area in which there is very low molecular density. Sound requires an elastic medium, which is provided in solids (such as steel, wood, or body tissue), in liquids (such as water), as well as in a gas (such as air).

The density of the material—"the number of molecules per unit of volume" —determines the velocity at which sound may be propagated. Sound travels faster in denser materials. For example, sound travels more rapidly through steel (about 15,000 feet/second) than through air (about 1100 feet/second), since steel

Figure 4.1

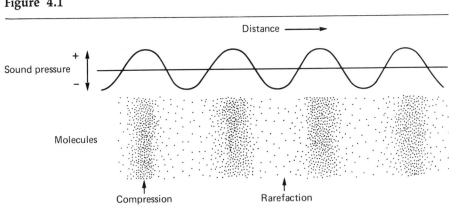

A graph of sound-pressure changes and alternating compression and rarefaction of molecules in sound propagation in air.

is denser than air. Compared to the speed of light (186,000 miles/second), sound travels very slowly. This comparison is apparent during a thunder storm, since lightning can be seen at a distance well before the thunder it produces can be heard.

Simple Harmonic Motion

Several acoustic properties need to be explained: **frequency, amplitude,** and **phase.** These characteristics can be defined and understood most readily in the context of **simple harmonic motion** (SHM). Consider the motion of a pendulum, as depicted in Fig. 4.2. The pendulum is at its position of rest, point A, when it is suspended vertically from its place of attachment. If a force is applied from the left, the pendulum is displaced toward the right, point B. The pendulum will return to its position of rest, but because of elasticity and enertia (the tendency to maintain a constant velocity, that is, stay at rest or in motion), it will pass through its position of rest and move a similar distance to the left, point C, as compared to the distance it was displaced to the right. In turn, it will move again

Figure 4.2

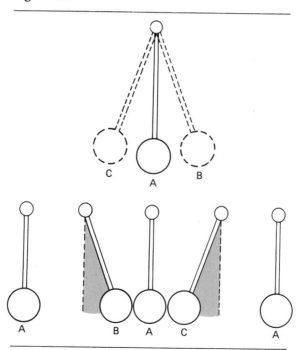

Simple harmonic motion, depicted by the motion of a pendulum.

83

to its position of rest, point A, which is the completion of one full cycle. Although this motion may repeat itself until it is halted by frictional forces, let us focus our attention on the motion that occurred in one complete cycle.

The time required for one complete cycle is referred to as the **period.** The number of complete cycles occurring within a given time interval, usually a second, is referred to as the *frequency of vibration.* By convention, the frequency, or number of cycles per second, is referred to as *Hz,* after the German physicist Hertz, who described periodic motion. Thus by this international convention 100 cycles per second, for example, would be referred to as 100 Hz. The period required for a complete cycle and the frequency of vibration are reciprocally related; thus 1/f equals the period, and 1/p equals the frequency.

The *amplitude* of vibration is the distance of displacement of the particle or vibrator from its position of rest or equilibrium. In Fig. 4.2, the distance the pendulum moved from its position of rest (point A) to the farthest lateral position (point B or point C) would be described as the amplitude, or distance of displacement. In general, the greater the applied force, the greater the amplitude.

The *phase* of vibration depicts exactly the position and direction of particle or vibrator movement and is often expressed in degrees. For example, in Fig. 4.2, the pendulum at its point of rest (point A) is at zero degrees phase; at point B, phase is 90 degrees; at its return to point A, phase is 180 degrees; at point C, 270 degrees; and after one complete cycle, it has traversed 360 degrees.

All of these characteristics of simple harmonic motion can be described accurately and conveniently by a function from trigonometry, the **sine wave** function, which is shown in Fig. 4.3. Thus SHM often is referred to as a sine wave. Note that time is depicted along the horizontal axis and that the time required for one complete cycle is the *period* of the particular frequency. The distance in the vertical direction, thus on the vertical axis, shows the amplitude at any given time within the period of vibration. Finally, any specific point on the sine wave indicates the phase, which reveals the position and direction of displacement.

It must be recognized that SHM, or the sine wave (sinusoid), describes a pure frequency, or vibration at a single frequency only. Pure frequencies rarely occur in nature, but are generated by tuning forks or pure "tone" audiometers, which will be discussed in Chapters 6 and 13. Most natural sounds are complex in their frequency and amplitude characteristics. Speech is indeed a complex sound, so we must consider this concept in detail.

Complex Sounds

Complex sounds are composed of many frequencies which may vary in phase and amplitude. Complex sounds may be classified as **periodic waves** or **aperiodic waves,** which implies that the sound-wave form either does or does not continuously repeat itself. For example, continuous vibrations such as vocal-fold vibrations are periodic, and random noises such as clicks are aperiodic. Is it possible,

Figure 4.3

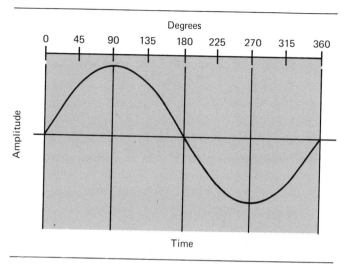

A sine wave used to describe simple harmonic motion.

then, to determine the frequency composition of a complex wave? Fortunately, this problem was solved for us by a brilliant French mathematician, Fourier, more than a century ago. Fourier demonstrated that all complex waves—periodic or aperiodic—are composed of the sum of a number of sine waves (sinusoids) of different frequencies, phases, and amplitudes. Figure 4.4 shows three different frequencies (A, B, C) which when summed would produce a periodic complex wave (D). Conversely, if the complex sound produced by waveform were analyzed, the components, or individual sinusoids, would be revealed to be A, B, and C.

Such an analysis reveals the **spectrum,** or the frequency and amplitude, of the components of the complex wave. The spectrum of a periodic complex wave is shown in Fig. 4.5. The frequency of the various components is shown on the horizontal axis, and amplitude is indicated by the height of the vertical line at each frequency. In the case of a pure frequency, or sinusoid, in SHM, of course, spectrum is indicated by only a single vertical line which appears at the respective frequency. The spectrum of a complex wave, however, includes many different frequencies.

We can further clarify our earlier distinction between periodic and aperiodic complex waves by considering differences in the spectrum of such waves. The spectrum of periodic waves, as shown in Fig. 4.5, will reveal that each component frequency is a whole-number multiple of the lowest frequency in the spectrum. The lowest frequency is referred to as the first **harmonic,** or more commonly as the **fundamental frequency.** For example, if the lowest frequency were 200 Hz,

Figure 4.4

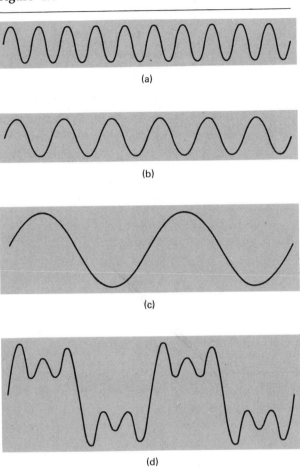

(a)

(b)

(c)

(d)

A periodic complex wave and its individual sine-wave components. (From The Speech Chain *by P. B. Denes and E. N. Pinson. Copyright © 1963 by Bell Telephone Laboratories, Inc. Reprinted by permission of Doubleday & Company, Inc.*

higher frequencies would be present at twice the fundamental frequency (400 Hz, or the second harmonic), three times the fundamental (600 Hz, or the third harmonic), and so forth.

Conversely, the spectrum of an aperiodic complex wave might reveal all or numerous component frequencies which bear no inherent relationship. Therefore, the spectrum of such waveforms would appear as a curve, as shown in

Figure 4.5

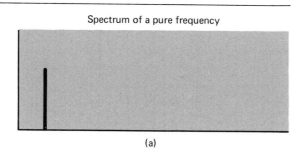

Spectrum of a pure frequency

(a)

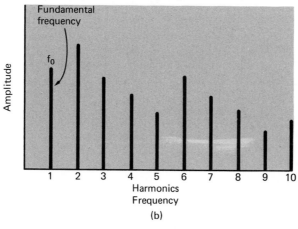

Spectrum of a complex periodic sound

(b)

The spectrum of (a) a single-sine wave and (b) a complex periodic sound.

Fig. 4.6, rather than as distinct vertical lines for each frequency. Amplitude is indicated in the spectrum of the aperiodic wave by the height of the curve at respective frequencies.

It is important to recognize the difference between periodic and aperiodic complex waves, since both waveforms are significant in speech acoustics and perception. In the production of a vowel sound, for example, the vocal folds vibrate periodically and thus produce periodic waves. In the production of consonant sounds, by contrast, aperiodic waves are introduced. Such differences are readily distinguishable by the human listener; for example, the sound "ah" is periodic and "sh" is aperiodic.

Figure 4.6

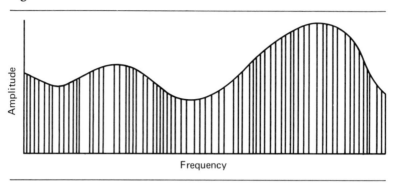

The spectrum of a complex aperiodic sound.

Resonance

The spectrum of an acoustic signal is influenced significantly by the acoustic environment in which the signal is generated and propagated. For example, the vibration of the vocal folds generates only a complex buzzing sound in isolation. In normal speech production, however, the vocal folds produce pressure changes which resonate in the throat, mouth, and nasal cavities (the vocal tract). As a result of this **resonance,** the quality of voiced sounds is quite different from that which would result from vocal-fold vibration alone.

Let us examine the concept of resonance. All objects or volumes of air in open and closed tubes and cavities vibrate more readily at some frequencies than at others. That is, all have certain natural frequencies of vibration and thus are more responsive to those frequencies. Therefore, when signals with a complex spectrum are generated, the frequencies in that complex will resonate more freely and thus with greater amplitude if they are the natural frequencies of a given object or volume of air.

The concept of resonance is of particular significance in the acoustics of speech. Since the vibration of the vocal folds is periodic, the acoustic spectrum of vocal-fold vibration contains a fundamental frequency with certain harmonics or overtones. Since the cavities of the vocal tract as resonators have certain natural frequencies, they will be responsive to some and not to other frequencies generated by the vocal folds. Also, as noted in Chapter 3, the cavities of the vocal tract are modified continuously during the production of speech, and thus the tract may assume different resonant frequencies.

Formant Frequencies

The resonances of the vocal tract are called **formants,** and the frequencies to which they are most responsive are called formant frequencies. Formant frequencies are most apparent in the spectrum of vowel sounds and are revealed as resonance peaks, that is, the peaks of maximum energy or amplitude at given frequencies. Since the configuration of the vocal tract must be changed to produce different speech sounds, different formant frequencies also occur. Recall that the fundamental frequency and resultant harmonics are produced by the vibration of the vocal folds. Formant frequencies result from changes in the vocal tract, and thus the resultant resonant frequencies are not the same as the harmonics produced by the vocal folds unless by coincidence (Denes and Pinson, 1973; Minifie, 1973). Figure 4.7 indicates a periodic signal produced by the vocal folds and the resultant harmonic spectrum, which reflects the fundamental frequency of vocal-fold vibration and the respective harmonics. It also indicates a vocal-tract configuration and the resonant or formant frequencies that occur as a result of vocal-tract resonance on the vocal-fold output.

As mentioned, vowels are characterized by periodic signals and resonant or formant frequencies; consonants typically are characterized by aperiodic signals

Figure 4.7

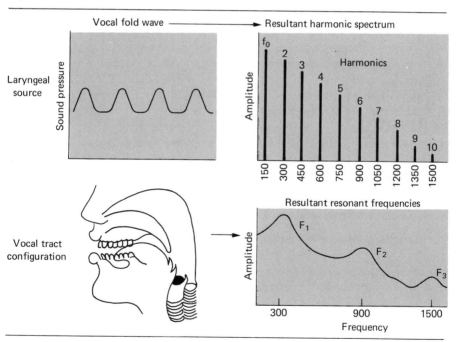

A periodic signal produced by the vocal folds and the resultant harmonic spectrum are shown in the upper portion. The vocal-tract configuration and the resultant formant or resonant frequencies are shown in the lower portion.

which may or may not include periodic information as a result of voicing. The voiceless consonant contains only aperiodic vibration, which results from air turbulence produced by changing and constricting the size of the orifice of the mouth and friction or interference in air flow by the articulators such as the tongue, teeth, and lips. Voiced consonants, of course, include the periodic vibration of the vocal folds and the aperiodic vibration described in voiceless consonants.

Speech Perception

Considerable acoustic information is generated by the speech mechanism, and as indicated in Chapter 1 speech is acoustic information which varies over time. Thus speech intensity, duration of speech sounds, and the frequency components of speech change continuously during spoken language. Obviously, the acoustic information that reaches the ear permits us to understand spoken language. In our study of speech perception, we wish to learn how this information is used, or at least to discover what information is important. Does understanding depend on receiving all of the acoustic information generated in speech production? We probably can determine from our own experiences that even though certain aspects of speech are lost or distorted in transmission or simply missed in listening, the message nevertheless is understood. If so, how can we determine the necessary conditions or characteristics for understanding?

One method might be to modify or eliminate certain characteristics of normal speech and see if speech intelligibility is impaired. In such an experiment listeners would report what they could or could not understand under given conditions. Another method might be to generate "speech sounds" artificially, known as synthetic speech, and, as in normal speech, modify or eliminate certain characteristics and study the effect on speech intelligibility.

Speech-Reception Threshold and Discrimination

Speech intelligibility can be measured in different ways, but there are essentially two primary measures. First, it is important to know how loud, or actually at what intensity, speech must be presented for a normal listener to hear and understand. This measure is referred to as **speech-reception threshold.** The speech-reception threshold usually is measured by the use of two-syllable words which carry equal stress on each syllable, such as *baseball* or *staircase*. These words are relatively homogeneous and are easily audible. Second, it is important to know how well speech can be discriminated when presented at a sufficient loudness or intensity level to be understood. This measure is referred to as **speech discrimination** testing. Speech discrimination usually is measured by the use of single-syllable words selected to reflect the frequency of particular sounds as they occur in spoken English. Such word lists are referred to as phonetically balanced, or PB, lists. Both of these measures are of fundamental importance in measuring hearing loss as well as normal hearing for speech and thus will be discussed further in Chapter 13.

Acoustic Characteristics and Perception

Since we have indicated ways in which we can measure speech intelligibility, we can now consider the effects of modifying the acoustic characteristics of which speech is composed: intensity and frequency.

Intensity Since intensity changes are the least complicated to study, let us consider the effects of intensity first. It is intuitively clear that speech must be sufficiently loud or intense to be understood. The intensity range among the various speech sounds of English is 680 to 1, or a range of 28 dB from the weakest to the strongest speech sound. (Decibel, a unit of sound energy or intensity stated in pressure or power, is abbreviated as "dB" and will be explained in greater detail in Chapter 6.) The energy or sound pressure of normal speech measured at one meter from the lips of the speaker is about 65 dB. If a person talks as loudly as possible, speech may reach a sound-pressure level of about 85 dB, and the softest speech is about 45 dB (Fletcher, 1953).

Vowel sounds derive their initial energy from vibration of the vocal folds. In males the fundamental frequency of the vocal folds is about 125 Hz and in females about an octave higher, or 250 Hz. Since vowel sounds are periodic signals composed of the fundamental and related harmonics of vocal-fold vibration, the primary energy in vowel sounds is of low frequency. Also, vowel sounds are known to carry most of the energy or power of speech and in addition are of longer duration than consonants. In fact, in spoken English, the frequencies below 500 Hz contain 60 percent of the power of speech but contribute only 5 percent to intelligibility. The frequencies above 1000 Hz contribute 5 percent of the power and 60 percent of the intelligibility. Thus the vowels, or low-frequency sounds, carry most of the power, and the consonants, or higher-frequency speech sounds, are much more important for speech intelligibility (Fletcher, 1953).

Effects of noise Heretofore, we have discussed the intelligibility of speech in quiet listening. In real-life situations, however, we frequently listen to speech in the presence of noise. In general, noise does not interfere seriously in understanding speech unless the noise and the speech occur in the same frequency range. This often does occur, however, and in these cases the relationship between the signal-to-noise intensities is critical. If speech is 100 times more intense than the noise, speech intelligibility is not affected. If speech and noise are of equal intensities, speech intelligibility may be reduced for word lists by 50 percent (Denes and Pinson, 1973). In many situations, however, speech may be understood even when it is of lower intensity than noise if the speech and the noise come from two different directions. This matter will be discussed further when binaural hearing is considered in Chapter 6.

Frequency The relationship between speech intelligibility and frequency pertains, of course, to the spectrum of speech sounds. The frequency range of speech sounds is from about 100 to 8000 Hz. As mentioned, most of the energy of speech occurs below 1000 Hz, and peak energy occurs at about 500 or 600 Hz. The influence of the frequency range of speech on intelligibility can be determined by the use of filters, devices which can be used to eliminate somewhat selectively certain frequency bands or ranges from a broader frequency spectrum. For example, filters can be used to eliminate high- and/or low-frequency bands and thus pass a selective midfrequency band.

Important findings have resulted from experiments in which filters were used. For example, speech intelligibility for one-syllable words is reduced only slightly when frequencies above 1600 Hz are eliminated. When filtering is extended downward to 800 Hz, 25 percent reduction occurs in intelligibility. Conversely, when frequencies below 1600 Hz are eliminated, intelligibility is not adversely affected. When all frequencies below 3200 Hz are filtered out, intelligibility is reduced again by about 25 percent.

This information reveals some important conclusions, then, about the relationship of frequency spectrum and intelligibility. First, it is apparent that speech can be rather well understood if we can hear only those sounds of speech below 1600 Hz; conversely, speech can be understood only if we hear those sounds of speech above 1600 Hz (Hirsh, Reynolds, and Joseph, 1954). Figure 4.8 shows the speech intelligibility in percentages for the two filtering conditions. Since it is apparent that we do not need all the low-frequency or all the high-frequency information to understand speech satisfactorily, we must determine just what frequency band is necessary to understand speech. Apparently it is some midfrequency band. A band-pass filter can be used to pass selective frequency bands so as to investigate their importance. In other words, the upper and lower frequency limits can be adjusted until satisfactory speech intelligibility is obtained. Such experiments have indicated that the most important range of frequency for speech intelligibility is about 300 to 3000 Hz (Davis and Silverman, 1970).

Segmental Analysis

A **segmental analysis** of vowel sounds reveals that the perception of vowels depends essentially on the respective formant frequencies of the sound. Such formants are shown in Fig. 4.9. It is interesting to note that even though different individuals have varying sizes of vocal mechanisms and vocal tracts, men, women, and children all use about the same vocal-tract configurations to produce the same vowel sounds. Although the formant frequencies may be higher or lower in different persons, the formant pattern or frequency ratio (relation-

Figure 4.8

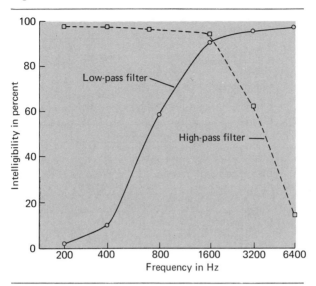

Speech intelligibility under two filtering conditions —low-pass filtering, in which energy below 1600 Hz was passed, and high-pass filtering, in which energy above 1600 Hz was passed. (Adapted from W. R. Hodgson, "Speech Acoustics and Intelligibility," in W. R. Hodgson and P. Skinner, eds., Hearing Aid Assessment and Use, Baltimore: Williams and Wilkins, 1977.)

ship among frequencies) is about the same, and thus the vowel is perceived to be the same even though produced by different speakers.

Many consonant sounds are classified as either *fricatives* (e.g., "s" or "sh") or *stops* (plosives) (e.g., "p" or "t") and are produced by constriction of the vocal tract (see Chapter 3). The constriction of the vocal tract results in a turbulent air stream which passes continuously through the tract. It is possible to distinguish among fricative sounds, essentially because of spectral or frequency differences. For example, "s" has little energy below 4000 Hz, with a resonance peak between 4000 and 7000 Hz. In contrast, "sh" has a significantly lower spectrum, with primary intensity at about 2500 Hz (Strevens, 1960; Fant, 1960). Stops, or plosives, result when the turbulent air stream is stopped by closure of the vocal tract and then released. In English, plosives occurring in the initial position of a word are "exploded" more strongly than are those occurring at the final position of a word; for example, the initial plosive "p" in the word "pop" is more forcefully exploded than the final plosive "p." Plosives are dis-

93

Figure 4.9

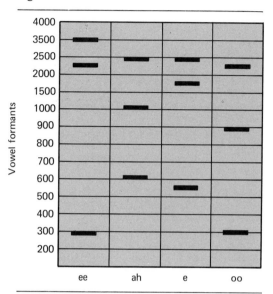

Formant frequencies for selected vowel sounds.

tinguished among one another and from other consonants as a result of spectral differences. For example, the voiced plosive "b" and its unvoiced cognate "p" have most energy between 500 and 1500 Hz. In contrast, "t" and "d" have a higher spectrum, with energy up to about 4000 Hz (Halle, Hughes, and Radley, 1957). The discrimination of a plosive, however, may be influenced significantly by its use in a word.

Coarticulation

The observation that the recognition of specific speech sounds, or phonemes, may commonly be influenced by associated or connecting sounds vastly complicates our efforts to understand speech perception (Curtis, 1970). Traditionally, speech has been considered to be composed of a sequence of distinctive, separate sounds—by analogy, "beads on a string." Although this may be essentially so in analysis of sounds in isolation, it indeed is not the case in an analysis of continuing, or "running," speech.

The interaction of associated sounds is referred to as **coarticulation.** As indicated in Chapter 3, coarticulation occurs because the vocal tract is continually in transition in the production of continuous speech, since its configuration for any given sound is influenced by the shape required for the previous sound and anticipatory movement for production of a following sound.

Spectrogram

The acoustic patterns of speech, which change continuously, can be observed by spectrographic analysis to reveal the effects of certain preceding and succeeding sounds on a given sound. A special electronic instrument, the speech spectrograph, can record and display the acoustic changes which occur in speech production over time. The resultant analysis is referred to as a **speech spectrogram** and is shown in Fig. 4.10. Frequency is represented on the vertical axis; time, on the horizontal axis. The effect of amplitude, or intensity, is indicated by the relative density or darkness of the pattern.

The speech spectrogram has been used as an aid for deaf persons to "read" speech by the visual patterns—"visible speech," so to speak (Potter, Kopp, and Green, 1947); however, it has proved to be more useful for acoustic analysis of speech. In recent times, the speech spectrogram has been used as a method to identify speakers as a "voiceprint"; however, this application is quite controversial. Some experts claim that individual speakers can be identified by "voiceprints," but most disagree.

As mentioned, the spectrograph has provided much useful information on the relationship between acoustic changes in transition among speech sounds and speech perception. It was noted earlier, for example, that the identification of plosives is influenced by associated transitional sounds. In synthetic speech,

Figure 4.10

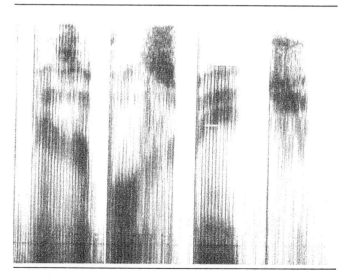

A speech spectrogram of the message "Visible Speech." (Type B/65 Sonagram® Kay Elemetrics Co., Pine Brook, N.J.)

if the "d" sound of the sound "du" is removed by cutting it from the "tape," the "u" will be perceived as the complete syllable "du." Similarly, if the "u" sound is removed and the "d" retained, again the full syllable will be perceived. If the "transitional pattern" or acoustic portion of the syllable between the "d" and the "u" is removed and a silent interval substituted, the perception of the sound "du" will be degraded significantly (Liberman *et al.*, 1967).

This discussion of coarticulation leads us to the realization that separate or segmental features of speech commonly do not provide independently or integrally the information necessary for their recognition or the perception of speech. Stated otherwise, the recognition or perception of continuous speech is determined also by **suprasegmental factors.**

Suprasegmental Factors

Many other factors influence the perception of speech, such as changes in intonation or "melody" of the voice, stress on syllables, rate of syllable utterance, and duration of syllables. The duration and stress of speech sounds often are critical in the perception of speech. For example, the word "OBject" may be used as a noun under certain conditions; the same word "obJECT" may be used as a verb under other conditions.

Other Factors

Clearly, many factors must be considered to understand human perception of speech. We have considered the acoustic, segmental, and suprasegmental aspects of speech and in so doing discovered the importance of "transitional patterns" of speech. We acknowledged further that despite individual differences in voice quality or speech acoustics and sex differences on speech frequency, the same speech sounds can be recognized. Moreover, humans have the capacity to perceive speech in the presence of noise and among competing messages which result in the loss of acoustic information. Finally, given the same information, machines engineered to recognize speech can do so only with vastly limited capacity as compared to human observers. Surely other factors must be considered.

Situational clues permit the listener to anticipate what might be or might have been said. When combined with prior knowledge about situations or various conversational subjects, one may be able to follow conversations with less than complete perception of all the acoustic information transmitted.

Language

Obviously, knowledge of the spoken language used is fundamental to speech perception. We must comprehend the speech code or its sound patterns, the words, the grammar, the syntax in order to understand the word order and semantics to derive meaning. With this knowledge, it is possible to anticipate what will precede and follow many words, be they perceived or missed. It is also possible to synthesize partial information to comprehend messages.

Conclusion

Although the study of speech acoustics is fundamental for an understanding of speech perception, many other factors are important as well. Moreover, the importance of certain acoustic information and linguistic and situational factors varies under different conditions. Indeed, the perception of speech is not a simple matter. The most elementary study of speech sounds in isolation or through segmental analysis is confounded seriously by coarticulation in "running speech." Suprasegmental analysis may be confounded by linguistic and situational factors. Nevertheless, the human brain apparently has an innate capacity to recognize spoken language. In addition, machines have been built which can recognize certain types of speech messages. Remarkable advances have been envisioned through speech control of machines which some day may be realized through the scientific study of speech acoustics and perception.

Glossary

Amplitude: The distance of displacement of a particle or vibrator from its position of rest.

Aperiodic waves: Random or nonrepetitive waves, such as a click. Vibration that does not repeat itself at a fixed or continuous frequency.

Coarticulation: The interaction of associated sounds which results from continuous changes in voicing and the vocal tract in the production of continuous speech.

Complex wave or sound: A sound composed of many frequencies which may vary in amplitude and phase.

Compression: The bunching together of molecules as a result of an applied force.

Elastic medium: In general, mass—be it air or solid—can be compressed or changed in shape. If it tends to retain its shape, it is elastic. If air molecules are expanded or compressed, they will spring back to their normal position.

Formants: The resonances of an instrument or the vocal tract. In speech, formant frequencies are the natural frequencies or resonance frequencies of the vocal tract.

Frequency: The number of complete cycles that occur in a given time interval.

Fundamental frequency: The first or lowest frequency in a periodic complex wave.

Harmonics: Whole-number multiples of a fundamental frequency. Also referred to as overtones which occur in a periodic complex wave.

Period: The time required for completion of one full cycle.

Periodic wave: A wave or sound that continuously repeats itself. The vibration of the vocal folds produces periodic waves.

Phase: An indication of the position and direction of particle or vibrator movement. Phase may be measured in degrees.

Rarefaction: The spread or thinning of molecules as a result of release of an applied force in the compression of molecules or a force exerted in an opposite direction.

Resonance: The natural frequency of vibration of solids or a volume of air.

Segmental analysis: An analysis of speech sounds in which sounds are studied either in isolation or when separated arbitrarily from other sounds in continuous speech.

Simple harmonic motion: Vibration at a single frequency.

Sine wave: A mathematical function that describes exactly the frequency, amplitude, and phase of simple harmonic motion.

Sound generation: Vibration of an object or volume of air as a result of an applied force.

Sound propagation: Transmission of pressure waves through a medium such as air or metal as a result of compression and rarefaction of molecules.

Spectrum: An analysis or graph showing all the frequency components of a complex wave and their respective amplitudes.

Speech discrimination: The ability to understand the various sounds of speech when speech is presented at an intensity level sufficient for speech to be understood.

Speech-reception threshold: The intensity of speech necessary for a listener to be just able to hear and understand speech.

Speech spectrogram: A visual display of speech sounds or acoustic changes that occur over time in the production of speech.

Suprasegmental factors: Characteristics of speech that are above or larger than the separate sound segments of speech. Factors such as melody or intonation of the voice, rate of syllable utterance, and stress.

Study Questions

1. What is required for the generation of sound?
2. How does sound travel through the air?

3. What is the difference between a sine wave and a complex wave?
4. What is the relationship between sine waves and a complex wave?
5. What is the difference between periodic and aperiodic sounds?
6. What is resonance and why is it important in speech?
7. What are formants and why are they important in the perception of vowels?
8. What is the relationship between frequency and the perception of speech?
9. What information has been learned about the acoustics of speech through segmental analysis?
10. Why is segmental analysis complicated by coarticulation?
11. How might suprasegmental factors influence the perception of speech?
12. Since acoustical information may be lost as a result of noise and competing messages, how is it possible to understand speech under such conditions?

Bibliography

CURTIS, J., "Segmenting the Stream of Speech," in J. Griffith and L. Miner, eds., *The First Lincolnland Conference on Dialectology*, Chapter 3, University: University of Alabama Press, 1970.

DAVIS, H., AND R. SILVERMAN, *Hearing and Deafness*, 3rd ed., New York: Holt, Rinehart and Winston, 1970.

DENES, P., AND E. PINSON, *The Speech Chain*, New York: Bell Telephone Laboratories, 1973.

FANT, G., *Acoustic Theory of Speech Production*, The Hague: Mouton, 1960.

FLETCHER, H., *Speech and Hearing in Communication*, Princeton, N.J.: Van Nostrand, 1953.

HALLE, M., G. HUGHES, AND J. RADLEY, "Acoustic Properties of Stop Consonants," *J. Acoust. Soc. Amer.* **29** (1957):107–116.

HIRSH, I. J., G. REYNOLDS, AND M. JOSEPH, "Intelligibility of Different Speech Materials," *J. Acoust. Soc. Amer.* **26** (1954):530–538.

HODGSON, W., "Speech Acoustics and Intelligibility," in W. Hodgson and P. Skinner, eds., *Hearing Aid Assessment and Use*, Chapter 6, Baltimore: Williams and Wilkins, 1977.

LIBERMAN, A., F. COOPER, D. SHANKWEILER, AND M. STUDDERT-KENNEDY, "Perception of the Speech Code," *Psych. Rev.* **74** (1967):431–461.

MINIFIE, F., "Speech Acoustics," in F. Minifie, T. Hixon, and F. Williams, eds., *Normal Aspects of Speech, Hearing, and Language*, Chapter 7, Englewood Cliffs, N.J.: Prentice-Hall, 1973.

POTTER, R., G. KOPP, AND H. GREEN, *Visible Speech,* New York: Van Nostrand, 1947.

STREVENS, P., "Spectra of Fricative Noise in Human Speech," *Language and Speech* **3** (1960):32–49.

VAN BERGEIJK, W., J. PIERCE, AND E. DAVIS, *Waves and the Ear*, Garden City, N.Y.: Doubleday, 1958.

CHAPTER 5
Overview

Necessary to understanding the role that hearing plays in the human communication process is a basic knowledge of how the ear receives sound from the environment and converts it to meaningful signals within the nervous system. The hearing mechanism is the most complex of all our sensory systems. This is true partly because of the tremendous range of intensities and frequencies that the ear must be able to respond to and partly because the tiny amount of energy that constitutes quiet sounds must be carefully preserved if it is to be heard. The ear takes energy from the air in the form of vibrations and converts that energy to several other forms in the process of creating nervous impulses. Each of these changes in the form of sound energy has to be accomplished very effectively so that a minimum amount of energy is lost in the process. In this chapter the anatomy and function of the ear are described by following sound energy on its journey through the ear and observing both its effects on the ear and the ways in which that sound energy is transformed by the ear.

K. D. McClelland, Ph.D.
University of Southern Mississippi

Hearing Mechanism

Introduction

The ear is a mechanism for gathering sound from the environment and changing it into a form that can be interpreted by the brain. This changing of sound energy into nervous energy—or, for that matter, the changing of any energy from one form to another—is called **transduction.** The overall function of the ear is to transform sound energy into nervous energy, but this transduction process has some important intermediate steps. As sound energy (see Chapter 4) passes from the ear canal into the middle ear, it is converted to mechanical motion. Energy is changed from mechanical motion to fluid displacement as it passes from the middle ear into the inner ear. Further intermediate transductions occur in the inner ear—some mechanical, some electrical—before the final transformation to nervous impulses takes place.

Although the events in the transduction process occur almost simultaneously, it is convenient to consider the anatomy and physiology of the ear in the natural anatomical sequence that sound energy follows in its journey through the ear mechanism. The *outer ear, middle ear,* and *inner ear* will be considered in that order (see Fig. 5.1).

Outer Ear

The **auricle,** the visible part of the ear, plays a very minor role in human hearing. In some animals the auricle is highly developed to collect sound and can be moved to help locate a sound source without turning the head. Rabbits, cats, and horses have this capability. In beavers, otters, and other swimming mammals, the external ear can be closed off to keep water and dirt out. Birds, reptiles, and amphibians do not even have an external ear, yet they hear effectively.

The relationships among the major anatomical features of the human ear are shown in Fig. 5.1. The **ear canal** (external auditory meatus) runs horizontally from the opening in the auricle toward the center of the head and is closed at its inner end by the **tympanic membrane.** The canal is about 2.5 cm long and varies in shape from individual to individual. It is lined with skin that is continuous with the surface of the auricle and contains stiff hairs and glands which secrete **cerumen** (ear wax) near its outer end. The hairs aid in keeping insects and foreign particles out of the ear. Cerumen, an effective insect repellent and an antiseptic, also serves to carry dirt and foreign particles out of the ear and helps to keep the skin of the ear canal from drying out.

Sound waves arriving at the **outer ear** are funneled down the ear canal to the tympanic membrane, which moves in and out in response to the pressure changes. As an acoustic resonator (see Chapter 4), the ear canal amplifies sound energy in the frequency range between approximately 1500 and 5500 Hz and by

Figure 5.1

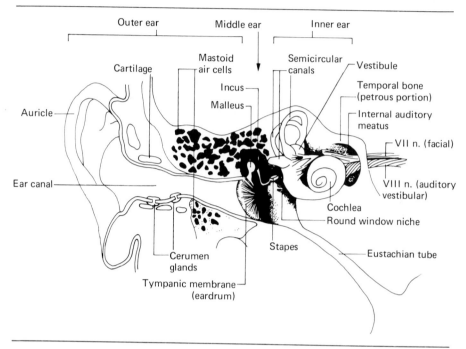

The ear. (From Hearing and Deafness, *Third Edition by Hallowell Davis and S. Richard Silverman. Copyright © 1947, 1960, 1970 by Holt, Rinehart and Winston, Inc. Adapted by permission of Holt, Rinehart and Winston.)*

so doing makes the ear about four times more sensitive to tones near 3800 Hz than it would be without the canal resonance (Wever and Lawrence, 1954).

Middle Ear

Components

The *tympanic membrane,* or eardrum, forms the lateral wall of the air-filled middle-ear cavity and separates the cavity from the ear canal. The **middle ear,** similar in size and shape to an aspirin tablet, is 15 mm in its vertical dimension, 10–15 mm in its anterior/posterior dimension, and about 4 mm wide. The middle-ear cavity lies between the soft, spongy part of the **temporal bone** called the *mastoid* and the inner petrous portion of the temporal bone which contains the inner ear and lies adjacent to the brain. ("Petrous" means rocklike, and the bone was given that name because it is the hardest bone in the human body.)

The **Eustachian tube,** a duct that opens into the middle-ear cavity (see Fig. 5.2), connects the air-filled middle ear to outside air. The Eustachian tube is normally closed, but opens and ventilates the middle ear whenever an individual swallows or yawns. Ventilation of the middle ear is necessary for two reasons. First, body tissues absorb air, and the middle ear would soon fill with fluid secretion if fresh air were not periodically introduced. Second, ventilation equalizes pressure differences between the two sides of the eardrum brought about by atmospheric-pressure changes, skin diving, flying, or mountain driving. Air-pressure differences between the two sides of the tympanic membrane limit its freedom to vibrate. Large pressure differences can rupture the eardrum.

The tympanic membrane is a thin, pearl gray, almost translucent cone-shaped membrane. The apex of the cone is pointed into the middle-ear cavity. The membrane consists of three layers and is attached to the wall of the ear canal by a thickened fibrous ring (an annulus) which fits into a groove in the bony canal wall.

Figure 5.2

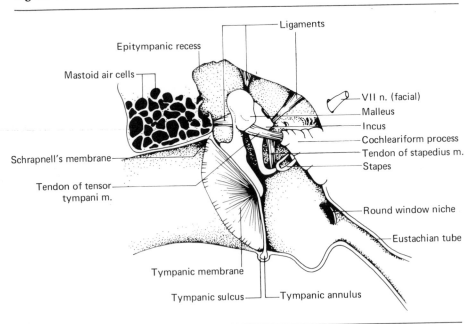

Structures of the middle ear. (Adapted from P. B. Denes and E. N. Pinson, The Speech Chain, New York: Bell Laboratories, 1963; and H. Davis and S. R. Silverman, Hearing and Deafness, 3rd ed., New York: Holt, Rinehart and Winston, 1970.)

Attached to the inner layer of the drum membrane is one of the three smallest bones in the body. It is the first of a series of three bones called the **ossicular chain,** and this chain conducts sound energy across the air-filled middle ear to the inner ear. The first of these bones, the hammer-shaped *malleus,* is firmly attached to the next member of the three-bone chain, the *incus.* A long arm of the incus curves down and medially to attach to the head of the last bone, the **stapes,** by means of a joint that permits some motion between the incus and stapes. Motion at this point is important because it allows the stapes to vibrate in one direction for low-intensity sounds and to change its direction of vibration for high-intensity sounds to reduce the amount of energy transmitted to the inner ear. The ossicles are held in place within the cavity by several ligaments and two muscles (the smallest in the body), called the **stapedius** and the **tensor tympani.**

Transduction Processes

When sound energy enters the middle ear, the first of several transduction processes occurs. Variations in pressure, which constitute sound in the ear canal, become mechanical motion of the ossicles. In the process of transferring vibratory motion from the tympanic membrane to the inner ear, the middle ear performs two major functions: (1) protection against excessively loud sounds, and even more important (2) **impedance matching,** or delivering sound energy from the eardrum to the inner ear with very little loss.

The most important function of the middle ear is to serve as a *mechanical transformer,* decreasing the amplitude and increasing the force of vibration of the stapes relative to the vibrations of the eardrum. Air through which sound is transmitted has very little mass compared with the inner-ear fluid to which vibration must be transmitted. This results in what engineers call a *mismatch in impedance* between the two media. The magnitude of this problem can be illustrated by stating that when sound is present in air adjacent to water, 99.9 percent of that sound energy will be reflected back into the air, and only 0.1 percent will enter the water.

Two mechanisms present in the middle ear act together as a mechanical transformer to match impedance. First, a small lever advantage gained by the bones of the middle ear is applied at the base of the stapes. Second and more important is the ratio of the area of the eardrum to the area of the **stapes footplate.** About two-thirds of the eardrum is effective in transmitting sound energy to the stapes. The footplate of the stapes has a much smaller area than the eardrum. The difference in area between the eardrum and stapes footplate results in a substantial pressure increase at the footplate. This pressure increase, together with the lever advantage provided by the arrangement of the ossicles, results in a good impedance match between inner-ear fluid and the air.

Protection and impedance matching might seem to be mutually contradictory tasks for the middle ear because one function (protection) involves reducing the amount of energy allowed to pass, whereas the other involves transferring energy as efficiently as possible. Protection is necessary only when sound levels are high; optimum transmission, however, is important at all sound levels and is especially important when the sound is weak.

Both protection against and optimum transmission of sound energy can be accomplished in the middle ear because different mechanisms perform the two functions. Two mechanisms help protect the inner ear by reducing the transmission of excessive intensities, and two other mechanisms provide for optimum energy transfer. One of the protective mechanisms is the **middle-ear-muscle reflex** (acoustic reflex). The two middle-ear muscles contract reflexively when loud sounds enter the ear. The contraction of the stapedius tends to pull the stapes out of the opening into the inner ear called the **oval window.** Movement of the stapes in the oval window moves the fluid in the inner ear, and this fluid motion transmits the sound energy from the middle ear into the inner ear.

Alongside the Eustachian tube lies the *tensor tympani.* Contraction of this muscle pulls the eardrum into the middle-ear cavity. When high-intensity sounds enter the ear, the stapedius and tensor tympani muscles contract, reducing the mobility of the ossicles. Since the two muscles act at about the same time in different (antagonistic) directions, their overall effect is to stiffen the ossicular chain and reduce its amplitude of vibration.

The second protective mechanism is the mode of stapes vibration. The stapes is able to vibrate in two different directions. When low- or moderate-intensity sounds enter the ear, the stapes moves in and out of the oval window, much like

Figure 5.3

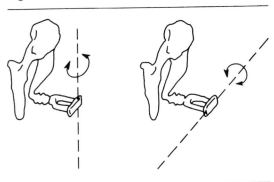

Modes of stapes vibration: (a) low to moderate intensities; (b) high intensities. (From The Speech Chain by Peter Denes and Elliot N. Pinson. Copyright © 1973 by Bell Telephone Laboratories, Inc. Reprinted by permission of Doubleday & Company, Inc.)

a gate swinging on a hinge located near its back edge. This mode of stapes vibration is efficient in transferring energy into the inner ear and thereby enhances hearing sensitivity. When the intensity of a sound exceeds a certain level, the stapes changes to its second mode of vibration, one that is less efficient in transferring energy to the inner ear. This new mode of stapes vibration causes the stapes to pivot on a horizontal axis located in about the middle of the stapes footplate. When the upper half of the footplate swings into the oval window, the lower half swings out simultaneously, substantially reducing the amount of fluid displaced (see Fig. 5.3).

Inner Ear

Components

The footplate of the stapes fits into an opening in the medial wall of the middle-ear cavity. This opening, called the *oval window,* is the path through which sound energy enters the fluid of the **inner ear.** The inner ear consists of a *labyrinth* of tubes and cavities hollowed out in the petrous portion of the temporal bone. Enclosed within the hardest bone in the body, the labyrinth is probably the best-protected structure in the body. Within the labyrinth are located the receptor organs for the senses of hearing and balance. The *vestibule,* an enlarged central portion of the labyrinth, opens into the oval window.

The hearing part of the inner ear is the **cochlea.** The word "cochlea" means "snail," and the cochlea does look like a snail shell. As Fig. 5.4 shows, the cochlea is like a cave or passages within the bone, like spaces rather than an object. To understand the anatomy of the cochlea more clearly, it is helpful to imagine it unrolled into a straight tube, as shown in Fig. 5.5. The basal end of the cochlea is adjacent to the vestibule and middle ear. The apical end, named for the apex (peak) of the coil, is the end farthest from the vestibule and oval window.

The cochlea is divided into two large fluid-filled cavities for almost its entire length. The dividing structure is a third fluid-filled space variously called the **cochlear partition,** cochlear duct, or scala media. Sound energy (vibration) passes through the oval window from the middle ear into the fluid-filled cavities of the cochlea. Pressure generated by the passage of vibration through the oval window into the cochlear cavities is relieved by the **round window.** This opening (see Fig. 5.5) is covered by a round, flexible membrane called the **secondary tympanic membrane.**

Functioning

Fluid displacement   Pressure generated in the cochlea by motion of the stapes causes the secondary tympanic membrane to bulge into the middle-ear cavity.

107

Figure 5.4

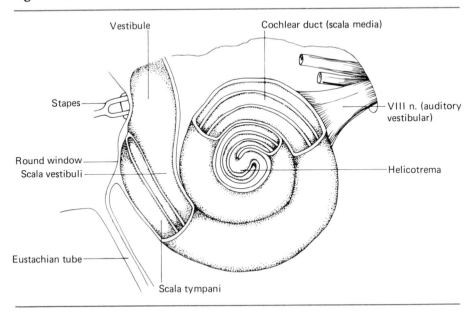

Cutaway view of the cochlea. (From The Speech Chain *by Peter Denes and Elliot N. Pinson. Copyright © 1973 by Bell Telephone Laboratories, Inc. Reprinted by permission of Doubleday & Company, Inc.)*

When the stapes moves back and forth rapidly, as it does in response to sound vibrations, fluid pressure causes the cochlear partition to be displaced. This bulging permits a more direct path for the sound energy to use in going from the stapes to the round window. The bulge created by fluid displacement then moves more slowly along the **basilar membrane,** which forms the floor, or base, of the cochlear partition. The basilar membrane becomes progressively more elastic toward the apical end of the cochlea. It takes as long as three milliseconds for the bulge to travel to the apical end of the cochlea.

The bulge that moves from the basal end of the cochlea toward the apex is called the **traveling wave.** A traveling wave will always move in this direction, regardless of how sound energy is introduced. Each portion of the membrane is most responsive to a particular range of frequencies and will respond to those frequencies with maximum amplitude. This relationship between frequency and place of maximum amplitude on the basilar membrane was observed in cochleas taken from human cadavers by Nobel Prize winner Georg von Békésy. In Fig. 5.6, the numbers along the border of the basilar membrane indicate the approximate location at which the frequency indicated will cause an amplitude maximum in the traveling wave.

108

Figure 5.5

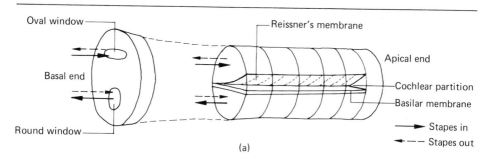

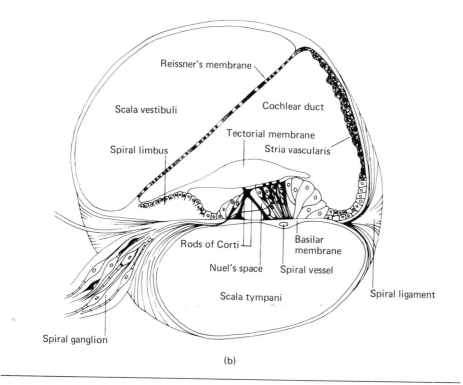

Diagram of (a) uncoiled cochlea; and (b) cochlear cross-section.

Because of the traveling wave, frequencies present in audible sounds are distributed along the length of the basilar membrane, with higher frequencies located nearer the basal end of the cochlea and lower frequencies located nearer the apex. This arrangement of sound frequencies according to specific anatomical location within the cochlea is continued as information about the sound is trans-

109

Figure 5.6

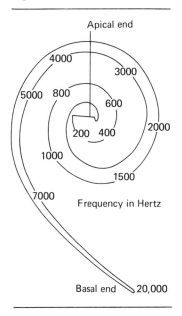

Apical end

4000

3000

5000 800

600

200 400 2000

1000

1500

7000 Frequency in Hertz

Basal end 20,000

Distribution of place of maximum amplitude on the basilar membrane. (From Hearing and Deafness, Third Edition *by Hallowell Davis and S. Richard Silverman. Copyright © 1947, 1960, 1970 by Holt, Rinehart and Winston, Inc. Adapted by permission of Holt, Rinehart and Winston.)*

mitted along the nervous pathways within the brain. The orderly arrangement of frequencies begun in the cochlea and preserved throughout the nervous system all the way to the **auditory cortex** is called **tonatopic organization.**

Although place representation of frequency in the brain has been demonstrated to exist in a general way, mechanical analysis in the cochlea is not precise enough to account for the human ability to discriminate one tone from another. Additional frequency analysis must take place in the auditory nervous system (von Békésy, 1960).

Basilar-membrane activity **Hair cells,** specialized sensory cells located on the basilar membrane, convert the mechanical motion of the basilar membrane into an electrical signal thought to be capable of stimulating auditory nerve endings. Each hair cell supports about 40 individual hairlike structures. The lower ends of these hairs are imbedded in a cuticular plate on the top of the cell. This part of the hair cell is more rigid than the rest of the cell and holds the hairs upright unless force is applied to them.

The organ of Corti, which rests on the basilar membrane, consists of the sensory hair cells and a complex arrangement of supporting cells and structures which limit deformation of the hair cells except at their hair-bearing ends. The approximately 3500 inner and 12,000 outer hair cells in humans are the actual sensory receptors for hearing.

110

The organ of Corti is bounded on the top by the **tectorial membrane,** which on its outer margin is relatively free (see Fig. 5.7). Firmly attached along one margin to a point well above the basilar membrane, the tectorial membrane will slide relative to the netlike structure supporting the hair cells **(reticular lamina)** and exert a shearing force on the hairs of the hair cells whenever the basilar membrane is moved by fluid displacement in the cochlea. When the basilar membrane moves in response to a traveling wave, the tectorial membrane and the reticular lamina tend to slide past each other, much as the two blades of a pair of scissors do. This shearing force bends the sensory hairs because they are located between and attached to the two sliding surfaces.

Electrical activity   The bending of the sensory hairs causes the hair cells to generate an alternating current whose waveform closely approximates the original acoustic pressure wave at the tympanic membrane. This electrical response of the organ of Corti to sound is called the **cochlear microphonic;** it is a summation of the electrical activity of all the hair cells responding to shearing pressure. The cochlear microphonic can be recorded by placing an electrode on the round window or by placing a pair of electrodes within the cochlea itself on either side of the basilar membrane.

The discovery of the cochlear microphonic is reminiscent of the invention of the telephone. Wever and Bray (1930), who had placed an electrode on the **auditory nerve** of a cat, reported that speech could be understood quite clearly when the signal from the cat's auditory nerve was amplified and fed into a loud-

Figure 5.7

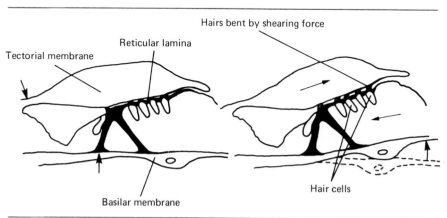

Hair cell shearing action. (Adapted from H. Davis and S. R. Silverman, Hearing and Deafness, *3rd ed., New York: Holt, Rinehart and Winston, 1970.)*

speaker. It was later discovered that the electrical signal they had recorded was actually the cochlear microphonic generated by the hair cells and not a nervous-system phenomenon, as they had first believed. Because body tissues are electrically conductive, the cochlear microphonic generated by the hair cells spreads outside the cochlea and can easily be recorded from nearby structures, such as the auditory nerve.

The cochlear microphonic is considered by some investigators (Gulick, 1971) to be the generator potential which causes the auditory nerve fibers to fire. The cochlear microphonic contains substantially more energy than is present in the acoustic signal and is believed to obtain its energy increase, or amplification, from a "biological battery" made up of two physiological voltage sources. A positive voltage, called the **endolymphatic potential**, is generated by the **stria vascularis**. A negative potential is present inside the hair cells. Current flow resulting from these positive and negative voltages is believed to be increased by the bending of sensory hairs in one direction and decreased by their bending in the opposite direction. These bending motions are accomplished by alternating shearing forces between the tectorial membrane and the reticular lamina. Substantial mechanical advantage is gained by the shearing action, and this contributes to the overall amplification obtained.

To summarize, at this point in the hearing process, acoustic energy has been transduced to mechanical energy by the eardrum. Mechanical energy has been transduced to hydraulic pressure by the footplate of the stapes. The resultant fluid displacement of the cochlear fluid has imparted mechanical wave motion to the basilar membrane. Basilar-membrane activity has resulted in shearing force being applied to the hairs on the sensory cells, and those cells have modified an available electric power supply to generate an electrical signal of considerably greater magnitude than the original acoustic signal.

Nervous-system activity   One further transduction must be accomplished before the information contained in sound can be used by the brain to generate perceptions. The nervous system can operate only in terms of nerve impulses which can travel along the nervous pathways of the brain and be analyzed by the various centers in the brain that process auditory information. Nerve endings surround the base of the hair cells. Most of these nerve endings are the dendritic, or "receiving" end of the **bipolar cells** which make up the auditory (eighth cranial) nerve. Eighth-nerve cells, or bipolar cells, are unlike most other nerve cells in the body. (See Fig. 5.8.) In the typical **nerve cell**, the receiving **dendrites** are attached to the cell body, and a long **axon** carries nerve impulses away from the cell's body. Eighth-nerve cells, by contrast, have a single axonlike structure going into the cell body from the dendritic endings, as well as a true axon. These nerve endings enter the cochlea and travel to the bases of hair cells in a variety of complex patterns which permit the possibility of many different kinds of neural analysis. A detailed description of the innervation patterns of the

Figure 5.8

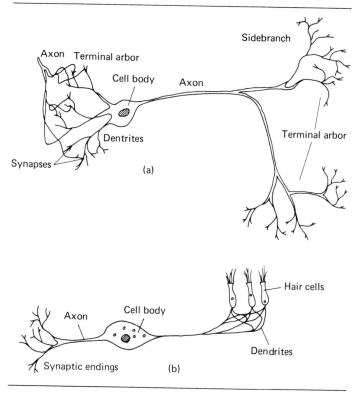

Axon Terminal arbor

Sidebranch

Cell body

Axon

Dentrites

Terminal arbor

Synapses

(a)

Axon

Cell body

Hair cells

Synaptic endings

(b)

Dendrites

*Two types of neurons: (a) typical nerve cell; (b) bipolar
cell (primary auditory nerve cell). (Adapted from W. A.
van Bergeijk, J. R. Pierce, and E. E. David,* Waves and the
Ear, *New York: Doubleday, 1960.)*

cochlea is beyond the scope of this text. We merely note that each nerve fiber
is attached to several hair cells, and each hair cell is innervated by several nerve
fibers. The cell bodies of the bipolar cells of the eighth nerve are contained
within the central core of the cochlea.

The "business" of a nerve cell is sensitivity, or irritability. Each nerve cell
has a cell body containing the nucleus, a dendritic, or input, end that is most
sensitive to stimulation, and an axon that carries the nerve impulse. The whole
cell is enclosed by a membrane that maintains an electrical difference between
the inside and the outside of the cell. This electrical difference, or **polarization,**
keeps the nerve cell more negative on the inside than on the outside while it is
"resting" and not conducting a nerve impulse. When a sufficiently stimulating or
irritating event occurs at the dendritic end of the cell, a local voltage is gen-

113

erated, causing the difference in voltage across the cell membrane to break down, or *depolarize.*

Because a flow of ions across the cell membrane represents a tiny local electric current, the depolarization moves along the nerve fiber from its point of origin to the end of the axon by a wave of progressive depolarization. Metabolic activity in the cell very quickly restores the resting potential after this depolarization wave, called an **action potential,** has passed. Hundreds of action potentials can be conducted by a single nerve fiber in one second. An action potential is very different from the cochlear microphonic generated by the hair cells. The microphonic reproduces both the frequency and amplitude of the sound stimulus which caused its generation. A nerve action potential occurs only when the stimulus at the dendrites exceeds a certain level, or **threshold.**

Threshold is the smallest stimulus intensity that will cause an action potential to occur. Any stimulation of less than threshold amplitude will have no effect, and any stimulus greater than threshold will cause an action potential. The only qualification is that a recovery period must pass after the nerve conducts an action potential before a succeeding one can occur, no matter how large a stimulus might occur during the recovery period. This recovery time is called the **refractory period** of the nerve.

At the end of each axon where the nerve transfers its information to the next neuron in the chain, there is a small space called the **synapse.** When a nerve impulse reaches a synapse, a chemical is released that causes depolarization and the initiation of a new nerve impulse in the dendrites of the following nerve fiber. An action potential takes about one millisecond to cross each synapse. Several synapses in a neural pathway cause a significant delay in the transmission of neural information.

The wealth of subtle information which we can glean from sounds in our environment must be represented and processed as patterns of sequential pulses by the nervous system. That the nervous system is equal to the task is demonstrated by the wealth of variety and subtlety that human beings are capable of perceiving in their sound environment.

Auditory Nervous System

Nerve information leaves the cochlea by way of the nerve endings at the base of the hair cells and travels via the cell bodies of the eighth-nerve fibers to the brain stem through a hole in the temporal bone. The length of the eighth nerve is about one-fourth of an inch.

Nuclei between the eighth nerve and the cortex process auditory signals and transmit them to higher levels. The first synapse in the **auditory pathway** occurs in the *cochlear nucleus* (see Fig. 5.9), located on the side of the brain stem. Out of the cochlear nucleus arise about three neurons for each eighth-nerve fiber entering it. Similar proliferation of the number of nerve fibers carrying auditory

114

Figure 5.9

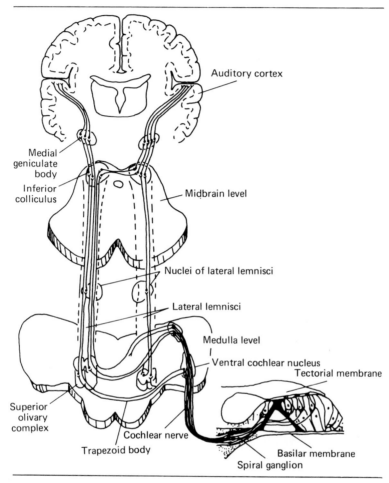

Auditory cortex

Medial geniculate body

Inferior colliculus

Midbrain level

Nuclei of lateral lemnisci

Lateral lemnisci

Medulla level

Ventral cochlear nucleus

Tectorial membrane

Superior olivary complex

Cochlear nerve

Trapezoid body

Basilar membrane

Spiral ganglion

The auditory pathway. (Adapted with permission from an original painting by Frank H. Netter, M.D., for The CIBA Collection of Medical Illustrations, *published by CIBA Pharmaceutical Company.)*

information occurs at the successive levels of the auditory nervous system so that about a million nerve fibers bearing information about sound reach the cortex of the brain.

In the **medulla,** or brain stem, are found most of the way-stations of the auditory pathway. These way-stations and the pathways that connect them are duplicated on each side of the brain. Additional pathways are also known, but they are not so well understood as the classical pathways shown in Fig. 5.9.

Numerous cross-connections present at several locations along the ascending auditory tract permit interaction of information from the two ears.

In addition to the 25,000 or more eighth-nerve fibers that carry auditory information *to* the brain (*afferent fibers*), about 500 *efferent fibers* descending from the *superior olive* (a brain-stem nucleus) regulate the amount of information that the ear is permitted to send to the brain. This group of descending control fibers is called the **olivo-cochlear bundle** because of its connections, and it has been demonstrated in animals that activation of this bundle can cause a substantial increase in the amount of sound pressure required for hearing. It seems that individuals have the capability of either consciously or unconsciously not listening or turning down the signals coming from the ear.

Most of the knowledge currently available about the **auditory cortex** was obtained from experimentation on cats (Neff, 1961). In the cat's brain, the so-called primary cortex lies in an area analogous to the human **temporal lobe.** In animal research, cortical areas responsible for processing sound were first delineated by stimulating the exposed brain of the waking cat and observing ear and eye movements similar to those made in response to sound. Subsequent investigations utilizing a variety of techniques have differed in detail about the exact boundaries of auditory cortex, but the general location of cortex responsive to sound remains in the temporal area of the brain.

Auditory cortex responds to tones varying from low to high frequency in an organized pattern; that is, the locations to which successively higher-pitched tones are directed occur at adjacent areas on the cortex. Recent research involving complex auditory stimuli and sophisticated experimental techniques suggests that auditory cortex is not critical to auditory sensitivity or the discrimination of pitch and loudness. Rather, the auditory cortex seems to be necessary for the processing of sounds with high information content. Auditory cortex simultaneously receives information about sounds in the environment, processes this input, sends the abstracted information to other cortical areas, and sends signals back to lower centers to modulate their activity (Ades, 1959).

Conclusion

The ear has been described as a series of transducers. Hearing has been described as a series of transductions, a process which provides an individual with information about a wide variety of events in his or her environment. The mechanical events that occur in the middle ear are well understood, as is most of the mechanical and hydraulic activity within the cochlea. The electrical events intermediate between mechanical distortion of the hair cells and the responses of auditory nerve fibers have been studied extensively. Although the major nerve pathways traveled by auditory information have been delineated, much remains to be learned about the processing and analysis of auditory signals within the brain. Finally, the means by which complex patterns of nervous activity become conscious perceptions of sound remain for the present, at least, a mystery.

Glossary

Action potential: A negative electrical potential of about one millisecond duration which results when the threshold of a nerve fiber has been exceeded.

Auditory cortex: A portion of the temporal lobe situated in the area of the sylvian fissure which receives auditory neurons from the thalamus.

Auditory nerve: That part of the eighth (VIII) cranial nerve which carries information from the cochlea to the brain stem. Consisting of approximately 30,000 individual fibers, the auditory nerve is the only nerve in adult humans that is made up of bipolar nerve cells.

Auditory pathway: Nerve tracts within the central auditory nervous system that carry signals from the ear to the various brain nuclei that process auditory information.

Auricle: Flap of skin and cartilage visible on the side of the head; colloquially call the "ear."

Axon: The output, or sending, branch of a nerve cell which carries nerve action potentials away from the cell.

Basilar membrane: The primary structure separating the two cochlear cavities; it forms the base of the cochlear partition and supports the organ of Corti on its inner service.

Bipolar cell: A nerve cell having two axonlike structures rather than an axon on its output end and branching dendrites on its input end. Bipolar cells are present only in the eighth cranial (auditory) nerve of adult mammals.

Cerumen: A substance (earwax) with antiseptic and insect-repellent qualities secreted into the ear canal.

Cochlea: The snail-shaped portion of the labyrinth which contains the organ of Corti.

Cochlear microphonic: An electrical signal generated by the hair cells which closely reproduces the waveform of the acoustic signal. The cochlear microphonic is considered to be the signal which activates the primary auditory nerve fibers.

Cochlear partition: A fluid-filled tube that contains the organ of Corti and separates the two main cochlear cavities.

Dendrites: Treelike branches which make up the receiving, or input, section of a nerve fiber.

Ear canal: An irregularly shaped passage approximately one inch in length extending from the side of the head at the auricle to the tympanic membrane.

Endolymphatic potential: A steady $+80$ millivolt DC potential present in the fluid of the cochlear partition but not present within the organ of Corti. The potential is the result of metabolic activity in the stria vascularis.

Eustachian tube: The duct connecting the middle-ear cavity with the naso-pharynx; normally closed, it opens periodically to ventilate the middle ear.

Hair cells: The sensory cells in the organ of Corti which transduce the mechanical activity of the basilar membrane to an electrical signal capable of stimulating the primary auditory neurons.

Impedance matching: Transfer of energy between two media which have different apparent resistances (with a minimum of loss).

Inner ear: The portion of the hearing mechanism contained within petrous temporal bone and consisting of the cochlea, vestibule, and semicircular canals.

Medulla: The widening continuation of the spinal cord forming the lowest part of the brain and containing nerve centers for the control of breathing and circulation. The majority of the cranial nerves enters and leaves the brain through the medulla.

Middle ear: An air-filled cavity containing the ossicles, the middle ear is approximately two cubic centimeters in volume and is bounded medially by the petrous portion of the temporal bone and laterally by the tympanic membrane.

Middle-ear-muscle reflex: Contraction of the stapedius and tensor tympani muscles reflexively in response to a loud sound. This muscle contraction reduces the amount of sound energy transferred by the ossicular chain. Most of the effect of the middle-ear-muscle reflex is believed to be due to stapedial contraction, and the reflex is sometimes called the stapedius reflex.

Nerve cells (Neurons): Cells specialized to be sensitive to stimulation and to conduct an electrical impulse when sufficient stimulation is received.

Olivo-cochlear bundle: The descending fiber tract whose fibers originate in the superior olivary complex and travel to the hair cells in the cochlea. These fibers control the input of auditory information from the hair cells to the brain. Descending fibers are known to originate at the cortical level and descend through the primary pathways, but they are not well understood.

Organ of Corti: A complex spiral structure supported by the basilar membrane and extending through almost the entire length of the cochlea. It consists of the hair cells and other cells whose primary function is to support the hair cells in the proper position for optimum stimulation.

Ossicular chain: Three small bones articulated so as to conduct sound vibration from the tympanic membrane across the middle-ear cavity to the oval window.

Outer ear: Consists of the auricle, ear canal, and tympanic membrane.

Oval window: The opening into the vestibule of the inner ear filled by the footplate of the stapes.

Polarization: The difference in electrical potential between two locations. Polarization of a nerve fiber refers to the electrical difference between the inside and outside of a nerve cell.

Refractory period: The period of time after the occurrence of a nerve action potential during which the nerve either cannot be made to fire or requires more intense stimulation.

Reticular lamina: A netlike structure extending across the organ of Corti which is perforated by and supports the upper ends of the hair cells.

Round window: An opening between the basal end of one of the cochlear cavities and the middle-ear cavity which is covered by the secondary tympanic membrane.

Secondary tympanic membrane: A flexible membrane that covers the round window and permits pressure variations within the cochlea to be released into the middle-ear cavity.

Stapedius: One of the two smallest muscles in the body, the stapedius originates in the posterior wall of the middle ear. Its tendon attaches to the head of the stapes. Contraction tends to pull the footplate of the stapes out of the oval window.

Stapes: The third in the sequence of bones in the ossicular chain in the middle-ear cavity. The footplate of the stapes transfers sound energy into the fluid of the inner ear.

Stapes footplate: The flat kidney-shaped part of the stapes that fits in the oval window and whose inner surface contacts the inner-ear fluid.

Stria vascularis: A layer of highly vascularized secretory epithelium which provides nutrition to the organ of Corti and maintains the endolymphatic potential within the cochlear partition.

Synapse: The junction between the axon termination of a nerve fiber and the dendritic receptor sites of a following nerve fiber. Transmission of a nerve impulse can occur in a forward direction only, is chemically mediated, and requires approximately one millisecond.

Tectorial membrane: A fibrogelatinous mass above the organ of Corti which contacts the upper ends of the hairs on each hair cell.

Temporal bone: One of the bones of the skull which forms part of the lateral and basal surfaces of the cranium and contains the organs of balance and hearing.

Temporal lobe: The lateral portion of the cortex which contains the cortical auditory receptive areas.

Tensor tympani: One of the two smallest muscles in the body, it lies in a bony canal above the Eustachian tube. Its tendon crosses the middle-ear cavity and inserts on the handle of the malleus. Contraction tends to pull the tympanic membrane into the middle-ear cavity.

Threshold: The statistical probability that a response will occur given a certain stimulus intensity.

Tonatopic organization: The relationship between the location at which each frequency maximally stimulates the basilar membrane and the location in the various cortical auditory receptive areas where nerve impulses corresponding to those frequencies arrive. Frequencies occurring sequentially along the basilar membrane elicit nerve responses in cortical nerve cells in an orderly spatial contiguity.

Transduction: The process of changing energy from one form to another.

Traveling wave: A bulge in the cochlear partition that originates near the basal end of the cochlea as a result of fluid displacement caused by stapes motion. It travels along the basilar membrane toward the apical end of the cochlea, reaching a maximum in amplitude at a location along the basilar membrane determined by the frequency of the sound initiating the disturbance.

Tympanic membrane: A cone-shaped membrane separating the outer ear from the middle ear.

Study Questions

1. What anatomical structures participate in the functioning of the ear in such a way as to increase hearing sensitivity?
2. What physiological processes contribute to the remarkable sensitivity of the auditory system?
3. What physiological processes occur in the functioning of the ear which tend to reduce hearing sensitivity?
4. Why is it necessary for the ear to be able to decrease its sensitivity to sound, when the primary function of the ear is hearing?
5. How does the fact that the ear has mechanisms for both enhancing and reducing hearing sensitivity affect the variety of different sounds that can be received?
6. What is the function of the auditory pathways in addition to providing a channel to carry auditory information from the ear to the cortex?
7. Why is periodic ventilation of the middle ear necessary even in the absence of pressure changes due to altitude changes?
8. How are the two middle-ear muscles able to work synergistically when their actions are in antagonistic directions?
9. How does the cochlea sort out the various frequencies within a complex sound?
10. Indicate the anatomical location of the energy transductions that occur as sound travels from the environment through the hearing mechanism and to the brain.
11. Describe the form of energy that represents the sound before and after each transduction.
12. How is it possible for the electrical response of the ear to a sound to contain more energy than the sound at the eardrum?

13. How are nervous impulses transmitted from one nerve cell to another?

14. What limits the rate of frequency at which a nerve can fire?

15. Why is the propagation of a nerve impulse called a "wave of progressive de-polarization"?

Bibliography

ADES, H. W., "Central Auditory Mechanisms," in J. Field, H. W. Magoun, and V. E. Hall, eds., *Section 1: Neurophysiology*, Vol. 1, Chapter 24, Washington, D.C.: American Physiol. Soc., 1959.

DAVIS, H., AND S. R. SILVERMAN, *Hearing and Deafness*, 3rd ed., New York: Holt, Rinehart and Winston, 1970.

DENES, P. B., AND E. N. PINSON, *The Speech Chain*, New York: Bell Laboratories, 1963.

FLETCHER, H., *Speech and Hearing in Communication*, New York: Van Nostrand, 1953.

GERBER, S. E., *Introductory Hearing Science: Physical and Psychological Concepts*, Philadelphia: Saunders, 1974.

GULICK, W. L., *Hearing: Physiology and Psychophysics*, London: Oxford University Press, 1971.

HIRSH, I. J., *The Measurement of Hearing*, New York: McGraw-Hill, 1972.

NEFF, W. D., "Neural Mechanisms of Auditory Discrimination," in W. A. Rosenblith, ed., *Sensory Communications*, Cambridge, Mass.: M.I.T. Press, 1961.

NETTER, F. H., *The CIBA Collection of Medical Illustrations: Neurons System*, Vol. I, New York: CIBA Pharmaceutical Company, 1962.

NEWBY, H. A., *Audiology*, 3rd ed., New York: Meredith Corporation, 1972.

PENFIELD, W., AND L. ROBERTS, *Speech and Brain Mechanisms*, Princeton, N.J.: Princeton University Press, 1959.

RASMUSSEN, G. L., AND W. F. WINDLE, eds., *Neural Mechanisms of the Auditory and Vestibular Systems*, Springfield, Ill.: Charles C Thomas, 1960.

STEVENS, S. S., F. WARSHOFSKY, *et al.*, *Life, Sound, and Hearing*, New York: Time Incorporated, *Life* Science Library, 1967.

TOBIAS, J. V., *Foundations of Modern Auditory Theory*, Vol. 1. New York: Academic Press, 1970.

TRAVIS, L. E., ed., *Handbook of Speech Pathology and Audiology*, New York: Appleton-Century-Crofts, 1971.

VAN BERGEIJK, W. A., J. R. PIERCE, AND E. E. DAVID, *Waves and the Ear*, Garden City, N.Y.: Doubleday, 1960.

VON BEKESY, G., *Experiments in Hearing*, New York: McGraw-Hill, 1960.

WEVER, E. G., AND C. W. BRAY, "Action Currents in the Auditory Nerve in Response to Acoustical Stimulation," *Proc. Nat. Acad. Sci.* 16 (1930):344–350.

WEVER, E. G., AND M. LAWRENCE, *Physiological Acoustics*, Princeton, N.J.: Princeton University Press, 1954.

ZEMLIN, W. R., *Speech and Hearing Science*, Englewood Cliffs, N.J.: Prentice-Hall, 1968.

121

CHAPTER 6
Overview

In Chapter 1 it was shown that the ear is a vital component of the speech and hearing system in the production of speech. In a general sense, we speak as we hear. If hearing is impaired prior to speech development so that speech is not heard correctly, the speech produced by the hearing-impaired person usually will be defective. Profoundly deaf persons who have not heard speech at all cannot produce speech unless they receive special training. It is important, then, for persons interested in human communication to gain an understanding of hearing.

The purpose of this chapter is to develop a general understanding of the decibel and to show how the decibel is used in the determination of normal hearing sensitivity. This determination, in turn, provides the basis for the audiogram, a graph designed to indicate the hearing levels of an individual. In this way hearing loss can be measured.

Finally, other relationships between certain characteristics of sound and hearing, such as intensity and loudness, frequency and pitch, are described under the title of "psychoacoustics." The importance of psychoacoustics for audiology and many other disciplines is explained.

The study of hearing gains significance as it relates to the previous chapter (5) on the hearing mechanism and its function, and to a later chapter (13) on hearing disorders and their diagnosis and treatment.

Paul H. Skinner, Ph.D.
University of Arizona

Hearing

Introduction

Hearing encompasses the relationship between acoustics and concomitant psychological sensations. This relationship is referred to as **psychoacoustics.** The interaction of sound and the hearing mechanism, discussed in the previous chapter, is referred to as physiological acoustics. The ultimate goal in the study of hearing is to understand how the ear works—what and how do we hear? The combined study of physiological and psychological acoustics enables scientists to build theories to answer these questions.

It is from this knowledge of normal hearing that one can describe hearing loss and impairment and what can be done about it. Thus the audiologist and other specialists who deal with hearing must gain a thorough understanding of the hearing mechanism and hearing. This chapter will present fundamental concepts as an introduction to the study of hearing.

The Decibel

Physics of sound were introduced in Chapter 4 on the acoustics of speech, and thus you may refer to that chapter for basic concepts of sound generation and propagation. Although the energy that produces sound can be measured in electrical power or acoustical pressure, the usual reference in hearing is acoustical pressure. Thus only **sound pressure** and its measurement will be considered in this chapter. It is clear that sound is generated and propagated by molecular vibration, be it in a gas (air), fluid, or solid. The molecular vibration that produces sound pressure results from an applied force (physical strength or energy) over a given area. Applied force can be measured in units referred to as **dynes.** The force of one dyne applied to an area of one square centimeter gives a measure of pressure (dyne/cm²). Common usage of the term "pressure" assumes a steady pressure, but as described earlier, sound is an alternating pressure. Although alternating pressure continually exerts pressure in opposite directions, both alternating and steady pressure can do work.

The human ear can perceive sound over a phenomenally large range from very low to very high sound pressure levels **(SPL).** The smallest acoustic pressure, which is barely audible, is about 0.0002 dyne per square centimeter, and a pressure of about 2000 dynes per square centimeter is painful. Thus a ratio of ten million to one exists from the faintest to the loudest perceptible sound. This range from decimal values to whole numbers in the thousands results in inconvenient calculations, most of which merely involve manipulating decimal points. For this reason, electrical and acoustical engineers adopted a more convenient scale, the **decibel** scale. The term "decibel" has come into common usage with increased public concern about noise pollution. Let us try to understand what decibels are.

The decibel scale was named in honor of Alexander Graham Bell. Thus when the term is abbreviated (dB), the B is capitalized. Originally this scale was labeled the Bel scale, but later the scale was modified and renamed the decibel scale.

The scale has two primary features which must be understood. First, the dB scale is based on ratios. Many scales start with zero, which often is interpreted to mean absence of a quantity, e.g., no weight or no length. In such measures one is dealing with absolute quantities or absolute scales. In other measures, such as pressure, there is no absolute zero or total absence of pressure. Thus pressure is expressed as a ratio between any given pressure and a specified reference pressure. A given pressure may be double (twice as much), triple, tenfold, hundredfold times a reference pressure.

Second, the scale is logarithmic. Logarithms are simple exponents* which are referred to a specified base number, usually base 10. In logarithms the base number is multiplied by itself the number of times indicated by the exponent. Thus in base ten, each logarithmic unit represents a tenfold increase. By the law of exponents, the logarithm of the number 1 to any base is zero. The logarithms of 10, 100, 1000 to the base 10, for example, are 1, 2, 3, respectively. In other words, the base 10 raised by the exponent equals the number: $10^0 = 1$, $10^1 = 10$, $10^2 = 100$, $10^3 = 1000$. Written in logarithmic convention, given base 10, $\log 1 = 0$, $\log 10 = 1$, $\log 100 = 2$, $\log 1000 = 3$. In this way, large changes can be expressed by small numbers; for example, the logarithm of 100,000 is 5.

It was stated previously that the decibel scale is based on ratios, since there is no absolute zero. In other words, a decibel is the logarithm of a ratio. A reference pressure must be expressed to permit a ratio. It then can be stated that any given sound-pressure level is so many times greater or less than the reference SPL, e.g., (2:1) or (10:1). The reference must be selected arbitrarily. In acoustics the most commonly used reference is the SPL of a 1000 Hz tone, which is just barely audible, about 0.0002 dyne per square centimeter. Other references can be used, but the reference must always be stated or understood. Since a reference SPL has been established (SPL will henceforth be used to imply the reference pressure of 0.0002 dyne/cm²), we can present the decibel formula for sound pressure as

$$N(\text{dB}) = 20 \log \frac{p_1}{p_2},$$

where N is the number of decibels, and p_1 and p_2 represent a pressure ratio. The reference pressure is p_2 and is taken to equal 0.0002 dyne/cm², whereas p_1 is taken to represent any given pressure. The value 20 is a somewhat arbitrary constant.

---

*   An exponent is a number superimposed above another number; for example, 4^2 indicates the times that an associated number (4) is multiplied by itself.

Table 6.1 Ratios expressed in dB SPL (reference .0002 dynes/cm^2).

RATIO	QUOTIENT	20 × LOGARITHM OF QUOTIENT	
$\dfrac{\text{given} \quad .0002}{\text{ref.} \quad\; .0002}$	1	20 log 1 = (20 times 0) =	0
$\dfrac{\text{given} \quad .0004}{\text{ref.} \quad\; .0002}$	2	20 log 2 = (20 times .3)* =	6
$\dfrac{\text{given} \;.002}{\text{ref.} \quad .0002}$	10	20 log 10 = (20 times 1)=	20
$\dfrac{\text{given} \;.02}{\text{ref.} \quad .0002}$	100	20 log 100 = (20 times 2) =	40
$\dfrac{\text{given} \;.2}{\text{ref.} \quad .0002}$	1,000	20 log 1000 = (20 times 3) =	60
$\dfrac{\text{given} \; 2}{\text{ref.} \quad .0002}$	10,000	20 log 10,000 = (20 times 4) =	80
$\dfrac{\text{given} \; 20}{\text{ref.} \quad .0002}$	100,000	20 log 100,000 = (20 times 5) =	100
$\dfrac{\text{given} \; 200}{\text{ref.} \quad .0002}$	1,000,000	20 log 1,000,000 = (20 times 6) =	120
$\dfrac{\text{given } 2000}{\text{ref.} \quad .0002}$	10,000,000	20 log 10,000,000 = (20 times 7) =	140

* $\log_{10} 2 = .3$

Ratios expressed in dB are shown in Table 6.1. If a given SPL equals the reference pressure, the ratio is 1, or 0 dB. Note that a tenfold increase in a given SPL equals 20 dB; a hundredfold increase equals 40 dB; a thousandfold increase equals 60 dB, and so forth. Also note that doubling SPL ordinarily does not double the number of decibels, since SPL is measured in dynes on a linear scale, and the decibel is based on a logarithmic scale. Therefore, doubling SPL results in a 6 dB increase. (A programed method for comprehending more fully and applying the decibel scale is available in Berlin, 1967.)

Hearing Sensitivity

Sensitivity is generally understood to imply responsiveness to stimulation, and this meaning is consistent with usage of the word in **audiology** and psychoacoustics. For example, it is common knowledge that dogs and bats hear sounds of higher **pitch** or frequency than humans do. Also, the ear cannot hear all sound frequencies equally well. In other words, the ear is differentially responsive to tones produced at different frequencies. As indicated earlier, the ear is most sensitive to tones produced at about 1000 Hz, meaning that a tone produced by this frequency can be heard at less intensity than other frequencies. As frequency is increased or decreased from 1000 Hz, acoustic signals must be increased in intensity in order to be audible.

If the SPL were plotted at which different frequencies barely become audible, the resultant graph would provide a frequency response curve, or sensitivity curve, for the ear. Such a sensitivity curve will receive further discussion later in this section. The average frequency range for the human ear is from about 20 to 20,000 Hz. The frequency range for bats extends upward from 80,000 to 120,000 Hz. Thus the two species clearly operate in different "bandwidths," or frequency ranges.

Also of interest is the range of intensity that the ear can perceive. It was stated earlier that the least amount of SPL that can be perceived is about 0.0002 dyne per square centimeter and that this reference in the decibel scale equals zero dB SPL. The ear can perceive and tolerate sound over a phenomenal intensity range, from zero to about 130 dB SPL. At this high level, the pressure exerted produces physical discomfort. The dynamic range of an instrument is taken as that range in which signals can be handled effectively. The dynamic range of the ear, then, is about 130 dB, since sound is barely audible at the lower limit of hearing and painfully loud at the upper limit.

In the measurement of hearing or hearing sensitivity, the intensity at which the various tones or frequencies can be perceived as barely audible must be specified precisely. Each of the frequency and intensity points so specified is a threshold value. The sensitivity curve of the ear, which is shown in Fig. 6.1, can also be described as the threshold curve for hearing. The **threshold of hearing** can be defined as the least SPL barely audible on about 50 percent of the trials at a given intensity and frequency. Normative threshold curves are based on the judgments of a number of young adults with normal ears tested under optimum listening conditions. The curve is taken to represent normal hearing.

The least SPL barely audible is about 0.0002 dyne per square centimeter at 1000 Hz, and more must be said about the conditions under which this value was obtained. Hearing may be tested without earphones by the use of loudspeakers, and this is known as "testing in the field." This manner of testing is valuable because it involves testing both ears simultaneously. This condition is comparable to the normal listening condition. If thresholds are determined in this manner under rigorously controlled conditions, the testing is known as "minimum audible field" **(MAF)**. Also, hearing may be tested with the use of earphones, which permits the audiologist to evaluate each ear separately. If thresholds are determined in this manner under rigorously controlled conditions, the testing is known as "minimum audible pressure" **(MAP)**. One difficulty in

Figure 6.1

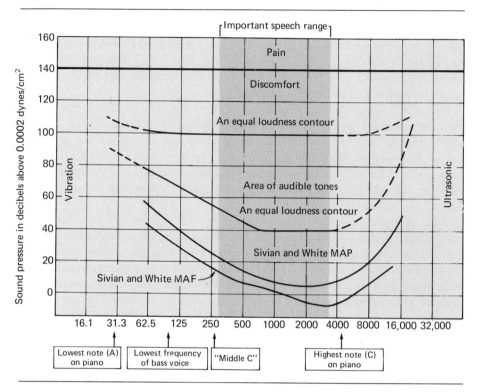

The range of human hearing. (Adapted with permission from H. Davis and
S. R. Silverman, Hearing and Deafness, 3rd ed., New York: Holt, Rinehart
and Winston, 1970; H. Newby, Audiology, 3rd ed., New York: Appleton-
Century-Crofts, 1972; and I. Hirsh, Measurement of Hearing, New York:
McGraw-Hill, 1952.)

determining threshold values by this method is that the acoustic pressure must
be measured that is developed under the earphone. These two methods for the
determination of hearing levels are illustrated in Fig. 6.2.

The primary concern in this discussion between MAF and MAP measurement techniques is a difference which occurs in the threshold values obtained.
When monaural listening is compared under both conditions, a significant discrepancy of about 6 dB exists. The earlier reference to normal threshold indicated a value of about zero dB SPL at 1000 Hz. This value was obtained from
MAF measurements. Normal threshold at 1000 Hz obtained under earphones* or

---

* The type of earphones used influences the SPL necessary to determine threshold.

Figure 6.2

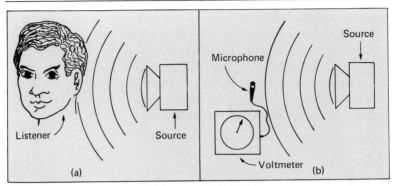

Minimum audible field

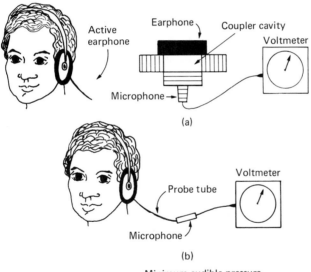

Minimum audible pressure

Demonstration of minimum audible field (MAF) and minimum audible pressure (MAP) measurement techniques. In MAF, the listener's hearing thresholds are determined (a), and the respective sound-pressure levels are determined by inserting a microphone in place of the listener's head (b). In MAP, the listener's hearing thresholds are determined under an earphone (a), and the respective sound-pressure levels are determined by a microphone connected to a probe tube placed under the earphone (b). (Adapted by permission from A. Small, "Psychoacoustics," in F. Minifie, T. Hixon, and F. Williams, eds., Normal Aspects of Speech, Hearing, and Language, *p. 368, Englewood Cliffs, N.J.: Prentice-Hall, 1973.)*

129

MAP measurements is about 6.5 dB SPL. This difference, in general, exists between MAF (monaural listening) and MAP (monaural earphone listening) measures across the audible frequency range. Since there is no satisfactory explanation for this difference, it is commonly referred to as the "missing 6 dB." This difference probably is a result of the effects of resonance and impedance differences imposed on the ear by earphones. The normal threshold curves for MAF and MAP conditions are shown in Fig. 6.1, and the "missing 6 dB" difference between these conditions is apparent. Again, observe that the normal threshold values vary in intensity with different frequencies.

The Audiogram

Clearly, if one wishes to be able to measure hearing loss, the first step is to determine and specify normal hearing. Since the concept of normal hearing has been developed, the information can be put to practical usage. Hearing loss is determined by pure-tone and speech **audiometry,** and these topics will be discussed in Chapter 13. In pure-tone audiometry, tones of different frequencies are generated at varying intensities by an electronic machine called an audiometer and presented through earphones. Normally, the lowest frequency used is 125 Hz, and this frequency is raised in octave (doubling in frequency) steps to 250 Hz, 500 Hz, and so on up to 8000 Hz. The intensity levels required to establish threshold for each frequency tested are recorded. Obviously, these recorded threshold values must be compared to normal threshold values to determine the amount of hearing loss, if any, measured for the patient being tested. This record of the patient's hearing is called an *audiogram.*

To facilitate pure-tone audiometric testing and simplify interpretation of the audiogram, pure-tone audiometers are calibrated so that the particular SPL in decibels required for normal threshold at each frequency is arbitrarily labeled zero dB on the audiometer. Thus the hearing-sensitivity curve shown in Fig. 6.1 is depicted as a straight line on the audiogram, with zero dB indicated as hearing level **(HL)**, or normal hearing. Since the reference on the audiometer and the audiogram is changed from SPL to HL, it is imperative that reference levels be indicated.

Consider that zero dB on the audiometer, or zero dB hearing level, at 1000 Hz is actually about 6.0 dB SPL as measured under earphones. Thus, for example, if the audiometer reads 20 dB HL at 1000 Hz, what is the actual SPL presented? Since 0 dB HL at 1000 Hz equals about 6.0 dB SPL, the total SPL is about 26.0 dB when the audiometer indicates 20 dB HL.

An audiogram based on audiometric zero, or hearing level, is presented in Fig. 6.3. Note that increased intensity or hearing loss is plotted downward on the audiogram to show less sensitivity, in contrast to the hearing-sensitivity curve shown in Fig. 6.1.

130

Figure 6.3

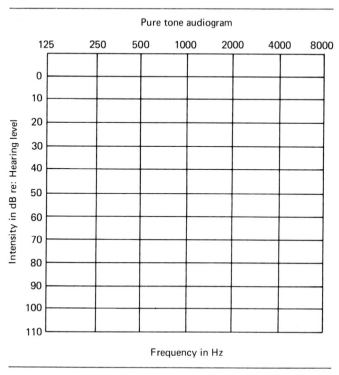

The audiogram.

Pure-tone audiometry provides a specific graph of one's hearing. This information is an important aid in determining types of hearing loss and provides a good index of one's ability to hear speech. The critical range for understanding speech is about 300 to 3000 Hz. Recall from Chapter 4 on speech acoustics that the energy dispersion in speech well exceeds this range. Nevertheless, speech can be understood quite adequately under ordinary circumstances within the range specified. Hearing loss for speech and speech discrimination are measured directly in speech audiometry and are discussed in Chapter 13.

Psychoacoustics

Sensory psychologists have been interested for centuries in the relationships between sensation and the physical stimuli which evoke them. This branch of experimental psychology is called *psychophysics,* and psychoacoustics is a branch of that broad discipline. Psychoacoustics is concerned with what the ear can hear. The sensations of **loudness** and pitch are common experiences in hearing. It is generally recognized that loudness is related to sound intensity and pitch to sound frequency. This is merely a starting point, however, for the scientist who wishes to explore psychoacoustics. Many questions follow: What is the faintest sound which can be heard (threshold)? Does this change with frequency? What is the loudest sound that can be perceived? What are the lowest and highest perceivable pitches (frequencies)? How well can pitch changes be perceived? The psychoacoustician studies all of these questions and many more. The psychoacoustician studies the relationship of auditory sensations to all the physical characteristics of acoustic stimuli: intensity, frequency, spectrum, and time.

Although interest in sensation was expressed by philosophers in early times, experimental psychologists developed the scientific study of sensation. These scientists developed the basic measurement techniques and information now used by audiologists, engineers, physicians, physicists, physiologists, and others. Engineers use such information for the development of communications systems. Engineers and physicists are concerned with the relationship between hearing and the acoustic energy created by various systems or machines. The field of audiology (described in Chapter 1) also has profited greatly from psychoacoustics. Experimental psychologists were concerned initially with normal hearing and its measurement; audiologists have adopted and adapted techniques and information to pursue the psychoacoustics of pathological auditory systems. Comparison of this information to that derived from normal ears has advanced significantly the fields of clinical audiology, aural rehabilitation, otological and neurological diagnosis, and assessment of treatment.

Although psychoacoustics historically is an area of psychology, it also must be considered an area of audiology. Audiologists must study and understand, along with acoustics, the psychoacoustics of normal and pathological auditory systems, as well as auditory physiology, pathology, and rehabilitation.

Temporal Factors

Sound or hearing occurs in the dimension of time, just as light or vision occurs in the dimension of space. Thus time, or duration, is an important parameter in psychoacoustics. Since frequency is a temporal phenomenon, it is difficult to separate the influence of time versus spectrum in pitch perception. Time, or temporal, factors also influence the perception of loudness, although quite differently from pitch perception. For example, the duration of an auditory signal up to 200 msec markedly influences the perceived loudness. Thus auditory threshold can be greatly affected by stimulus duration. Also, it is known that speech is an acoustical signal that fluctuates over time. The duration of certain speech sounds or intervals between speech sounds influences the intelligibility of speech. Differences in the arrival time of signals at the two ears are important in sound localization.

Loudness and Intensity

Loudness is the psychological counterpart of sound intensity. It will be shown that the study of the relationship between loudness and intensity has been of great importance to audiology, engineering, and otology. Several basic concepts are important: What is the softest sound that can be heard (threshold)? What is the intensity of sound at a most comfortable loudness level, or a maximum tolerance level? At what intensity does sound become intolerable or produce pain? The limits of this range were pointed out earlier as 0 dB SPL (threshold) to about 135–140 dB SPL (pain). It is important to realize that the maximum SPL that can be tolerated generally does not increase with hearing loss. Since there are no pain cells in the inner ear, pain results from pressure imposed on the outer and middle ear.

Although the ear is differentially sensitive to frequency (hears some frequencies at lower intensities than others), the growth of loudness from threshold to pain gradually equalizes or flattens out among different frequencies at the upper limits of hearing. This phenomenon is described by equal loudness contours, as shown in Fig. 6.1. The growth of loudness is known to increase with increase in intensity. Loudness growth rises steeply at low-intensity levels, then gradually tempers its rise toward the upper limits of hearing. This relationship can be described mathematically, and scales based on direct measurements of loudness have been devised.

The term **phon** (rhymes with "gone") is used to describe a level of loudness. The reference level of the phon scale is the loudness of a 1000-Hz tone at 40 dB SPL. This loudness level is taken as 40 phons. Thus for a 1000-Hz tone only, the number of phons equals the number of decibels. All other tones or sounds equal 40 phons when they are judged to be equal to the loudness of a 1000-Hz tone of 40 dB SPL. The equal loudness levels, or contours, shown in Fig. 6.1 have been determined in this manner. All the frequencies shown on the same loudness level, or contour, are equal in phons or loudness level, even though they may differ in dB SPL. These loudness, or phon, levels provide the basis for sound-level meters, which are used to relate industrial noise, for example, to perceived loudness. It must be noted, however, that the phon scale does not measure subjective loudness; rather, it merely equates the loudness of different sounds to a reference level in decibels. A scale has been devised, however, to measure subjective loudness directly.

The term **sone** (rhymes with bone) was proposed to describe a unit or scale of loudness developed by a noted psychophysicist, S. S. Stevens. One sone is arbitrarily defined as the loudness of a 1000-Hz tone at 40 dB. From this reference point, direct judgments of the magnitude of loudness of tones of the same frequency are made. The task of an observer is to adjust the intensity of a variable tone, so that it is some ratio of the loudness of the reference tone, e.g., the variable equals half or twice the loudness of the reference tone. If the variable tone is judged to be equal to one half of the loudness of a reference tone of one sone, the variable tone has a loudness of one-half sone. Numbers on the sone, or loudness, scale are related to one another in the same way as the psychological magnitudes they represent.

The previous discussion focused on judgments of the magnitude of loudness. It is also important to consider judgments of loudness differences. Just-noticeable differences, or **difference limens*** for intensity (DLI), indicate the amount of intensity change which produces a change in loudness. Although the decibel scale does correspond somewhat to the way loudness is perceived, the decibel is not a loudness-difference limen. The decibel is a physical scale, not a psychological scale. The DLI varies with frequency and intensity from about 5 dB near threshold to about 0.5 dB at high intensities. Recall, however, that since the decibel scale is logarithmic, the range of pressure in dynes grows continually larger as intensity increases. Thus the pressure range encompassed by a decibel is much greater at higher intensities.

Knowledge of the relationship of loudness to sound intensity is of great importance to the audiologist. The audiologist must use this information to determine comfort and tolerance levels in selection and use of hearing aids, to gain insight about the nature and cause of hearing loss, and to study the effects of noise on hearing.

Adaptation and Fatigue

Our interest in loudness logically entails other concerns in psychoacoustics. An auditory stimulus of a sufficient duration will achieve full loudness, then decay in loudness slightly and persist at that level of sensation. This process is common in sensory systems and is known as *adaptation*. Abnormal adaptation also occurs in auditory pathology; the loudness of tones may drop dramatically or even completely.

The auditory system fatigues when exposed to intense or prolonged sound levels. These changes are measured as shifts or increases in hearing. Gradually, with relief from exposure, this **temporary threshold shift** (TTS) diminishes, and threshold returns to normal. Temporary threshold shift and subsequent recovery after different time intervals are shown in Fig. 6.4. Overexposure to sound or exposure to very intense sounds often results in a permanent threshold shift (PTS) or hearing loss. Such a loss results from nerve damage and is not amenable to medical or surgical treatment.

Our society has become a particularly noisy one. The effect of noise, in addition to annoyance, often is permanent hearing loss. This menace to society

---

*   "Limen" is another word for "threshold," but will be used only to refer to just-noticeable differences among stimuli.

Figure 6.4

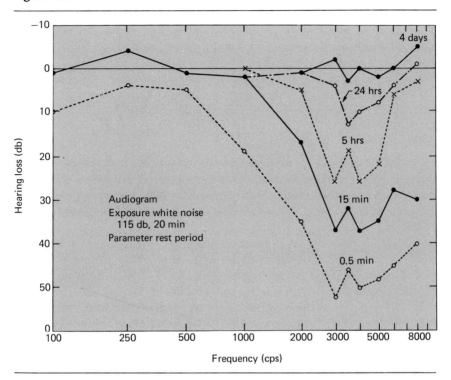

Audiograms determined at different time periods after the cessation of continuous exposure for 20 minutes to a white noise of 115 dB. (Figure 16, p. 72, from L. J. Postman and J. P. Egan, Experimental Psychology: An Introduction, *New York: Harper & Row, 1949. Reprinted by permission.)*

appears in many forms: from industrial noise to modern music. Rock-and-roll devotees, as well as the musicians themselves, routinely are exposed to noxious sound levels produced by electronically amplified music. The study of psychoacoustics in relation to noise pollution has come from relative obscurity to the forefront among our concerns.

The general public and government, as well as audiologists, otologists, and acoustical engineers, are becoming increasingly concerned with these problems. The relationship between sound intensity and hearing is an important subject in research. Scientists interested in this problem are concerned with (1) annoyance and speech-interference levels, and (2) **damage-risk criteria.** The latter requires explanation. Since there are no pain cells in the inner ear where nerve damage presumably occurs as a result of noise exposure, other warning indicators are necessary. Damage-risk criteria have been established which specify sound-

135

intensity levels and durations which may not be exceeded without the risk of hearing loss.

As a result of government regulations, industry is giving increased attention to hearing-conservation programs for employees. The audiologist will be called on to assume greater responsibility in the emerging field of industrial audiology. This field involves periodic hearing testing, measuring noise levels, recommending safe noise levels for personnel, and use of appropriate ear-protective devices. These programs are vitally needed throughout the country.

Masking

Quiet, it will be discovered, is indeed a very relative matter. In quiet, one might be awakened by a dripping faucet. This disturbance, however, is easily lost in the background of other noises. Quiet for audiometric testing requires that ambient (surrounding) noise not interfere with the determination of one's lowest or best threshold. An acceptable noise level for audiometry may not exceed about 30–40 db SPL. If the noise level increases above these levels, audiometric thresholds will be increased. The effect of a background noise to render an audible sound inaudible is referred to as **masking.** Masking is a common occurrence in everyday listening; for example, a truck or airplane noise may mask out a speech message. Masking is a valuable tool for the audiologist to exclude one ear while testing the other. This is accomplished by feeding noise through an earphone into the ear not being tested. In this case, the relationship of the intensity and frequency band width of the masking stimulus to a test tone or speech is critical.

Any auditory signal can be masked by tones, as shown in Fig. 6.5, and by a broad-band white noise,* if the noise is sufficiently intense compared to the signal. It can be demonstrated, however, that the frequency band width of the noise can be greatly reduced or narrowed with no effect on the masking of the signal as long as the band width of the noise encompasses the signal. In other words, only the relatively narrow band width of the noise surrounding the signal actually contributes to the masking of that signal. If the noise is narrowed beyond that band width, the effective, or actual, masking is reduced, and the signal becomes audible.

The ear may be likened to a system of resonators or filters that pass or analyze information in certain frequency band widths only. This analysis is perhaps the most important and unifying concept in hearing and is known as *critical band theory.* Thus although the simultaneous occurrence of sounds may cause distraction, they do not actually mask one another unless they occur in the same band width or frequency range. When different signals occur in the same band width, the loudest one will prevail.

---

* White, or thermal, noise is loosely defined as a noise spectrum that includes all frequencies at equal average intensities. White noise sounds much like the hissing produced by the release of steam or a prolonged "sh" sound.

Figure 6.5

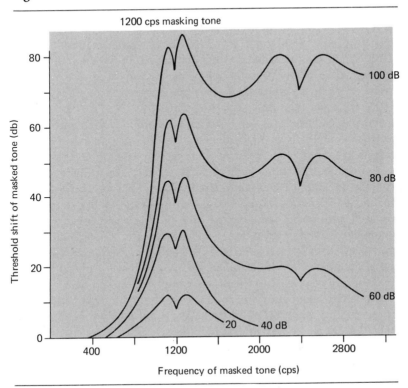

Masking of one tone by another tone of 1200 Hz. Note that the masking by the tone spreads upward into higher frequencies as the intensity of the masking tone is increased. (Adapted from R. Wegel and C. Lane, "The Auditory Masking of One Pure Tone by Another and Its Probable Relation to the Dynamics of the Inner Ear," Phys. Rev. 23 (1924):266–285.)

Pitch and Frequency

Pitch is the psychological counterpart of sound frequency. The lowest perceptible pitch occurs from a tone or frequency of about 20 Hz to the highest pitch from a tone of about 20,000 Hz. Again, these values are based on averages, and the upper limit of the frequency range varies widely in human listeners. As one may not speak of decibels of loudness, neither may one speak correctly of frequency of pitch. Pitch, like loudness, has been scaled directly. In fact, some musicians are reported to have absolute pitch, or the ability to produce or identify a given musical note (tone) in isolation. Since there is a general awareness of musical scales, the concept of a pitch scale may be more easily comprehensible than a

137

loudness scale. In addition to musical scales, there is another scale of pitch, known as the **mel** scale. The mel scale is a direct measure of pitch magnitude; however, it has no relationship to musical intervals. It is the pitch counterpart of the sone scale of loudness and was devised in the same manner. Arbitrarily, a value of 1000 mels was assigned to the pitch of a 1000 Hz tone of 40 dB. Numbers are assigned to other tones in some ratio of the pitch of a reference tone. For example, a pitch of 500 mels is half the magnitude (half as high) as the pitch of 1000 mels and twice the pitch of 250 mels.

Just-noticeable differences, or difference limens, for frequency (DLF) have been determined in pitch as in loudness. The DLF is remarkably small in the lower frequencies, about one-half cycle per second at about 250 Hz to about 20 cycles at about 8000 Hz. Pitch acuity* varies widely among listeners. Thus far, only the pitch of simple tones—pure frequencies—has been discussed. Indeed, this is an unusual listening experience in nature. Most of the sounds of nature, such as speech and music, are complex sounds. The ear possesses the ability to analyze complex sounds which are not harmonically related. Harmonic complexes, however, usually are perceived as having a single pitch related to the fundamental frequency of the complex. Many fascinating phenomena occur in the ear's perception of pitch, but they exceed logical inclusion here.

The physiological substrate for loudness seems to be rather well understood, but pitch perception has proved to be vastly more elusive. Perhaps this is the reason that the "lion's share" of auditory research has been conducted in pitch perception. Knowledge of pitch perception has some practical value for musicologists and speech pathologists who work with voice problems, but only limited practical implications for audiologists.

Binaural Hearing and Localization

Perhaps the topic of **binaural hearing** should have come first rather than last among the selected topics in psychoacoustics, since binaural hearing is of considerable interest. The localization of sound in space may be enhanced through binaural hearing. In the animal kingdom, this may mean survival. Localization is also of interest in studying the orientation of humans to their environment. Normally, localization is based on binaural processing of information—a comparison between ears. Localization usually is determined by loudness and arrival time differences between the two ears. Localization favors the ear in which the signal is louder or which precedes in signal arrival. Also, localization can be accomplished with one ear (monaurally) based on experience in judging the quality or distance (by loudness) of a sound. Head movement is very important for the

---

* Acuity has been used traditionally in psychology to imply the perception of differences among stimuli, as distinct from sensitivity used to imply responsiveness to stimulation.

localization of sound in the environment. Otherwise in humans, since the pinna (outer ear) is not mobile, sound localization can only be determined to be to the right or left within a sound rotational cone (see Fig. 6.6).

Binaural hearing also can result in lateralization of sound in the head. High-fidelity enthusiasts are familiar with the enrichment of stereophonic sound. One may establish internal lateralization (fusion or separation of sounds in the head) of signals with headphone stereo listening. This is accomplished most readily by adjusting for greater loudness in one ear than in the other. If the two ears re-

Figure 6.6

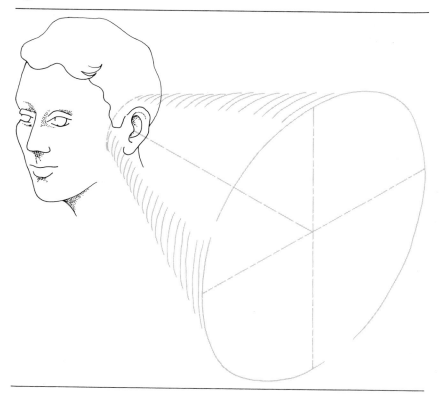

Localization of sound within a rotational cone can provide only right- or left-side orientation unless head movement is possible. (From P. Skinner, "Relationship of Electro and Psycho Acoustics Measures," in W. Hodgson and P. Skinner, eds., Hearing Aid Assessment and Use in Aural Rehabilitation *(Baltimore: Williams & Wilkins, 1977). Adapted from A. Mills, "Auditory Localization," in J. Tobias, ed.,* Foundations of Modern Auditory Theory, *Vol. 2, Chapter 8, New York: Academic Press, 1970.)*

ceive signals that differ in loudness or spectrum, each signal will be lateralized at the ear. If the signals are identically perceived, the unified signal is fused and located in the center of the head. It is possible to experience lateralization at each ear and in the center of the head (so-called phantom effect, or channel) simultaneously in earphone stereophonic listening.

It has been demonstrated in laboratory studies that binaural fusion enhances listening in noise or among competing messages, the so-called "cocktail party effect." In real-life listening situations, however, such effects are difficult to demonstrate and may not be a significant advantage of binaural hearing.

Both external localization and internal lateralization are important in communications, engineering, and ecology, as well as in audiology. Audiologists are vitally concerned with binaural hearing in order to understand normal hearing and assess auditory pathology. Also, the role of binaural hearing is of considerable interest in the selection and use of hearing aids, particularly in speech perception in noise and among competing messages.

Conclusion

Chapters 5 and 6, on the structure and function of the ear and on hearing, respectively, provide a necessary background for Chapter 13, on disorders of hearing. The discussion of the decibel, hearing threshold, and the audiogram introduces information of fundamental importance for the audiologist and speech pathologist, as well as persons in many other related professions.

Glossary

Audiology: The study of hearing, including hearing disorders and nonmedical rehabilitation.

Audiometry: The measurement of hearing and hearing loss.

Binaural hearing: Hearing with two ears simultaneously.

Damage-risk criteria: Specified intensity, frequency, and durations of sound which may cause hearing loss.

Decibel: The logarithm of a ratio of pressure in which a reference pressure is expressed.

Difference limen: A just-noticeable difference or change in pitch or loudness. "Limen" is another word for "threshold."

Dyne: A unit used to measure force which, when applied to a given area, produces pressure.

HL: Hearing level is used to indicate that audiometric zero or normal hearing is the reference level.

Loudness: The psychological sensation or counterpart of sound intensity.

MAF: The technique of determining hearing threshold values in a free field.

MAP: The technique of determining minimum audible pressure in the ear canal sufficient to elicit threshold responses.

Masking: The use of one sound or noise to render another sound inaudible.

Mel: A unit of pitch magnitude determined directly in pitch. Arbitrarily, 1000 mels is defined as the pitch of a 1000 Hz tone at 40 dB. Thus 2000 mels would be twice as high as the pitch of 1000 mels.

Phon: A unit of loudness level. The reference level for the phon scale is the loudness of a 1000 Hz tone at 40 dB SPL. All other tones or sounds equal 40 phons when they are judged to be equal to the loudness of the 40-phon reference.

Pitch: The psychological sensation or counterpart of sound frequency.

Psychoacoustics: The relationship between acoustics and concomitant psychological sensations which deals with what and how we hear.

SPL: Sound-pressure level is used to indicate a direct pressure reference and commonly is taken to represent 0.0002 dynes/cm^2.

Sone: A unit of loudness magnitude measured directly in loudness. One sone is arbitrarily defined as the loudness of a 1000-Hz tone at 40 dB. Two sones would equal twice the loudness of one sone.

Sound pressure: Molecular vibration in a gas or solid produced by an applied force on a given area.

Temporary threshold shift: Temporary hearing loss as a result of auditory fatigue.

Threshold of hearing: The intensity of a tone or frequency perceived as barely audible.

Study Questions

1. Why is the decibel based on ratios of sound pressure?
2. Why are logarithms used in the decibel scale?
3. What is the significance of the ear's differential sensitivity to frequency as it pertains to determining the frequency response curve of the ear?
4. How is threshold determined by the MAF technique?
5. How is threshold determined by the MAP technique?

6. What are the significant differences in the results and interpretation of MAF to MAP measures?

7. How are phons and equal loudness contours determined?

8. What is meant by temporary threshold shift, how is it caused, and how is it determined?

9. What are damage-risk criteria, and how are they determined?

10. What is masking and how is it used?

11. In general terms, what is the relationship between intensity and loudness and between frequency and pitch?

12. What clues or differences in sounds arriving at the two ears are used to localize sounds in the environment?

Bibliography

BERLIN, C., *Programmed Instruction on the Decibel in Clinical Audiology*, rev. ed., New Orleans: Louisiana State University School of Medicine, 1967.

DAVIS, H., AND S. R. SILVERMAN, *Hearing and Deafness*, 3rd ed., New York: Holt, Rinehart and Winston, 1970.

GERBER, S., ed., *Introductory Hearing Science: Physical and Psychological Concepts*, Philadelphia: Saunders, 1974.

GREEN, D., *Introduction to Hearing*, New York: Wiley, 1976.

HIRSH, I. J., *The Measurement of Hearing*, New York: McGraw-Hill, 1952.

HODGSON, W., AND P. SKINNER, eds., *Hearing Aid Assessment and Use in Aural Rehabilitation*, Baltimore: Williams and Wilkins, 1977.

MINIFIE, F., T. HIXON, AND F. WILLIAMS, *Normal Aspects of Speech, Hearing and Language*, Chapter 9, Englewood Cliffs, N.J.: Prentice-Hall, 1973.

NEWBY, H., *Audiology*, 3rd ed., New York: Appleton-Century-Crofts, 1972.

POSTMAN, L. J., AND J. P. EGAN, *Experimental Psychology: An Introduction*, New York: Harper, 1949.

TOBIAS, J., ed., *Foundations of Modern Auditory Theory*, Vol. 2, Chapter 8, New York: Academic Press, 1970.

VAN BERGEIJK, W., J. PIERCE, AND E. DAVIS, *Waves and the Ear*, Garden City, N.Y.: Doubleday, 1958.

WEGEL, R., AND C. LANE, "The Auditory Masking of One Pure Tone by Another and its Probable Relation to the Dynamics of the Inner Ear," *Phys. Rev.* 23 (1924):266–285.

Disorders in Speech, Language, and Hearing

PART TWO

This chapter proposes that the scientific study of disordered communication processes complements the study of "normal" processes and that the information derived from the research of speech and hearing scientists forms the foundation for clinical practice. Although clinicians and scientists share many common interests and concerns, differences in their primary professional responsibilities occasionally result in disagreements and misunderstandings.

The clinical work of all health professions can be traced to religious practices among primitive human societies. With the passage of time, however, these professions have come to rely more and more on the findings of science. The clinical intervention practices of speech pathologists and audiologists are described in terms of three major aspects: scientific, artistic, and humanistic.

Speech pathologists and audiologists are trained to provide a range of comprehensive services to the communicatively handicapped and their families, e.g., identification or prevention activities, evaluation, treatment, and counseling. The four major clinical management strategies discussed cast the clinician in the role of a facilitator for changing patient behavior. These strategies focus on the development of requisites essential to oral communication, the removal of barriers to the acquisition of oral communication, the modification of specific communication behaviors, and the acceptance of impaired communication.

Clinical intervention procedures which implement these management strategies are either indirect

Disordered Processes and Clinical Intervention

or direct. Indirect management procedures attempt to modify communication problems by changing the client's environment, personality, or other behavioral aspects. Direct management procedures focus on the modification of the client's communication behavior through assessment, response development, generalization, and automatization.

Standards of quality are usually established and monitored by the professions providing the care, and the clinical audit process is an important mechanism for evaluating and improving the quality of care of speech pathologists and audiologists. This chapter concludes with a brief preview of the chapters in Part Two.

Richard Curlee, Ph.D.
University of Arizona

Marcia Campbell, M.A.
University of Arizona

Introduction

As noted in Chapter 1, speech and hearing scientists frequently try to understand the "abnormal" in terms of the "normal." An understanding of the acquisition and maintenance of normal communication assists in developing a more profound understanding of impaired communication. By the same token, the study of disordered processes complements our studies of "normal" communication processes. Much of our knowledge about speech, hearing, and language has been derived from investigations of disordered communication. Clinical material is used to gain a better understanding not only of the communication impairments under study, but also of the functioning of unimpaired processes. The results of these clinical investigations are used to buttress the informational foundations of basic speech and hearing scientists.

In general, **speech pathologists** and **audiologists** seem to be more interested in processes lying immediately behind behaviors than in the behavior itself. That is, we are more concerned with hearing thresholds than we are with hand signals given 50 percent of the time in response to a **pure-tone stimulus.** We are more interested in the learning of general articulation skills than we are in noting changes in performance from 25 percent to 90 percent correct articulation on a list of 20 words. We are usually interested in a child's score on a vocabulary test to the extent that the score is an indication of some of the child's receptive language abilities. In short, we are interested in hypothetical constructs—hearing thresholds, learning of articulation skills, receptive language abilities.

Clinical research in speech and hearing is extremely difficult because of the complexity of human behavior and of the multiple interactions of a multitude of variables. Adequate isolation of independent variables and experimental control of other variables is extraordinarily difficult to achieve. As a result, scientific study of communication problems, of the clinical process, of clinicians, of patients, of treatment outcomes is not as well controlled as is laboratory research. Clinical research usually involves a number of compromises from laboratory standards in quantification, measurement, and experimental control.

The scientific method may not be as powerful or as useful a tool for the behavioral sciences as it is for the physical sciences. Problems of measurement and of isolating and controlling relevant variables in human beings seriously weaken our inferential abilities as scientists and clinicians. The ease with which variables may be observed and measured in human beings seems inversely related to their meaningfulness and utility. For example, such concepts as anxiety, intelligence, and language have yet to be quantified in a satisfactory manner. Nevertheless, scientific evidence is more valuable than any other kind of information, and over time it has systematically increased our ability to work more effectively with the communicatively handicapped.

Both scientists and clinicians are concerned about adequate explanations of human behavior. This mutual concern and interest, however, sometimes results

147

in misunderstandings between these two groups. As noted by Dews (1962), clinical practitioners are responsible for making decisions about their patients that usually cannot be based solely, or even primarily, on available scientific evidence. It is the clinician's responsibility to make decisions on the basis of all available information. It is equally apparent that the researcher must not make decisions until sufficient scientific evidence justifies it.

It is likely that these differences in the responsibilities of clinicians and basic scientists have contributed to the perennial antipathy some members of these two groups have for each other. Some clinicians accuse scientists of being so vague and noncommittal that they are of little or no help in the management of real, everyday clinical problems. Some scientists, on the other hand, view clinicians as making decisions that are not scientifically defensible and, if not ignorant, as having little understanding of the nature of science. Undoubtedly, some clinicians do not appreciate the rules of evidence required by scientists. At the same time, some scientists do not appreciate the necessity for making clinical decisions. It is important that clinicians do not confuse the necessity for making a treatment decision with a belief that their decision was correct once it has been made. The need to make clinical decisions on the basis of insufficient evidence fosters errors and continues to be a likely source of tension between scientists and clinicians.

Clinical Intervention

Historically, clinical intervention strategies and procedures have been imbued with a certain "mystique." Some of this aura of mystery may result from its roots in religious practice. Originally, treatment of all illnesses, infirmities, and problems were viewed by human societies as religious functions. Demons were cast out, sins were forgiven, and devils were exorcised by the spiritual healers of a particular community. In some relatively primitive cultures, the title of the religious leader embodied this function—witch doctor. With the passage of time, however, the responsibility for providing healing functions passed from the religious institutions into secular hands in most cultures.

First, a group of secular practitioners began to assume responsibility for problems of the body, for the life and death of their patients. Later, other kinds of practitioners assumed responsibility for problems of the mind, behavior problems, hearing problems, speech problems. During this period, clinical intervention strategies and procedures for all professions came to rely less on metaphysical principles and traditions and more on empirical, observable phenomena. In many respects, speech pathologists and audiologists have marched in the vanguard of professions that view clinical practice as the application of scientific principles to human problems.

Speech pathologists and audiologists are independent practitioners. By virtue of their education and professional training, they are qualified to evaluate speech, hearing, and language problems, establish a plan of treatment, and direct that treatment. Speech pathologists and audiologists collaborate with their colleagues in basic speech and hearing science in adding to their professions' knowledge bases. The systematic application of that knowledge base to problems of human communication can be viewed as the scientific aspect of clinical intervention. Because our knowledge is not yet complete, however, there are also artistic aspects of clinical intervention as well as humanistic aspects.

Scientific Aspects of Clinical Intervention

Speech pathologists and audiologists carefully observe their patients during assessment and treatment and adhere to many of the principles and procedures followed by their laboratory colleagues, basic speech and hearing scientists. For example, both agree that the principle of controlled observations must be followed in order to identify reliably those processes involved in speech, hearing, and language problems. With the assistance of sound-treated rooms, precisely calibrated equipment, and well-established psychophysical methodology, audiologists evaluate their clients' hearing thresholds. And as described in Chapter 13, they are able to describe quite clearly the nature and severity of their clients' hearing impairments as well as provide important information on the probable anatomical location of the breakdown in the hearing mechanism. Differences in the nature of speech and language processes as contrasted with hearing processes do not permit us to assess speech and language as precisely and reliably as we measure hearing. Nevertheless, standardized tests and established evaluation procedures are used by speech pathologists to obtain controlled observations of their clients' communication behavior.

Both scientists and clinicians adhere to the principle of repeated observations. This ensures that adequate samples of the behavior under study have been observed. For the clinician, evaluation of a client's problem behavior extends from the formal evaluation session throughout treatment. As a result, speech pathologists and audiologists obtain a more profound, detailed understanding of a particular client's problem. Continued systematic evaluations permit clinicians to assess their clients' progress in treatment and provide a basis for modifying their treatment approach as necessary. In addition, of course, these procedures document clients' and clinicians' judgments about terminating treatment.

Another principle that guides the professional endeavors of both scientists and clinicians is the principle of consistency. This means that their conclusions must be consistent with all known information available about their area of study and their client. Clinical management decisions frequently have to be made on a tentative basis, and when in doubt, prudent clinicians pursue a conservative course of action. Treatment options are kept open, and evaluations continue until conclusions are consistent with all of the available evidence about the client. For example, it is not uncommon to find **hypernasality** and **nasal emission** of the breath stream in some children who also present a normal-appearing and functioning velopharyngeal mechanism. Most speech pathologists will see this type of child for a trial period of remediation and continuing evaluation before recommending that surgical or prosthetic approaches be considered.

In addition to their allegiance to many of the same principles, clinicians and scientists usually follow many of the same general procedures in their work. As noted by McDonald (1965), the organization of a research project is directly applicable to clinical evaluations and treatment. First, the problem must be defined. For clinicians, this usually means analyzing case-history information obtained from client or parent interviews, medical records, and other sources. From these "data" the clinician usually generates a series of alternative hypotheses to be evaluated. These hypotheses may concern the general nature and severity of the communication problem; the specific speech, hearing, and language behaviors likely to be involved; potential etiological factors that need to be screened; prognostic signs to be looked for; and treatment options to be assessed. After formulating these tentative hypotheses or questions to be investigated, the clinician must devise a plan for evaluating them. Screening procedures frequently permit clinicians to "rule out" some of the possible alternatives rather quickly. For example, if a client successfully passes a hearing screening, one can usually conclude that impaired hearing acuity does not contribute to the client's problem. Other tests enable clinicians to determine which language skills of an aphasic client remain relatively unimpaired (see Chapter 12) or if particular patterns of articulation errors suggest the possibility of velopharyngeal incompetence (see Chapter 8).

The data collected during the interview, formal testing, and clinical observation provide the clinician with a basis for supporting or rejecting his or her initial hypotheses. The experienced clinician looks for the kinds of information that would disprove initial hypotheses as well as support them. Ideally, sufficient evidence is available to support only complementary hypotheses. If sufficient evidence is not available or if all of the hypotheses generated must be rejected, it is obvious that further study and evaluation are needed. In many instances, it is at this point that speech pathologists and audiologists seek the consultative assistance of other professionals.

Artistic Aspects of Clinical Intervention

One of the goals of science is prediction and control. The more complete our scientific understanding of a phenomenon, the easier it is to manipulate and control. The less we know, the more unpredictable our attempts to control a phenomenon become. Currently, our understanding of normal processes of communication as well as of disordered processes is incomplete and imprecise. As a result, clinicians must be skilled in what we have chosen to call the artistic aspects of clinical intervention.

Given sufficient understanding of human behavior in general and communication behavior in particular, it would be possible to prepare a "Communication Disorders Recipe Book." One could scan the table of contents for the problem of concern, locate the proper recipe, and begin preparing the solution. A number of operant programs, in fact, have been developed in recent years to assist clinicians in working with communication problems. Although operant programs demonstrate the value of developing explicit treatment plans with explicit objectives and criteria for making clinical decisions, in most instances there is not an appropriate recipe available for a specific client. As a result, the clinician usually must rely heavily on personal clinical artistry. Guided by the information that is available, supplemented by those ill-defined processes frequently referred to as clinical judgment and clinical intuition, the clinician creates a treatment program and initiates clinical intervention.

The artistic aspects of clinical practice probably spring from the intuitive, creative processes common to everyone. Undoubtedly, these processes have been shaped and molded to some extent by the clinician's education, training, and past experience. As a result, each clinician's intuitive components are likely to be somewhat different from those of every other clinician. It is not surprising that each clinician's appraisal, treatment plan and approach for a specific client are different in many ways from other clinicians'. It is as if a number of architects were told to design a building that meets a limited number of specifications. There is only a small chance that any two buildings would be exactly the same. This diversity in clinicians and clinical approaches will continue until research with communication problems can specify what clinical procedures work best with what clients. Until then, each clinician's competence will be partly determined by those clinical hunches and impressions we see as reflecting artistic, creative processes.

Humanistic Aspects of Clinical Intervention

Experienced clinicians establish a relationship with their clients that facilitates changes in the clients' behavior. In effect, the clinician attempts to communicate the treatment plan in a way that is most effective for that particular client. In some cases, the clinician need be concerned only with providing remedial instruction and practice in a traditional manner. In others, the clinician must deal with client depression or anxiety, poor motivation, hyperactive behavior, or related family problems. To meet the problems encountered in dealing with people who have problems, clinicians must be adept in handling the humanistic aspects of clinical intervention.

Some writers have approached these humanistic aspects by discussing the clinician's personality. Van Riper (1972) described a number of traits necessary for a successful clinician. He included patience, a sense of humor, and social poise on his list, but emphasized the importance of empathy. Among physicians, these humanistic aspects probably contribute to what has been called "bedside manner." Among speech pathologists and audiologists, the word "rapport" is often used to describe the creation of a seemingly understanding, accepting, warm relationship with a client. Although it is widely accepted that it is important to establish some special kind of clinical relationship with clients, the essential elements of that relationship have not been identified by clinical research. Nevertheless, it is apparent that effective clinicians must be able to relate to both children and adults who present a diverse range of communication problems in a manner that permits reliable evaluation and efficient remediation.

Because speech pathologists and audiologists deal with people who have communication problems, they are frequently confronted with additional problems and needs associated with clients' reactions to their problems as well as their families' reactions. The desire to communicate is strong in most of us. A large number of individuals with communication problems appear to suffer deeply from their disability. Imagine the despair of someone whose larynx has been removed because of cancer and whose initial attempts to speak are accompanied by no sound except the rushing of air from a hole in his or her neck. Or, imagine the desperation of a stutterer who arises in the morning afraid of speaking and trying to think of ways to avoid speaking so as to avoid stuttering.

An aphasic patient (see Chapter 12) with whom we worked described his feelings after he had suffered a stroke:

I realized that I was having problems with speaking, although I could understand most of what people were saying to me. Then the clinician came in to see me. She asked me to say "ah." It seemed such a simple thing to do. I opened my mouth and nothing happened. Panic hit me. If I could not even say "ah," how would I ever talk again?

Families of individuals with communication problems may also express their fear, hurt, or disappointment. They too have needs that must be met. The experienced clinician recognizes these aspects of communication problems and meets these related needs in the most humanistic manner possible.

Continuum of Services

The role of the speech pathologist and the audiologist in clinical intervention is not limited to providing "therapy." There is a continuum of services to be provided: prevention-identification, evaluation, treatment planning, direct clinical management, counseling, and consultation.

Prevention-Identification

Prevention of communication disorders is based on the concept of early identification of problems and potential problems, followed by referral to an appropriate treatment source. It is believed that problems that go untreated become more severe, more handicapping, and more difficult to treat. Therefore, prevention programs focus on limiting the number of untreated cases. For example, hearing screenings identify children with hearing loss. Children with recurring **otitis media** (middle-ear infections) (see Chapter 13) should be under the care of and checked frequently by a physician if permanent damage is to be avoided. Many disorders of phonation (see Chapter 9) might be prevented were the individuals identified promptly and counseled concerning misuse of their voices. Early recognition of a change in voice quality may prevent, with prompt treatment, the development of vocal nodules, polyps, or contact ulcers (see Chapter 9). Treatment of disorders of articulation, fluency, and language in children may be facilitated by early intervention and dissemination of information. In general, the sooner a communication problem is identified, the better the prognosis for that problem. The two-year-old who has not said any words or the three-year-old whose speech is not readily understood about 90 percent of the time needs attention.

Evaluation

Evaluation should provide an "in-depth" study of the client's problem, potential etiological and maintenance factors, and the client's potential for habilitation. It includes parent/client interviews, medical and case histories, and formal and informal testing. An evaluation may or may not result in a diagnostic label, but it should identify a set of problem behaviors to be modified.

Occasionally, an evaluation may lead to the identification and exploration of a more serious problem. Audiometric testing may reveal the possibility of an acoustic tumor. With some neurological diseases, such as multiple sclerosis or amyotrophic lateral sclerosis, speech may be the first behavior noticeably affected. The clinician must be knowledgeable concerning the signs of these disorders and how they affect speech and hearing so that a prompt referral to a neurologist may be made.

Treatment Planning

Once an evaluation has been completed, a plan of treatment must be developed. This plan may include a statement of prognosis, long- and short-range objectives, specific techniques to be employed, supplemental consultation with other professionals, and, possibly, a referral to other agencies. Treatment planning should never be limited solely to the individual's speech problem. It is always necessary to consider the client's social, family, medical, and physical needs in planning an effective, comprehensive, habilitative program.

153

Treatment

Therapy involves the implementation of the treatment plan, and speech pathologists and audiologists employ a number of different treatment procedures and techniques, depending on the client, the problem, the client's age, and the clinician's training and background. Because many aspects of the treatment process are discussed in more detail later in this chapter, here we will note only that therapy comprises the largest portion of the work of most speech clinicians and of those audiologists engaged in rehabilitation.

Counseling

The clinician frequently becomes a counselor. Indeed, the very closeness of the clinician's contact with the client and the client's family often seems to create a counseling situation. Also, severe problems affect not only the client, but also others. Boone (see Chapter 12) emphasizes the importance of a family's understanding the condition of **aphasia** and of being given reading materials prior to counseling. Even with less severe problems, such as a mild articulation problem, some families may need to be assured that they are not responsible for the client's problem. The clinician's goal is to make certain that persons concerned with the client understand the nature of the disorder. In some instances, family members may need assistance in modifying their attitudes. Frequently, the family should be apprised of what they can do to help achieve the desired changes in the client's communication behavior.

Consultation

It is not unusual for clinicians to consult with other professionals about their patients. Because a communication disorder may be the problem that is most apparent, speech pathologists or audiologists can be the first professionals to see the patient. Therefore, they need to be aware of related professions and the services they can provide in the total habilitation and rehabilitation of communication-impaired clients. Experienced clinicians evaluate whether these services are likely to be of real benefit to the client or whether they may simply result in added expense with little effect on the client's problem. In many instances, a decision to refer to other specialists is a simple one. The child who has insufficient **velopharyngeal closure** because of a short velum (see Chapter 9) needs to be seen by the plastic surgeon and prosthodontist to determine whether surgical procedures or being fitted with a speech appliance may correct the problem. Likewise, the rare child who has a malocclusion that is interfering with the production of certain sounds in a normal manner needs the services of an orthodontist. Other problems, however, may be more subtle, and the clinician must exercise good judgment in deciding which referrals, if any, are appropriate.

Clinical Management Strategies

Clinical management strategies should be thought of as general approaches for attacking a communication disorder. In general, these strategies express a clinician's philosophy of treatment; basic knowledge of normal speech, hearing, and language processes and their impairments; and understanding of a client's problems. Speech pathologists and audiologists usually employ one or more of four general treatment strategies: (1) facilitation of acquisition of the prerequisites to oral communication; (2) facilitation of the removal of barriers that preclude development of normal oral communication; (3) facilitation of the modification of specific communication behavior; and (4) facilitation of acceptance of limited communication performance. In succeeding chapters these general strategies are exemplified by the treatment procedures described for the disordered communication processes under discussion. First, however, we will summarize the primary rationales for each strategy and illustrate how they are commonly applied.

Facilitate Development of Prerequisites

This strategy is based on the observation that speech and language development occurs in a relatively predictable sequence. Further, it is presumed that speech and language behaviors developed later in this sequence are dependent, to some degree, on the development of earlier forms of speech and language behavior. Thus these earlier forms may be viewed as prerequisites to subsequent normal development of oral communication.

If there is no evidence of an anatomical or psychological basis for a client's delay in speech and language development, a clinician may adopt a strategy of optimizing the child's environment for speech and language development. The clinician evaluates the client's environment outside the clinical setting in order to assist in shaping that environment so that it will be conducive to the development of oral communication. Hubbell (see Chapter 11) points out that in order to talk, a child must have something to talk about. Some children lack an appropriately stimulating environment at home, and the parents may need counseling. In some cases of delayed speech, analyses of conversations between parent and child show the parent to be primarily asking questions or giving commands, rather than feeding information to the child. It is as if the child were being tested, not taught. This strategy may incorporate referral to a child-development group or the use of speech-improvement programs, such as that presented in Margaret C. Byrne's *The Child Speaks* (1965).

Facilitate Removal of Barriers

In the presence of anatomical or psychological anomalies, any strategy for clinical intervention should include the removal or alleviation of these barriers to achieving oral communication. A hearing aid may be of significant value to those individuals with a loss of hearing sensitivity (see Chapter 13). Individuals with orofacial deviations that interfere with the production of speech often need to have these corrected before direct therapy is begun. Disorders of fluency and phonation may be improved by reducing accompanying anxiety or tension. This strategy is based on the belief that when there are barriers that prevent the client from achieving appropriate communication, they must be removed.

Facilitate Modification of Communication Behaviors

Following an evaluation, a clinician sets up a program for modifying a client's problem speech and language behaviors. Many of the procedures for doing this are discussed in more detail later in this chapter. They include such things as articulation training, speech reading and aural rehabilitation, selection and habituation of **optimum pitch,** conditioning of stuttering, and retrieval of language in aphasic patients. This strategy is based on selecting impaired communication behaviors and assisting the client to modify them in a planned, systematic manner. When people think of speech and hearing therapy, most are thinking of the treatment procedures founded on the strategy of direct management of speech, language, and listening behaviors.

Facilitate Acceptance of Limited Communication Performance

Clinicians must recognize that some clients cannot be helped. There are instances when no matter what clinical procedures are used or how skillfully they are carried out, there will be little or no improvement. With such persons, the clinician should have the integrity to acknowledge these limitations and to assist the client and his or her family in accepting the communication problem and adjusting to it. This strategy, then, is based on the belief that the client's communication potential has been achieved and that personal and family acceptance of that potential must occur for successful rehabilitation of the client. The parents of a child severely handicapped by a hearing loss or by brain damage must be guided by the clinician in the acceptance of the child's limited communication. Such problems need to be met with honesty and empathy on the part of the clinician. It is rare that this can be done in just one or two sessions. "We hear what we want to hear," and it takes a skillful clinician to assist parents to acknowledge and accept their handicapped child's condition.

With adults, the problem may be even more severe. The client may be the "breadwinner" of the family, and roles may have to be changed. The person whose larynx has been removed needs to recognize that although talking can be relearned, speech will never be the "same." Adults who suffer speech and language impairments associated with brain damage and resultant aphasia (see Chapter 12) should be encouraged to emphasize what they can still do rather than what they can no longer do.

We are now working with a young woman, 27 years old, who has a language impairment as a result of a "stroke" following open-heart surgery. Prior to this she showed promising artistic talent. At the present time, she has probably recovered as much speech and language as possible. Although she is now independent communicatively, she is still too impaired to be employed in most jobs. She has been encouraged in her sketching and painting and has recently been commissioned to paint three pictures. She has expressed an interest in fabric weaving, and arrangements have been made for her to take instruction in this art. The treatment strategy focuses on helping her accept her communicative limitations and become independent through the development of her other skills.

Clinical Intervention Procedures

Once an intervention strategy has been selected for providing habilitation services to a specific client, a number of procedures may be used for clinical intervention. Traditionally, some procedures are associated with some intervention strategies more than others. For purposes of discussion we have chosen to divide these strategies into two categories: indirect management and direct management procedures.

Indirect Management

Indirect management procedures attempt to treat speech, hearing, or language problems by modifying the client's environment, personality, or some other aspect of behavior thought to be related to the problem. Most often, the focus of attention is some factor believed to cause or maintain the communication problem. For example, if a child is not speaking in sentences and also has a marked deficiency in auditory sequential memory abilities, some clinicians would advocate remedial training on auditory memory rather than direct work on sentence production (Kirk and Kirk, 1972). Three of the four intervention strategies discussed in the previous section typically employ indirect management procedures.

Counseling/consultation Perhaps the most commonly employed indirect management procedure is counseling/consultation. We use the word "counseling" to describe information sharing with patients and their families and the word "consultation" to denote information sharing with other professionals responsible for the client's care. In both instances, the goal of speech pathologists and audiologists is to communicate their findings and recommendations in a manner that results in more effective management of the client's problem. With few exceptions, counseling with parents constitutes part of the clinical management strategy for all children with communication problems. It is also a common element of many treatment plans for adults. For example, in Chapter 13, Hodgson describes the need to counsel hearing-impaired clients and their friends and relatives about the effects of hearing loss on communication and personality.

Consultation with other professionals usually is determined by the specific needs and circumstances of the client. Teachers may be contacted to ensure that hearing-impaired children receive preferred seating in classrooms; social workers may become involved in the coordination of outpatient restorative services needed by an aphasic person; or the progress of a voice client may be reviewed regularly with the physician. Although counseling and consultation are employed in some way with all patients, their effectiveness as intervention procedures has not been well studied and for all practical purposes is unknown.

Psychotherapy   Psychotherapy, as an indirect intervention procedure, may be distinguished from counseling by its goals—to change those aspects of personality believed to be related to the client's communication disorder. Several decades of research (Goodstein, 1958; Bloch and Goodstein, 1971) have failed to identify any consistent relationship between personality variables and speech, hearing, and language disorders. Nevertheless, psychotherapy is often the treatment procedure of choice with stutterers, some individuals with voice problems, and other patients whose communication disability is thought to be a symptom of a psychogenic problem. Indeed, some speech pathologists have received extensive training in psychotherapy and limit their caseloads to patients they view as needing this kind of care. Measures of personality are notoriously unreliable, and research methodology may have obscured subgroups of people with communication disorders that are related to personality problems. Even so, the few published treatment-outcome studies of clients with communication problems who have received psychotherapy and presumably were selected on the basis of an apparent need for this type of treatment do not indicate that psychotherapy is effective in alleviating communication disorders.

Relaxation   The third and final indirect intervention procedure we will discuss is relaxation. Relaxation exemplifies a number of procedures currently in use that attempt to modify specific behavioral functions and processes thought to be barriers to the client's development of normal communication. Relaxation, like psychotherapy, is frequently used with stutterers and with those voice cases exhibiting hyperfunction of the vocal mechanism. Training in relaxation is used to reduce muscle tension, anxiety, or both, and to facilitate greater fluency or a more efficient voice. The conceptual strategy of relaxation is similar to that of providing swallowing training to clients with frontal lisps and overbite, tongue exercises to clients with dysarthria, or respiration exercises to patients with Parkinsonism or other neurological diseases that affect vital capacity. That is, the clinician attempts to modify nonspeech behavior in order to produce desired changes in speaking behavior. However, none of these approaches has demonstrated its clinical effectiveness with satisfactorily controlled research.

Direct Management

Direct management of communication disorders usually consists of four overlapping stages of treatment. These stages can best be described in terms of their goals: assessment, response development, generalization, and automatization. In the following paragraphs we will focus on some of the common features of these stages of treatment.

Assessment   Assessment is the initial stage of clinical intervention. It also overlaps with all succeeding stages as the clinician evaluates the client's progress and thereby the effectiveness of the intervention techniques being employed. Initially, clinical assessment attempts to answer the following questions: Does the client have a problem? If so, what is the nature and severity of the problem? Are there any associated problems needing further evaluation or referral? Does the client have the necessary prerequisites for achieving normal communication? What clinical management strategies seem most appropriate to the client's problem? What specific clinical techniques should be employed? What is the client's potential for improving communication skills? On the basis of the information obtained, the clinician determines if the client has a problem and should be seen for treatment. If so, an individualized treatment plan is established, based on the client's abilities and deficits.

In general, speech pathologists and audiologists can reliably identify people with speech, hearing, and language problems. To a lesser degree, but certainly with satisfactory reliability, we can determine the severity of most problems. We continue to have some trouble in differentiating among those clients who will (1) benefit from treatment; (2) achieve normal communication without clinical intervention; and (3) not benefit from traditional treatment or whose limited communication potential is not recognized until progress in treatment stops. Unfortunately, clinical research has not established the relative effectiveness of different treatment techniques for the various disorders, the rate of clinical success or failure among these disorders, or the average duration of treatment by type of disorder or by type of treatment.

Response development   We have called the goal of the second stage of direct clinical management "response development." The procedures used in this stage are determined by the client's competencies and deficits identified during assessment. The procedures utilized include: prerequisite development, shaping, stimulus manipulation, and reinforcement. Some clients need all four procedures, others fewer. Usually, a combination of procedures is employed, although we discuss them separately for the sake of clarity. Throughout this section, we use the language of operant conditioning to describe the response-development procedures usually employed by speech pathologists and audiologists. Essentially, this reduces various treatment approaches to a common behavioral dimension and permits the commonalities and differences among therapies to become more apparent. We do this for the convenience of discussion only.

Prerequisite-development procedures are designed to assist the client in acquiring abilities that are necessary for developing better communication skills. In some instances, however, these procedures are used to train the client in behaviors essential to the treatment plan. For example, Shriberg (1975) identified the following as prerequisites for his /ɝ/ evocation program.

1. Ability to move the body of the tongue grossly on command.
2. Knowledge (by pointing with finger) where one's tongue tip is.
3. Knowledge (by pointing) where the **alveolar ridge** ("bumpy place behind the teeth") is.
4. Ability to lift one's tongue tip to alveolar ridge.
5. Ability to sustain elevation of the tongue tip for several seconds (a nominal training time is five seconds) without the tongue tip roving around.
6. Ability to move tongue body and tip forward and backward without jaw motion.
7. Ability to move and tense one's tongue independent of phonation and jaw movement.

In other instances, prerequisite training typically focuses on specific behavioral or perceptual abilities integral to the communication process. As Shelton points out in Chapter 8, auditory-discrimination deficits may contribute to the problems of some people with articulation disorders. In these instances, some clinicians initiate clinical intervention with discrimination training before beginning phonation training. Similarly, some cases of vocal abuse related to inappropriate habitual pitch may benefit from pitch-discrimination training. Often, distractible, hyperactive children may need assistance in maintaining their attention on their treatment tasks.

Most young children seen for direct modification of their speech and language need some kind of concrete reinforcement in order to be sufficiently motivated to participate in their treatment. Traditionally, speech pathologists and rehabilitative audiologists have integrated their treatment procedures into game-like activities for young children. More recently, some clinicians present redeemable tokens, "M&Ms," or other tangible rewards whenever their young clients produce a correct response. Both approaches encourage the client's active participation in the treatment procedure.

Shaping is a clinical procedure that gradually modifies an existing inappropriate response toward a correct response. For example, a child may substitute a /d/ sound for the /tr/ blend. Consequently, the child may say "duck" instead of "truck," "dip" instead of "trip." With appropriate auditory stimulation, the child may repeat "tuck" instead of "duck," and the clinician may choose to reward that production for a while because it more closely approximates the correct response. This procedure is usually employed when a client does not appear to have a correct response in his or her behavioral repertoire under any condition.

On the basis of their assessment, clinicians select a response that has one or more properties of the desired response, provide both production instructions and appropriate acoustic models, and reinforce successive approximations of the desired response. Often, clinicians begin with a response that closely approximates the correct response unless it is the response habitually substituted for the correct response. Then it may be best to approach the desired response in a manner distinctly different from the error response. Frequently, clinicians find that shaping correct responses is expedited by pairing the client's responses with conditions that seem to facilitate the production of correct responses.

Stimulus-manipulation procedures are commonly employed with those clients who can produce the desired response correctly under certain conditions. Therefore, one of the clinician's assessment tasks may be to determine if there are stimuli that facilitate correct responses. If so, the clinician can manipulate these stimuli gradually from one context to another until the client produces the response correctly in all appropriate contexts. For example, some clients who distort the /s/ phoneme in most phonetic contexts may produce it correctly following the /t/ phoneme, as in "cats." McDonald's *Deep Tests of Articulation* (1964) systematically manipulate the phonetic contexts of phonemes to assess articulation and assist the clinician in developing an appropriate treatment plan.

A number of treatment programs employ the principles of stimulus manipulation to modify communication behavior. A task-continuum program for clients with **apraxia,** proposed by Rosenbek *et al.* (1973), involves stimulus-manipulation procedures: the clinician moves from auditory and visual stimulation followed by simultaneous production with the client, to the client's imitating the clinician after a delay, to an eighth step in which the clinician and friends role play everyday speaking situations with the client. Other treatment programs that incorporate stimulus-manipulation principles include the paired-stimulus technique for articulation, most treatment programs for stutterers that employ metronomes, **delayed auditory feedback** and shadowspeaking, and the association of muscle relaxation with phonation for vocal hyperfunction. Indeed, these procedures may be limited only by the clinician's ingenuity in identifying conditions that facilitate a client's correct response.

Reinforcement is the last response-development procedure we will discuss. The word "reinforcement" is usually associated with operant-conditioning procedures. We use it here to describe the responses of clinicians to the things their clients say and do. Consequences of a response that result in subsequent increases in the frequency of that response are said to be reinforcing. Conversely, consequences of a response that produce a decrease in its frequency are viewed as punishing.

In the clinical setting we are most often concerned with *positive reinforcement*, the presentation of a positive stimulus, such as tokens or verbal praise, contingent on a correct response. Occasionally, *punishment* procedures, such as reclaiming previously earned tokens or saying "no" or "wrong," are made contingent on undesirable responses. The selection of a specific consequence should be based on observations that it increases the frequency of correct responses. The consequences should be made immediately contingent on the target response, with as little time lag as possible. Usually reinforcement or punishment is made contingent on every target response at the beginning of training and becomes increasingly intermittent as training proceeds. Reinforcement procedures are frequently used when the client's communication problem is not consistent. Correct productions may be reinforced, and at times incorrect productions may be punished.

An alternative approach to punishment in eliminating unwanted behavior is *counterconditioning*. These procedures involve the client's being reinforced for producing responses incompatible with the unwanted behavior. For example, clinicians who employ relaxation training with stutterers in order to reduce their anxiety and excessive tension are attempting to condition a response that is incompatible with anxiety and tension. A third alternative in eliminating unwanted responses is *extinction*. Theoretically, all behavior must be reinforced some of the time, or it will disappear. Extinction procedures, therefore, systematically exclude potentially reinforcing stimuli from being contingent on an unwanted response. For example, people who respond to a little girl's lisp as being "cute" are probably reinforcing it, and clinicians frequently must enlist parents' help in eliminating such inappropriate rewards.

Generalization   The goal of the third stage of direct clinical management is transferring the responses learned in the clinic to everyday speaking situations. In many instances, progress achieved through training and practice in the clinic is extended to everyday living situations with no apparent problems. There are frequent problems with stuttering, however, and generalization problems are not unusual for some clients with voice disorders and with some adults who have a long-standing history of articulation problems.

The usual approach to generalization problems utilizes the same principles employed with stimulus-manipulation techniques described earlier. Because the client produces the desired response in some situations but not in others, generalization training frequently involves modifying the treatment situations and tasks so they gradually approximate the client's everyday life situations. For example, the client's treatment tasks may be gradually modified from saying single words and short phrases to general social conversation with the clinician. Friends or relatives of the client may attend and participate in the treatment sessions. The clinician may visit the client in some situations where generalization is not occurring appropriately and develop specific treatment plans to assist the client in generalizing the behavior developed in treatment. Some generalization problems appear to be related to insufficient positive reinforcement for the new correct response; strong, incidental reinforcement of the old, inappropriate responses; or everyday speaking conditions so dramatically different from the treatment environment that the new, correct responses do not compete successfully with the inappropriate response habit.

Automatization   The goal of the final stage of direct management is what we choose to call automatization. We use this term to refer to the client's ability to produce the correct response without conscious, volitional effort. In many instances, clients with articulation, voice, or stuttering problems produce the desired responses as long as they think about it. When they are not consciously attempting to speak correctly, however, they appear to lapse into old, inappropriate patterns. This problem seems particularly acute under conditions of heightened emotionality.

Currently, the automatization stage of clinical management usually emphasizes increased amounts of volitional practice until habitual patterns of the correct behavior are established on an automatic basis. Although this general practice appears to be reasonably effective with most communication problems, stutterers and some voice clients seem particularly vulnerable to relapse. In many instances, they seem unable to establish correct patterns of speaking behavior on an automatic basis.

Clinical Audits

Within recent years, a number of clinicians have proposed that systematic reviews of clinical intervention are an important aspect of providing quality speech pathology and audiology services. They believe that regular, continuing evaluations are essential components of effective treatment intervention. They advocate more rigorous monitoring of the patient's progress so that treatment effectiveness, or its lack, can be observed and modified when appropriate. Ideally, treatment is terminated when the patient reaches his or her communication potential, thereby avoiding unnecessary treatment and expense. Traditionally, assessment data have been employed only to assist clinicians in making patient-care decisions about individual clients. The information stored in individual patient records has seldom been used by our professions to monitor the patterns of care provided and improve the overall quality of patient care. Perhaps, as some clinicians claim, the information contained in current patient records is not adequate for this task. Siegel (1975), among others, has voiced his concern that the proponents of accountability may stultify the creative clinician and divert time away from the important tasks of serving the clients. This does not mean, however, that he and other concerned clinicians don't support the need for critical and reasoned self-evaluation by clinicians. They are concerned whether or not implementation of patient audits may inadvertently do harm.

The use of information collected and stored in patient records to study patterns of care provided selected groups of patients is not new. It has been employed for a number of years by physicians in medical audits. Only recently have speech pathologists and audiologists and other health professionals, such as physical therapists, nurses, occupational therapists and psychologists (Goran et al., 1975), begun to explore the audit process as a quality-assurance mechanism.

The audit process is not another name for clinical research, although both rely on clinical data. The audit process is not intended to identify practitioners providing substandard levels of care for disciplinary actions, although the quality of care is evaluated. The audit process does not attempt to compare the care provided by a group of practitioners to standards of care established by recognized authorities in the field. Rather, the audit process is intended to assist a group of practitioners study the patterns of care they provide in terms of the standards they agree must be met and to help them improve the quality of care they provide.

The audit process may be summarized as follows. First, a topic is selected for audit. Often this is done by a committee representing the total group of practitioners whose services will be audited if the number of practitioners is very large. The topic selected usually is one which the committee suspects may involve problems of providing appropriate care. At the same time, the committee identifies approximately four to eight criteria it believes are critical indicators of the quality of patient care. The criteria developed must be stated in objective, verifiable terms. They may be *process criteria,* which identify clinical procedures provided by the practitioners, or *outcome criteria,* which are measures of the patient's response to the care provided. Next, the committee decides how frequently clinical performance may deviate from each of these criteria. These expected levels of performance can be viewed as thresholds for action, since it is agreed that if the audit reveals actual levels of care below these expected levels of performance, action must be taken to correct the performance deficit. Next, the committee submits its work to the total group of practitioners for ratification. The criteria and levels of performance are discussed and modified until every practitioner approves each criterion and each expected performance level. At this point, patient records are reviewed and actual levels of performance are compared with expected levels of performance. Performance deficits are identified, and an analysis of the identified deficits begins. On the basis of its problem analyses, the committee develops plans for remedial action and a reaudit. It also reports their findings and recommendations to the total group of practitioners. Remedial action is implemented, and after an appropriate interval a reaudit is conducted to determine how effective the remedial program has been in eliminating performance deficits.

This audit cycle continues until identified patient-care deficits are remedied. Then new audits are begun on different topics. Systematic reviews of clinical intervention through the audit process can play an important role in improving the quality of care among speech pathologists and audiologists. Our history of professional self-regulation of standards of care will likely continue only if meaningful commitments are made by speech pathologists and audiologists to work for increasingly more effective methods of clinical care. Although the data are limited and may not be applicable, the audit process does appear to improve the quality of medical care among physicians.

Preview of Remaining Chapters

Disorders of communication may be classified in a number of ways. Many classification systems have been used, and different systems serve different purposes. Early clinics frequently classified communication disorders in terms of the complaints or problems presented by their clients. For example, patients seen for communication disorders accompanying cleft palate, cerebral palsy, hearing loss, autism, mental retardation, or neuromuscular disturbance were often placed in categories bearing those very names. The patients in each of these taxonomic cubicles, however, might present a diversity of communication disorders. Communication disorders that were not known to be accompanied by other problems often were called functional disorders.

Clinicians and scientists have sometimes used classification systems based on something other than the communication characteristics of the client. Some systems have been based on theory underlying a particular treatment. Psychoanalytic, **cybernetic,** or stimulus-response constructs have been outlined, developed, and then applied to disorders of communication. As a result, the disorders themselves have sometimes received relatively little attention.

Currently, some speech pathologists and audiologists contend that linguistic and psycholinguistic concepts should play a prominent organizational role in the study and treatment of communication disorders. Many clinicians have had the good sense to ignore explanatory, theoretical conflicts between linguists and stimulus-response (S-R) psychologists and to utilize linguistic information in deciding what to teach a person with a language disorder while at the same time utilizing S-R information to determine how to teach it. We now seem to be incorporating cognitive theory into the equation. For example, although reinforcement contingent on response is considered to be a basic clinical tool, we now seek active, cognitive participation on the part of the client, whereas previously we may have been content to have the client serve as a passive recipient of a bombardment of stimuli.

Substantive and theoretical information from linguistics and from learning, cognitive, and personality psychology must be utilized if communication disorders are to be understood. To adopt one or more of those viewpoints, however, shifts the focus of attention from the communication disorders inappropriately. Consequently, Part Two of this book is organized in terms of the communication behaviors that are disordered. This replaces a classification system based on associated etiological factors, such as cerebral palsy or hearing loss. Rather, following chapters are directed to articulation disorders, voice disorders, fluency disorders, hearing impairment, language disorders in children, and language disorders in adults.

This classification is not entirely satisfactory, because two or more of these disorders occur frequently in the same patient. For example, children who misarticulate may present problems in other aspects of language. Similarly, some aspects of motor learning may be equally applicable to articulation and voice. Consequently, there is some overlap in the chapters that follow.

The organization we have chosen is used in many university training programs. It has the distinct advantage of being compatible with a great deal of clinical research and knowledge that has been obtained by speech pathologists and audiologists. It also permits organization and presentation of information that has been accumulated by these specialists and is used in their daily work. Furthermore, it allows coverage of all communication disorders and the integration of information from other fields to improve service for the individual with a communication disorder.

Glossary

Alveolar ridge: The upper or lower gum ridge containing the rows of sockets that enclose the teeth.

Aphasia: Loss or impairment of speech and language due to brain injury.

Apraxia: Loss of the ability, due to brain injury, to execute simple voluntary acts.

Audiologist: A professional engaged in the study of the field of hearing.

Cybernetics: Comparative study of the automatic control system formed by the nervous system and brain and by mechanical-electrical communication systems.

Delayed auditory feedback: A delay of the speaker's voice returning to his or her ears by way of headphones when he or she talks.

Hypernasality: The quality of voice that occurs when there is excessive nasal resonance.

Nasal emission: The escape of air through the nose during speech because of malfunction or deficit of the soft palate.

Optimum pitch: The pitch range at which a given individual may phonate most efficiently.

Otitis media: Inflammation of the middle ear.

Pure-tone stimulus: A stimulus consisting of a periodic sound wave of the sinusoidal type that has no partial or overtone.

Speech pathologist: A professional engaged in the study of speech disorders.

Velopharyngeal closure: The shutting off of the nasal passage from the oral passage.

Study Questions

1. In what ways can speech pathologists and audiologists be viewed as clinical scientists?
2. What are the artistic and humanistic aspects of clinical intervention?
3. How may clinical management strategies be distinguished in terms of their rationales?
4. In what ways can you characterize speech pathologists and audiologists as providers of a comprehensive range of services?
5. How do clinical audits promote improved patient care?
6. In what ways can the audit process be viewed as an educational process?
7. What are the major goals of speech pathologists and audiologists in assessment procedures?
8. Differentiate between the rationale for indirect clinical management and direct management of a communication problem.
9. Describe the primary procedures employed in the response-development stage of treatment.
10. In what ways can speech pathologists and audiologists be described as behavioral scientists?

11. What are the goals of generalization and automatization procedures?
12. What kinds of problems do speech pathologists and audiologists have to work with?

Bibliography

BLOCH, E. L., AND L. D. GOODSTEIN, "Functional Speech Disorders and Personality: A Decade of Research," *J. Speech Hearing Dis.* **36** (1971):295–314.

BOONE, D. R., *The Voice and Voice Therapy*, Englewood Cliffs, N.J.: Prentice-Hall, 1971.

BYRNE, M. C., *The Child Speaks*, New York: Harper & Row, 1965.

DEWS, P. B., "Psychopharmacology," in A. J. Bachrach, ed., *Experimental Foundations of Clinical Psychology*, New York: Basic Books, 1962.

FAIRBANKS, G., *Voice and Articulation Drill Book*, New York: Harper & Row, 1960.

GOODSTEIN, L. D., "Functional Speech Disorders and Personality: A Survey of the Research," *J. Speech Hearing Res.* **1** (1958):359–376.

GORAN, M. J., J. S. ROBERTS, M. KELLOGG, J. FIELDING, AND W. JESSEE, "The PSRO Hospital Review System," *Medical Care* **13,** 4 (Supplement) (1975):1–33.

JOHNSON, W., F. DARLEY, AND D. SPRIESTERSBACH, *Diagnostic Methods in Speech Pathology*, New York: Harper & Row, 1963.

KIRK, S. A., AND W. D. KIRK, *Psycholinguistic Learning Disabilities: Diagnosis and Remediation*, Chicago: University of Illinois Press, 1972.

LONDON, P., *The Modes and Morals of Psychotherapy*, New York: Holt, Rinehart and Winston, 1964.

MCDONALD, E. T., *A Deep Test of Articulation*, Pittsburgh: Stanwix House, 1964.

———, *Articulation Testing and Treatment: A Sensory-Motor Approach*, Pittsburgh: Stanwix House, 1965.

ROGERS, C., "The Necessary and Sufficient Conditions of Therapeutic Personality Change," *J. Consulting Psychology* **21** (1957):95–103.

ROSENBEK, J. C., *et al.*, "A Treatment for Apraxia of Speech with Adults," *J. Speech Hearing Dis.* **38** (1973):462–472.

SHRIBERG, L. D., "A Response Evocation Program for /ɝ/," *J. Speech Hearing Dis.* **40** (1975):92–105.

SIEGEL, B. M., "The High Cost of Accountability," *ASHA* **17** (1975):796–797.

SLOANE, H., AND B. MACAULEY, eds., *Operant Procedures in Remedial Speech and Language Training*, Boston: Houghton Mifflin, 1968.

STRUPP, H., "Patient-Doctor Relationships," in A. J. Bachrach, ed., *Experimental Foundations of Clinical Psychology*, New York: Basic Books, 1962.

VAN RIPER, C., *Speech Correction: Principles and Methods,* Englewood Cliffs, N.J.: Prentice-Hall, 1972.

VAN RIPER, C., AND J. IRWIN, *Voice and Articulation,* Englewood Cliffs, N.J.: Prentice-Hall, 1958.

WOLPE, J., AND A. LAZARUS, *Behavior Therapy Techniques,* New York: Pergamon Press, 1966.

CHAPTER 8
Overview

Articulation is the production of speech sounds (consonants, vowels, and diphthongs); disordered articulation is the distortion or omission of sounds or substitution of one sound for another. These errors, which usually involve consonants, are likely to call attention to themselves, and they can make speech difficult to understand. In our word-oriented society, these differences can be handicapping. Misarticulation may result from organic pathology, as in cleft palate or dysarthria, but it may also be presented by persons for whom no causal factors are evident. Both kinds of articulation problems are considered in this chapter.

The clinical evaluation of an individual who misarticulates is likely to involve assessment of hearing, language, and other variables as well as articulation itself. Variables that coexist with disordered articulation are of interest to the speech pathologist because they may have caused the articulation problem, or their manipulation may contribute to change in articulation. Articulation tests, which may be used to identify and describe disordered articulation, help sample a speaker's production of sounds under different stimulus conditions and in different speech units, including words and connected speech. Prediction of future articulation behavior, plans for remedial work, or both may be based on knowledge of the number of sounds misarticulated, the consistency with which they are misarticulated, the influence of neighboring sounds on the sound of interest, and the way in which a sound is misarticulated.

Disorders of Articulation

Articulation remediation is discussed in terms of (1) dealing with conditions underlying the articulation disorder, and (2) directly training the individual to articulate better. Training procedures may be directed to acquisition of the ability to produce a sound and to the automatic usage of good articulation in spontaneous speech. Important components of articulation remediation include the use of principles of learning in the development of step-by-step programs to accomplish training goals, use of parents or other aides to assist in the clinical process, tailoring treatment to the client through continuing assessment of the client's progress, and relating to each client in open, supportive ways.

Ralph L. Shelton, Ph.D.
University of Arizona

Introduction

When the Vice-President saw Leggett, the smile widened. "Mr. Leggett." The small hand darted forward; touched Leggett's hand; was swiftly withdrawn (the professional politician's way of avoiding having his hand crushed). "How does Mr. Bryant?" Yes, Van Buren lisps; he also speaks with a slight Dutch accent . . .

Abruptly Van Buren said something to me in Dutch. A long sentence in which the lisp was not apparent. Then not waiting to see if I understood or not, the small golden historic figure moved away from us, leaving me bewildered and Leggett furious. "What's the good of being a Dutch oaf if you can't speak the . . . language?"**

This chapter will focus on articulation disorders as observed by the speech pathologist using various articulation testing and sampling procedures. Attention will be given to the nature of disordered articulation and to variables related to articulation. The evaluation and remediation of articulation disorders will be especially emphasized.

Articulation involves use of respiratory and oral movements to produce the speech sounds which comprise words and which are organized into categories called **phonemes** (see Chapters 2 and 3). In a phonetic alphabet, a distinctive symbol is assigned to each phoneme, and these symbols may be used for transcribing articulation. The words *pie, apple,* and *cup* each contain **phones** (sounds) which are members of the /p/† family, or phoneme. The word *cat,* when correctly articulated, consists of three phones—/k/, /æ/, and /t/—each of which belongs to a different phoneme. The speech pathologist concerned with articulation will focus attention on the client's production of various speech sounds—especially consonants, because they are misarticulated more often than vowels are. Those sounds may be observed isolated from context and in syllables, words, reading, and conversation.

Description of Disordered Articulation

Articulation errors involve the omission of speech sounds from words, the substitution of one sound for another, and the distortion of sounds. Occasionally, a

---

*   Gore Vidal, *Burr,* New York: Random House, 1973. Reprinted by permission.
†   Symbols representing sounds are usually enclosed in slashes (/ /) when the transcriber is concerned with the sound's contribution to meaning, and brackets ([ ]) are used when the symbol represents sound production without consideration of semantic distinctiveness. Here only slashes are used, whether the text reflects concern for meaning, sound production, or both.

DISORDERS OF ARTICULATION

speaker will insert an extra sound into a word. Such an error is referred to as an *addition*. The child who says "boo" to refer to a boot is making an *omission error*, having omitted the /t/. The child who says "wed" to refer to the color "red" is making a *substitution error*—a /w/ phone for an /r/. A lateral lisp is an example of a *distortion;* the speaker with a lateral lisp substitutes a slushy-sounding phone for an /s/ phone. This error is called a distortion rather than a substitution because the sound produced resembles /s/ more than any other phoneme. However, the sound produced is in some way nonstandard. In the lateral lisp, the tongue tip typically contacts the alveolar ridge more firmly than do the sides of the tongue (McGlone and Proffit, 1973). Consequently, the sound is produced by air which leaves the mouth lateral to midline.

Whether or not an articulation error constitutes a disorder depends on the number of sounds involved, the age of the speaker, and whether the errors call attention to themselves or interfere with the **intelligibility** of speech. A mispronunciation does not constitute an articulation error. For example, one young child said "mazagine" for "magazine," but each sound was correctly articulated and he made few such errors.

Articulation problems range widely in severity. A person may misarticulate phones from one phoneme, often /s/ or /r/, or from many phonemes. A person may misarticulate each /s/ phone that occurs or only some of them, and any such inconsistency in misarticulation may be a function of the phonetic context in which a sound appears (McDonald, 1964a). That is, a sound may be correctly articulated when it is adjacent to one sound but not another. Some speakers may be unintelligible to the listener because of their articulation errors, whereas others may present articulatory errors that are readily observable but which interfere little with intelligibility. Generally, the number of phonemes from which sounds are misarticulated serves as an index to the severity of any articulation disorder (Templin and Darley, 1969). However, a lisp involving only /s/ can be a source of embarrassment to a speaker. A child in the play *Music Man* portrayed despondency resulting from embarrassment about a lisp.

Whether or not misarticulations presented by an individual are considered to be outside the range of normal speech is influenced by the age of the speaker.

►

Normative articulation data. The left-hand margin of each bar represents the age at which 50 percent of the children in a normative study used the sound specified correctly. The right-hand margin shows the age at which 90 percent of the children used the sound correctly. Data reported in the lower bars are from Sander (1972). Data in the black bars are from the work of Hedrick, Prather, and Tobin (1975). Children appear to be developing speech sounds at earlier ages than in the past. (Adapted by permission from E. M. Prather, D. L. Hedrick, and C. A. Kern, "Articulation Development in Children Aged Two to Four Years," J. Speech Hearing Dis. 40 (1975):179–191.)

Figure 8.1

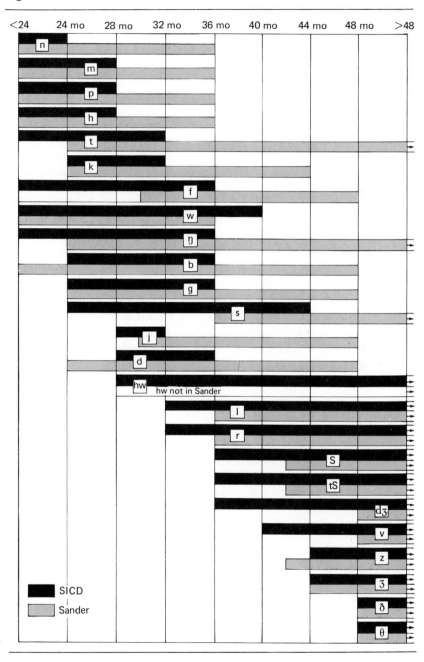

Because many children under eight years of age make articulation errors, normative data, such as those of Prather, Hedrick, and Kern (1975), are often utilized by the speech pathologist in the evaluation of articulation behavior (Fig. 8.1).

Various segments of the population of the United States speak different **dialects,** and at least some of those dialects have distinctive articulatory patterns. Many persons in the Northeast, for example, drop /r/ when it occurs after a vowel; similarly, the English spoken by a bilingual ethnic group tends to differ from standard English in orderly ways. Also, some black Americans speak a dialect called black English.

Although it is often advantageous for a person who speaks a dialect to acquire proficiency in the use of standard English, articulatory differences associated with use of a dialect are not disorders. Indeed, speech clinicians working in communities where dialects are spoken must distinguish between articulation characteristic of the dialect and articulation that is unacceptable in the dialect. Even aside from dialect differences, a particular articulatory pattern might be acceptable within one community but not another. For example, two adolescent boys who had undergone surgery for **cleft palate** made similar, moderate articulation errors that did not interfere with intelligibility. The father of one of the boys was a professional person actively seeking political office and the other father was a farmer. One father was satisfied with his son's articulation, and the other sought out surgery and speech training for his son. An unrepaired palatal cleft is shown in Fig. 8.2. In summary, whether or not the production of sounds in speech constitutes a problem depends on the values of the speaker, whether the sounds are noted as errors by a listener, and on interference with speech intelligibility.

Etiology and Related Variables

Some articulation disorders appear to be the direct result of physical disability. Others are observed in persons who are free from identifiable pathology. Persons in the latter category are frequently said to have functional articulation disabilities. Both organic and functional articulation disorders will be discussed in this section.

Organic Articulatory Disorders

Many physical disabilities may be accompanied by characteristic patterns of articulation. The organic condition is assumed to have caused the articulation problem if the two form a logical pattern. For example, a high-frequency hearing loss is likely to account for the misarticulation of consonants, such as /s/, which involve high-frequency sound vibrations, since they must be heard correctly to be produced correctly. This inference would be especially compelling if no other causal explanations were available, but **etiology** is difficult to establish with cer-

Figure 8.2

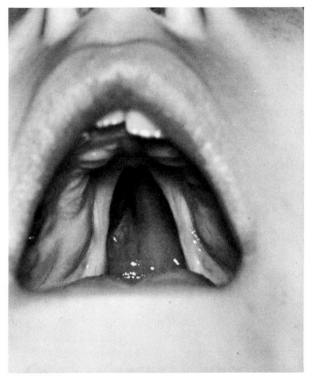

Cleft of the soft and hard palates in a boy. The cleft structures failed to develop normally during embryonic development.

tainty. Other organic conditions that influence articulation may involve anatomy of the speech mechanism, as in cleft palate, which is discussed below, or **glossectomy** (removal of tongue tissue in the surgical treatment of cancer). We have worked with patients who suffered the excision of moderate amounts of tongue tissue (partial glossectomy) with little effect on articulation; however, others who required removal of greater amounts of tissue suffered severe articulation and intelligibility impairment.

Organic conditions may also involve the physiology of the speech mechanism. For example, a boy whose facial nerves had failed to develop (Moebius syndrome) was unable to move his facial muscles and consequently was unable to smile, close his eyes, or purse his lips to drink from a straw. The boy also misarticulated sounds that required lip closure (/p/, /b/, and /m/) or contact between the lips and teeth (/f/ and /v/). However, he substituted phonetically similar sounds (for example, /t/ for /p/ and /θ/ for /f/) for the sounds he was unable to produce (see Table 3.1 for phonetic symbols and sound classifications), and his speech was quite intelligible.

Damage to the nervous system may impair motor function, sensation, or both, and the disability may cause misarticulation. Let us briefly consider cleft palate as an example of structural impairment of articulation and **dysarthria** and **apraxia** as examples of pathologies that interfere with the physiology of articulation.

Structural articulation impairment The normal American speaker uses the soft palate **(velum)** and pharyngeal (throat) walls to close the passage between the oral and nasal cavities during the production of all sounds except nasal consonants and also vowels adjacent to nasal consonants (Fig. 8.3). Failure to produce this velopharyngeal closure during speech will impair articulation in characteristic ways. Air pressure developed during speech production may escape through the nose—perhaps producing unwanted noise (nasal emission). Air pressure in the mouth may be insufficient for the production of normal **stop** and **continuant consonants,** and the voice may be hypernasal (see Chapter 9).* Clefts of the palate and lip may occur in various combinations, including soft and hard palate (Fig. 8.2), soft palate only, lip only, and soft and hard palate and lip combined. Clefts of the palate impair speech as described above, whereas defects of the lip involve only a few consonants. Speech problems resulting from inadequate velopharyngeal closure may also be observed in patients who present short palate, unusual pharyngeal depth, or other structural malformations, including defects beneath the mucosa that covers the palate. Surgical removal of oropharyngeal tissue in the treatment of cancer may result in velopharyngeal closure deficits, and the velopharyngeal mechanism may malfunction in the neurological deficits that are discussed in the next section.

Palatal clefts are usually closed by plastic surgery; however, even with surgical repair, the closure mechanism may not function properly. If the initial surgery allows continued leakage of air from the nose during speech, **secondary palatal surgery** may be undertaken. Also, prosthodontic dental appliances may be used to fill the space between the soft palate and the pharyngeal walls, thus providing velopharyngeal closure. These appliances are constructed to take advantage of the movements of the soft palate and pharyngeal walls that do occur.

---

* Patients with palatal defects may substitute easily produced nonstandard sounds for sounds that require good anatomical structure. For example, some individuals substitute sounds produced at the vocal folds or at the site of tongue-pharyngeal wall approximation (a throat-clearing sound) for front-of-the-mouth continuants (/s/, /z/, and /ʃ/) that require oral air pressure and hence velopharyngeal closure. Speakers who use proper articulatory placements but reduced oral air pressure avoid audible nasal escape at the cost of some intelligibility loss resulting from weak production of consonants. Sometimes their /b/ and /d/ consonants sound like /m/ and /n/.

Figure 8.3

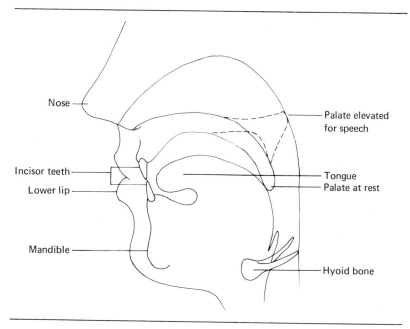

X-ray tracing of a normal speaker, showing the palate at rest (solid line) and elevated for speech (dashed line). During normal speech, the palate and the walls of the pharynx make contact during most sounds, thus closing the passage into the nose and preventing escape of air through the nose during speech.

Thus at rest, the passage from mouth to nose is open, allowing nasal breathing, but during speech the muscles move against the **prosthetic speech appliance,** thus closing the velopharyngeal port.

Sometimes the adenoids fill the space between the palate and the walls of the pharynx in persons with marginal velopharyngeal closure deficits, and speech is free from nasality or audible nasal escape of air so long as the adenoids are undisturbed. If a health problem makes removal of the adenoids necessary in such patients, a speech disorder will probably result. If the adenoids are too large in a person with an otherwise normal mechanism, they may make it impossible to open the passage into the nose satisfactorily. This may interfere with the production of /m/, /n/, and /ŋ/, which require nasal resonance (Chapters 4 and 9), and a resonance defect termed "denasality" results. Unfortunately, both speech pathologists and physicians occasionally mistake hypernasality for denasality, and as a result a few persons have had adenoids removed to help speech, when actually the presence of the adenoids was contributing to speech.

The role of the speech pathologist in working with cleft palate patients includes evaluation of the adequacy of the speech mechanism for producing good speech. Also included is training the patient to speak well after surgical and dental treatments have provided a suitable speech mechanism.

Velopharyngeal closure deficits for speech may be inferred from speech errors involving nasal air escape. Various instruments may be used in speech evaluation of the closure mechanism; for example, articulation-testing materials may be employed that are loaded with consonants requiring oral pressure, or instruments may be used to measure the air flow that escapes from the nose during speech. Velopharyngeal closure may be directly observed by X-ray techniques (especially those involving motion picture filming), and the speech pathologist participates in X-ray examination in terms of selecting utterances for the patient to produce as the X-ray film is exposed and observing the speech behaviors filmed. Direct observation of velopharyngeal closure by X-ray or by use of **endoscopes** placed in the mouth or nose and inference of closure from observation of speech are supplementary diagnostic procedures.

Whether or not either speech training or therapeutic exercise will improve velopharyngeal closure is a controversial issue, but if training procedures correct velopharyngeal closure deficits, that effect has not been well documented. In recent research speakers have been provided with biofeedback regarding the performance of their velopharyngeal muscles during speech. Although the results are encouraging, much more data are needed to determine whether and under what circumstances poor velopharyngeal closure can be corrected by behavioral methods. Speech training following successful surgical or prosthodontic treatment of the velopharyngeal closure mechanism is usually similar to that provided to individuals presenting functional disorders of articulation, voice, or both.

Often, speech-pathology services are delivered to cleft palate patients as part of a team effort. Teams may consist of plastic surgeons, orthodontists, **prosthodontists,** audiologists, otolaryngologists, psychologists, special educators, pediatricians, and other specialists as well as speech pathologists. A plastic surgeon's viewpoint of the team effort follows, and team efforts are considered later in the section on evaluation.

What is the goal of treatment for a patient with a cleft lip, cleft palate, or other oro-facial defect? A group of health professionals experienced in providing care for individuals with these deformities has defined the goal as development of an "individual who, for reasons which relate to the cleft defect, does not differ significantly from his peers in health, education, or vocational opportunities, and the ability to communicate and interact with others." * *This is a much more*

---

* Unpublished data, Conference on the Development of Norms, Standards and Criteria for Quality Assurance for Persons with Cleft Lip and Palate, Wheaton, Maryland, June 1975.

180

complex objective than that commonly sought by the plastic surgeon who attempts to remove diseased tissue, reconstruct anatomical structures, and provide normal appearance. Although a number of disciplines may participate in the total evaluation and treatment of the patient with the plastic surgeon, two disciplines, speech pathology and dentistry, are particularly important.

Ideally, each clinician should examine the patient and carry out diagnostic studies in the most convenient manner and setting. Each should formulate a tentative treatment plan. At the time of the initial evaluation and at intervals determined by significant events in the course of treatment, however, such as performance of surgery or fabrication of a prosthesis, or when failure to attain treatment objectives becomes apparent, consultation among the disciplines with staffing of the patient in a joint conference is almost essential. Although plastic surgeons are skilled in physical examination of the oro-facial area and may have considerable experience in judging the quality of speech, the need to distinguish speech dysfunction due to correctable physical defects from faulty articulation or other speech disorders not amenable to surgery may require a speech pathology consultation. The speech clinician may utilize a battery of articulation tests, manometry, pressure-flow studies, and other observations to contribute the needed information. Similarly, study of the cleft patient by the dental specialist is needed to assess facial development and estimate the potential for growth in the face and jaws, and the extent to which malocclusion and face and jaw deformity may be correctable by nonsurgical means.

Identification of patients who will benefit from surgery and the type of surgery most likely to achieve optimum habilitation of the patient are not enough. Treatment by several disciplines demands agreement among these disciplines in priorities, timing, and an awareness of the extent to which the treatment plan of one specialist may interfere with treatment by another. Failure to coordinate interdisciplinary management may needlessly prolong treatment and fail to achieve as successful habilitation as possible.

Finally, as pointed out by Kernahan,* evaluation of the results of surgical treatment by the surgeon alone, no matter how critical, is subject to bias. The careful longitudinal recording of physical and physiological data and the effects of treatment upon these measurements are essential in determining whether surgery, or any other treatment for that matter, has achieved its objectives. In fact, if stated objectives have not been achieved, was failure related to the

---

*   D. Kernahan, L. N. Monn, and C. F. T. Snelling, "Normality," in "Cleft Palate Speech: A Comparison of the Cleft Palate Population and Normal Controls at the Age of 7 to 9." Paper presented at the Annual Meeting of the Association of Plastic Surgeons, April 28, 1975.

surgery performed? Interdisciplinary observations are required to answer these questions.

William C. Trier, M.D.
Professor of Surgery and Dental Ecology
University of North Carolina at Chapel Hill

Physiological articulation impairment Injury and various illnesses may damage or interfere with the nervous system, which in turn may affect speech. For example, motor impairment resulting from brain damage prior to, during, or soon after birth is called **cerebral palsy.** Each of several categories of cerebral palsy, including athetosis and spasticity, is characterized by distinctive motor impairments. Persons with severe athetosis or spastic cerebral palsy are likely to present unintelligible speech and to be limited in the speech improvement they make with speech training.

Speech disorder caused by damage to the central or peripheral nervous system and resulting muscle weakness or disturbance of muscular control of the speech mechanism is called *dysarthria* (Darley, Aronson, and Brown, 1969, 1975). Dysarthria must involve articulation and may also involve phonation, **prosody** (speech rhythm), and respiratory function for speech; dysarthric articulation errors tend to involve slighting, distorting, and omitting sounds.

Darley, Aronson, and Brown (1969) studied the speech of persons presenting one of seven neurological disorders. A statistical analysis of the speech data identified several different patterns of dysarthria, and the authors concluded that dysarthric speech patterns are distinctive for different categories of neuroanatomical and neurophysiological pathology. Dimensions of speech impaired in dysarthria include pitch, loudness, voice quality, respiration, prosody, and articulation. For example, the authors found that the speech of patients with one neurological disorder, bulbar palsy, was characterized by hypernasality, imprecise consonants, breathy voice, monopitch, and to a lesser extent nasal emission of air, audible inspiration, harsh voice, short phrases, and monoloudness. They interpreted their observations to indicate that the vocal folds of these patients did not open or close properly and that their velopharyngeal and oral ports malfunctioned. The neurological impairment that causes dysarthria influences involuntary or reflexive movements as well as the voluntary movements of speech.

A second neurologically based articulation disorder is speech apraxia, which is thought to result from damage to Broca's area of the cortex, which programs or sequences speech-production movements (Darley, Aronson, and Brown, 1975). Speech apraxia involves an inability to make articulatory movements, even though involuntary movements of the speech mechanism occur normally. The apraxic patient may use the mouth normally for swallowing but make articulatory errors during speech, and these errors are likely to involve sound repetitions and additions and substitutions of some sounds for others. The more deliberately this patient tries to speak, the more difficulty he or she has with speech,

182

but the error pattern is variable with repetitions of the same utterance (LaPointe, 1975). Apraxia in adults has been described by Johns and Darley (1970) and in children by Yoss and Darley (1974). These conditions are discussed further by Boone in Chapter 12 because they occur in some stroke patients who may also present aphasia.

The concept of speech apraxia just outlined is controversial in that some authors think that motor-programing impairment and aphasia may not be distinguished and that linguistic variables not involving neuropathology may influence speech production (Martin, 1974). Winitz (1975) questioned the applicability of the speech-apraxia concept to children. Speech apraxia is easier to conceptualize in adults who present known brain damage (abrupt onset of disorder; medical evidence regarding site of lesion) than in children who appear to be developing normally except that they misarticulate. However, perhaps some small percentage of the children who misarticulate do have defects of that portion of the brain that programs speech production.

The speech pathologists' work with patients presenting dysarthria will include observation and description of articulation and other aspects of speech. If articulation testing shows some capacity for speech that the patient doesn't utilize, treatment will be planned to develop that capacity. Treatment will very likely be directed to intelligibility, and the clinician will utilize rate, rhythm, intensity, articulation, gesture—whatever is available—to help the individual express himself or herself. Netsell and Cleeland (1973) were able to help a patient with Parkinson's disease to reduce unwanted lip contraction. To do this they used instrumentation to record electrical activity in the muscle responsible for the contraction and to display that activity to the patient auditorily. The patient was able to use this biofeedback to modify her use of the muscle—in this case to turn the muscle off. Mysak (1963) discussed means of extinguishing unwanted reflexes that interfere with speech in persons with some kinds of dysarthria. For persons with severe dysarthria, conversation boards are sometimes devised. Words and pictures are arranged on the board to allow an individual to communicate by pointing. These boards are used as supplements to or substitutes for speech.

Remediation procedures for apraxia are undergoing development. Rosenbek et al. (1973) described a continuum of tasks intended to improve the speech of the apraxic adult. The continuum consisted of stimuli used to obtain speech from the patient. Initially the patient is asked to watch and listen to the clinician and to repeat speech units after the clinician. As the patient advances through the training, he or she is asked to read, produce speech in response to questions, and finally talk in a role-playing situation. More applied research is needed to develop effective remedial techniques for dysarthria and apraxia and to learn the conditions under which those treatments are effective.

The presence of a physical disability in company with an articulation disorder does not necessarily mean that the physical deficit is the cause of the articulation problem. Learning and other behavioral variables are also operative in persons with organic disability. For example, children born with cleft palate may have articulation problems that are caused by something other than the palatal defect (Van Demark, 1966). In the next section, the etiology of functional articulation disorders will be considered, and learning variables are discussed as they relate to functional articulation problems.

Functional Articulation Problems

Persons who make substitution, omission, and distortion articulation errors and who appear to be free from organic disability are frequently said to have *functional articulation problems*. Some, but not all, will present related problems, such as language disorders. Some will be concerned about their articulation problems, and others will not be aware of them. Few are likely to show deficits in respiration, phonation, or prosody. In clinical usage, the term *functional* has often served a "waste basket" function of collecting articulation problems of unknown causation.

Relationships   Various attempts have been made to discover the causes of functional articulation problems. For example, articulation measures have been correlated (studied for statistical relationship) with other measures in the hope that the resulting patterns might provide clues to causation. Articulation measures have been studied for relationship with measures of speech-sound discrimination, sex, motor skills, sibling status, **kinesthesis, tongue thrust,** socioeconomic status, handedness, personality, language, dentition, and educational achievement, among others (Winitz, 1969, Chapter 3). Most of the variables that have been studied have not been strongly related to disordered articulation.

One relationship that has achieved statistical significance in a number of studies involves articulation and speech-sound discrimination. Persons who misarticulate phones from a particular phoneme have been shown to have difficulty discriminating between correct and incorrect productions of those same phones. However, McReynolds, Kohn, and Williams (1975) demonstrated that the percentage of items misarticulated is much higher than the percentage of items incorrectly discriminated.* The role of auditory processing in understanding articulation and other communication disorders is controversial. Rees (1973) reviewed literature which indicated that auditory-processing information has been overemphasized and misused by persons attempting to manage and understand communication disorders. However, other viewpoints which stress the role of auditory processing in explaining and treating communication disorders have been developed (Rampp, 1972).

---

*   These authors presented syllables to misarticulating subjects that had been produced by other persons. A speaker's awareness of his or her own errors may be more important than awareness of other persons' errors.

Phonology, which is concerned with the nature and development of articulation, is considered in linguistic theory to be one of four major language categories (see Chapter 2). Some writers currently think that if articulation is one aspect of language, articulatory development should coincide and correlate with development of other aspects of language.* Accordingly, children with articulation defects should show problems in syntax and semantics. There is evidence that language problems sometimes accompany articulation problems (Panagos, 1974); however, the relationship is not invariant. Language deficits are especially likely to be observed in preschool children with severe articulation problems; however, articulation problems are also seen in persons skilled in language —teachers, statisticians, politicians, and others. This articulation-language relationship is currently receiving much research as well as speculative attention. Winitz (1969) suggested that we move on from a preoccupation with variables that correlate with articulation status and search for variables that correlate with indices to peoples' responses to articulation treatment. Information of that kind can be used to improve treatment effectiveness.

Causation   Presence of a relationship, or correlation, between two variables— for example, articulation and speech-sound discrimination—does not mean that one caused the other. However, since no one variable is present in all persons with articulation disorders, we can conclude that no single variable is responsible for all articulation disorders. Indeed, research is being conducted to identify clusters of misarticulating persons who may be quite distinctive. Arndt *et al.* (1977) identified clusters of misarticulating school children who performed very well on measures of school achievement and psycholinguistic ability, and they found other clusters whose members performed poorly on the same variables. Presumably, members of these two clusters need different speech and educational services.

Winitz (1969, 1975) has integrated data and theoretical constructs in an attempt to explain disordered articulation in physically normal persons. He distinguished between phonetic and phonological articulatory development. Phonetic development concerns the speaker's acquisition of the ability to produce speech sounds. Phonological development concerns acquisition of the phoneme system of one's language, including the learning of the acceptable phoneme sequences. Through processes that may involve innate capacity and discrimination learning, the child acquires rules which govern the distribution of sounds in speech. By two and a half to three years of age, most children can produce most sounds in their language. However, many do not complete mastery of the proper use of those sounds until they are approximately eight years old. Even if able to

---

*   The conceptualization of the relationship between speech and language is still under development (Cutting and Kavanagh, 1975).

produce all of the sounds of his or her language, a child may have an articulation problem if a sound is used correctly only part of the time.

Explanations of disordered articulation should be evaluated with reference to hypotheses and theories from linguistics, psychology, and physiology as well as speech pathology. Attempts to build theoretical explanations for "functional" articulation problems are in their infancy. For now, we recommend the explanatory hypothesis stated by Winitz (1969): "When obvious physical and mental impairments are not present, articulatory errors represent the incorrect learning of the phoneme system of the community language, which in some cases may have been partially a result of incorrectly learned phonetic production." That is, the phoneme system the child has learned is incorrect. This is not to say that learning variables are not involved in the speech of individuals with organically based articulation problems. Nor does it explain why incorrect learning occurred.

Although learning is important to functional articulation disorders, additional variables are undoubtedly involved in their etiology. Scientists are seeking evidence of hitherto unidentified oral sensory or oral motor deficits in persons categorized as having functional articulation problems (Bosma, 1970). Articulation errors may result from the presence of several factors, no one of which by itself could have caused an articulation disorder (McDonald, 1964a), and etiological factors may precipitate articulation problems only in persons who have a predisposition to those problems (Powers, 1971). Furthermore, the presence of additional variables may be necessary to perpetuate the articulation problem.

The search for variables related to articulation change in response to treatment may indeed be more important than the search for causes. The search for causes of "functional" articulation disorders hasn't been very fruitful, and many workers have concluded that we should shift our attention from cause-based explanation of articulation disorders to behavioral considerations that focus on remediation (Irwin, 1970). Articulation disorders of unknown origin are a frequently occurring communication disorder, and their evaluation and treatment usually progress in a satisfactory manner. The following consideration of evaluation and remediation emphasizes principles and procedures usually applied in working with persons whose misarticulations are either "functional" or organic in origin.

Evaluation

Evaluation of a person thought to present an articulation disorder involves observing, testing, and decision making. Much more is involved than counting the number of correct responses to articulation test items and comparing the results with **normative data.** However, the first decision to be made is whether a given individual needs a speech evaluation. Often that decision is made by someone other than the speech pathologist; for example, parents may be concerned that their preschool child is not developing speech normally and may seek a speech evaluation. Or a physician or teacher may refer a child about whom he or she is concerned. Older persons sometimes refer themselves for speech consultation. In school districts, speech pathologists often do screening testing to identify persons who may have articulation or other communication problems and therefore require evaluation services. The Templin-Darley Articulation Screening Test (Templin and Darley, 1969) is one instrument used for that purpose. Children are asked to name pictures, and a record is kept of their articulation of test sounds. The number of test sounds that are correctly articulated is compared with normative information, and if the number is too small, an evaluation is scheduled. Irwin (1972) devised a screening procedure to allow the speech pathologist to screen school-age children for articulation, language, voice, and fluency in a matter of minutes. Screening for misarticulation may simply involve listening to a sample of conversation. Regardless of the methods used, persons identified as presenting questionable articulation will be scheduled for more detailed evaluation.

In conducting an evaluation, the speech pathologist will gather information helpful in describing and classifying a person's articulation. If a problem is found, the clinician will need information to establish a prognosis and to guide any treatment that may be offered. The clinician attempts to discover the etiology of any problem that is identified. However, it is often impossible to be sure what caused an articulation disorder. The evaluation process will now be discussed in some detail.

Background Information

The speech pathologist will be especially interested in the viewpoint of the client or of the client's parents about the presence or absence of a speech disorder and about the nature of the problem if a problem is thought to be present. If a problem is identified that warrants speech remediation, that work will be facilitated if the clinician and the client or parents have a degree of mutual understanding about the problem. The speech pathologist must be able to relate to and communicate with persons who range widely in age, socioeconomic status, and communication ability. The client's cooperation is essential, because the clinician cannot examine speech or language that is not displayed. A key clinical evaluation error occurs when the clinician mistakenly considers a poor or inappropriate but atypical response to represent an inability to respond correctly.

A patient history is important, especially for the identification of variables that concern the client. It may also identify variables that have contributed to the communication problem. Such variables may or may not be active in maintaining the disorder at the time of the evaluation. Reports from dentists, psychologists, teachers, physicians, nurses, social workers, and other specialists may help the speech clinician understand a client and his or her disordered speech.

187

These specialists may provide information about variables that will restrict the amount of improvement that can be expected with articulation training. Also, the speech pathologist's evaluation may contribute to decision making by persons in other fields. For example, occasionally a classroom teacher will wonder whether an articulation error represents a word-recognition deficit in reading. Information from the speech clinician can help resolve that question, thus contributing to the teacher's lesson-planning process. Sometimes the speech evaluation is a part of a team effort wherein the client is studied by several of the specialists noted above. When their examinations have been completed, the specialists meet to discuss their findings and to plan a program for the individual. Since the client may require treatment for problems in addition to the communication problem, schedules and priorities must be established. Thus in addition to relating to clients and their families, the speech pathologist must establish and maintain effective working relationships with members of other professions.

Testing Variables Related to Articulation

The speech pathologist will test variables that are important to the understanding of any articulation problem that is present. He or she will either screen the child's hearing or make certain that it is tested by an audiologist (see Chapter 13). Failure to identify hearing loss has resulted in poor service to many children with articulation problems and sometimes in the misclassification of children as mentally retarded or aphasic. The clinician will also want information about the client's language—use of syntax and vocabulary and ability to communicate meaning. Some children have good language ability, but fail to use it to communicate with family or friends. Again, preschool children with severe articulation problems are especially likely to have problems with language. A linguistic analysis of an extensive recorded sample of a child's speech is too time consuming and costly to be used routinely in clinical practice. However, published tests which are less time consuming are available for use in language assessment, and we can expect reliable tools with greater validity to be available in the future. Tests in current use measure vocabulary, syntax, comprehension, expression, and psycholinguistic variables underlying language.

As was mentioned earlier, speech pathologists have been especially interested in whether a child can differentiate between one speech sound and another. At present, some clinicians record the individual's speech and attempt to determine whether the client can discriminate between sounds from a given phoneme that she or he has articulated correctly and those that were misarticulated.

Frequently clinicians inspect the client's oral cavity to identify any structural or physiological differences that may interfere with articulation. For example, effective diagnostic routines for evaluation of velopharyngeal closure adequacy for speech have evolved through research (see Chapter 9). That information is available in more advanced sources (McWilliams and Wertz, 1973).

The face and oral cavity are often inspected even in persons who are thought to be free from organic disability. No standard routine has yet been adopted for this purpose. However, the clinician may make observations to determine whether the speed with which a child can repeat series of syllables (diadochokinesis) meets norms for the individual's age (Fletcher, 1972). Certainly, the oral examination should include careful observation of the movements used in the production of various sounds. The clinician may learn, for example, that a child places the tongue against or between the teeth when it should be placed slightly farther back. Such information can be used in planning articulation lessons so that training directed to one or two sounds results in generalization to and improvement of sounds not directly trained. A young girl evaluated recently protruded her tongue for /s, z, ʃ, l, t, d, and tʃ/. Correction of one or two of those sounds may result in generalization of correct tongue usage to the other sounds.

Some persons believe that a condition termed "tongue thrust" exerts tongue pressure against the teeth, contributing to (1) malocclusion, (2) relapse to malocclusion following orthodontics, and (3) articulatory disorders. Tongue thrust involves placement of the tongue against or between the teeth during swallowing (Mason and Proffit, 1974; Hanson, 1976), and tongue posture at rest and during speech may also exert pressure on the teeth. This condition is observed in persons with articulation problems, malocclusion, or both, but it is also observed in individuals with normal speech and dentition. Some speech pathologists and orthodontists assume that tongue thrust is a habit to be corrected through training, whereas others contend that such training has not been demonstrated to have any beneficial effect. Also, tongue thrust may reflect the presence of an organic condition, such as obstruction of the upper airway. If so, training would not be expected to correct the condition. The Joint Committee on Dentistry and Speech Pathology, which is supported by the American Speech and Hearing Association and the American Association of Dental Schools (1975), has recommended that tongue-thrust treatment be considered an experimental procedure not for routine use. The tongue-thrust problem is thought to involve large numbers of children, and we expect that the recommendation of the Joint Committee will result in research that will provide a better basis for decision making by orthodontists, speech pathologists, and others who are involved.

In examining the mouth, speech clinicians sometimes observe nonspeech movements (such as the ability to position the tongue tip behind the upper central teeth) as well as structure and articulatory motions. However, observation or training of nonspeech movements appears to be of little value in persons with articulation disorders, since the cerebral innervation of those movements is different from that controlling speech (Hardy, 1970). Certainly no one has demonstrated that predictions about spontaneous speech improvement or speech change in response to treatment can be made from observation of nonspeech oral movements. However, this criticism is also true of many procedures used in speech evaluations.

189

Articulation Assessment

A major portion of the speech evaluation for a person with an articulation problem will be devoted to examination of articulation itself. Instruments such as the Templin-Darley Articulation Tests (Templin and Darley, 1969) consist of materials for eliciting articulation responses, recording the clinician's assessment of those responses, and analyzing and classifying articulation errors that are observed. Responses to these tests may be obtained from young children by asking them to name pictures or to imitate the examiner. Older persons may be asked to read test material aloud. The examiner must be trained to judge articulation responses accurately. Usually, word-size units are used in administering the Templin-Darley Tests, and the examiner focuses attention on one phone or on a blend or cluster of phones, such as /sl/ in sled. The examiner may indicate on a record sheet whether the phone or blend of interest was correctly or incorrectly articulated, and for incorrect phones the clinician may attempt to specify the nature of the error. That is, he or she may note whether the sound was distorted or omitted or whether another phone was used in its place. If the sound was distorted, the clinician may attempt to describe characteristics of the sound that was produced. Judgments of whether a given response is correct or incorrect are usually more reliable than judgments about the nature of errors made (Philips and Bzoch, 1969).

The heart of articulation testing is in organizing articulation observations into a meaningful and useful pattern. The Templin-Darley score sheet helps the clinician to organize a description of the client's articulation and to utilize the articulation information in a decision-making process. The clinician will probably examine the testing record to determine whether the client failed to produce any phones correctly from a particular phoneme. Such a failure would suggest that the client lacked the phonetic ability to produce sounds from the phoneme involved. Various patterns of disordered articulation exist, and the articulation test should help the examiner to identify them. A pattern wherein certain sounds are produced correctly sometimes and incorrectly at other times suggests to some clinicians that the child has not mastered the rules that govern mature articulation, even though his or her phonetic- or sound-production skills are apparently satisfactory. Preschool children who are slow in speech and perhaps language development often omit consonants at the ends of words. They are likely to articulate correctly sounds that appear early in developmental schedules (see Fig. 8.1), especially when those sounds start words. Older children with articulation problems usually misarticulate sounds from only one or two phones. The most frequently misarticulated sounds are /s/ and /r/.

The Templin-Darley Tests include a screening test, a diagnostic test, tests for particular sounds, such as /r/ and /s/, the Iowa Pressure Test, and other tests. Each test has age norms. The screening and diagnostic tests sample phones from many phonemes as they initiate and terminate words. The /s/ and /r/ sub-tests of the Templin-Darley Tests sample phones from those phonemes as they appear in many contexts. The Iowa Pressure Articulation Test is used to evaluate the adequacy of velopharyngeal closure for speech. It samples the articulation of consonants with high oral breath-pressure requirements. Persons with velopharyngeal closure deficits have been found to do poorly on this test, and it was, of course, designed to identify such persons. Nevertheless, errors on the articulation items may be made for reasons other than poor closure.

Many other articulation tests are available. The Goldman-Fristoe Test of Articulation (1969) samples the examinee's articulation in story-telling activities as well as in words and syllables. Comparison of performance under these different speaking conditions provides information about the consistency and therefore the severity of any misarticulation that is present. Differences in performance across the conditions can help the clinician to decide on activities to employ in remedial work.

McDonald (1964b) developed articulation tests which sample articulation of phones from a given phoneme as they occur in many phonetic contexts; that is, as they are preceded and followed by various consonants and vowels. Use of these tests enables the examiner to determine how consistently a client misarticulates a given sound. Phonetic contexts may be identified in which a given sound is articulated correctly. This information may be utilized in remediation so that a client may be helped to generalize from contexts in which a sound is correctly articulated to other contexts wherein it is misarticulated. McDonald's articulation tests are called "deep tests" because of the frequency with which phones from a given phoneme are examined.

Other procedures that the speech pathologist may use in evaluating disordered articulation include scaling of articulation adequacy, testing speech intelligibility, and phonological analysis. In scaling, the examiner listens to the child's speech and assigns a number—perhaps from 1 to 7—reflecting the severity of any disorder present. The number "1" would reflect normal articulation, "7" severely disordered articulation. These numbers provide an index to severity of misarticulation. Intelligibility testing involves recording the speaker's words or other units and playing the tape to judges. Intelligibility is defined in terms of the number or percentage of spoken units that were understood by the judges. Phonological analysis requires that the examiner prepare a phonetic transcription of lengthy speech samples and then process the transcription to identify linguistic patterns. Here, in contrast to articulation tests, every phone that the speaker utters must be transcribed. This task is much more time consuming than articulation testing; however, it may contribute to the discovery of rules that describe a child's articulation pattern. This represents the clinical application of a method used by linguists to study the speech of normal individuals who use different languages. Fisher and Logemann (1971) have devised a test for studying articulation that retains the convenience of articulation testing while providing some of the information that would be obtained through phonological analysis.

Speech sounds are frequently considered as bundles of **distinctive features** which may be described in physiological or acoustical terms. Physiological features pertain to placement of the articulators; for example, a sound may be classified as high or low depending on tongue position. Acoustical features involve such variables as presence or absence of voicing or nasalization. McReynolds and Engmann (1975) devised a method for organizing articulation test data in terms of the distinctive features found in a child's misarticulated sounds. If a child misarticulates sounds from several phonemes, a clinician might choose to train one or two phonemes that contain a feature that is present in several misarticulated phonemes. This can result in a generalization process whereby improvement is made not only for the phonemes that are taught, but also for other phonemes that share a feature or features with the phonemes taught.

Prognosis

The speech pathologist will want to predict future articulation performance by the person found to have an articulation problem. The evaluation process is reliable in the sense that different clinicians making independent observations tend to agree with one another about classification of disorders and identification of individuals in need of remedial service. However, clinicians frequently do not attempt to make very precise predictions about the future status of clients' articulation. Treatment decisions, therefore, are more likely to be based on theoretical viewpoint than on data-based predictions about how the individual's speech will develop either with or without remediation.

In making a predictive (prognostic) statement, the clinician will consider changes that may be anticipated. An individual whose articulation problem was caused by serious biological defect may be unable to improve his or her speech, regardless of the services received. The speech pathologist seeks to use evaluation information to identify discrepancies between how the individual talks and how he or she is capable of talking. To do this, the clinician is likely to compare a client's articulation of sounds from a given phoneme as they are elicited by different methods. For example, the clinician may be interested in articulation of a sound as it is produced in a word imitated after an examiner, as it is used spontaneously as the speaker names pictures, and as it is used in conversation as the speaker recounts an experience or tells a story. If a person is not observed to produce a sound correctly in words regardless of the stimulus condition, the speech pathologist may be interested in whether the individual can imitate the isolated sound or the sound in syllable context. Some individuals are so responsive to evaluation stimuli that the clinician will conclude that they are likely to improve their speech without remedial training. This often occurs in young children who misarticulate but who are free from biological deficits.

Many variables have been studied to determine whether they would be useful in the prediction of articulation improvement. Characteristics of articulation itself provide the best basis for prediction (Winitz, 1969). Persons with articulation problems are considered to be good candidates for improvement if their imitation of speech sounds is superior to their spontaneous articulation and if their articulation errors are inconsistent; that is, if sounds that are misarticulated are sometimes used correctly. A client's responsiveness to treatment during early lessons can also provide information predictive of future success in articulation training (Arndt, Shelton, and Elbert, 1971). Van Riper and Erickson (1975) developed a test for use by school speech clinicians to identify first-grade children who are unlikely to correct their articulation problems spontaneously.

Nonarticulatory variables, e.g., intelligence and socioeconomic status, have not proved to be good predictors of articulation change (Winitz, Chapter 3, 1969). Age, however, is an important variable. Lenneberg (1967) developed a hypothesis that a person's critical period for speech and language development exists and extends from about age 18 months to puberty. This hypothesis implies that speech and language disorders should be relatively difficult to correct beyond puberty. Indeed, treatment of functional articulation problems is often scheduled when children are in second or third grade, and many clinicians recommend training for preschool children. Little spontaneous articulation improvement is observed in children beyond the fourth-grade level (Powers, 1971), and clinical experience indicates that articulation change with therapy often is difficult with adults. Again, **stimulability,** or the ability to produce better articulation on an imitative basis, is an important predictor. Motivation to change articulation is especially important for adults who present long-standing articulation disorders. They must be ready to work actively and hard at improvement and to accept and use changes that are made. A willingness to have one's speech changed by the clinician is not sufficient. Rather, the client—especially the adult—must understand that improvement is dependent on his or her active efforts to improve speech.

Speech remediation should be directed to those who need it to improve and who can profit from it. In working with young children, the clinician may place special emphasis on individuals whose speech intelligibility is poor or who are embarrassed by their articulation errors. If a client appears to have a good prognosis for spontaneous articulation improvement and if the articulation problem is not a source of great distress, the speech pathologist may decide not to schedule the child for treatment, but rather to retest in a period of a few months. If the child makes the anticipated improvement, the clinician will retest again at a later period. This process will continue until articulation is no longer a problem. If, however, a child is scheduled for remedial work, the clinician will observe progress during early lessons in order to estimate future improvement with treatment.

The Evaluation Report

The evaluation report (see the evaluation report at the end of this chapter) serves as a record of information gathered during the evaluation process, and it should function as a tool in the planning of remedial services when they are required. A speech evaluation report should summarize (1) the problem of concern to the client, (2) history plus reports from other professionals, (3) the examiner's observations, and (4) findings from the various tests administered. The report should indicate whether the client's articulation was found to be disordered, and if so, a description of the articulation observed should be included. The examiner might attempt to infer the etiology of the problem, to predict future articulation behavior, and to make specific recommendations regarding speech training if needed. Impressions and decisions about these matters will be reconsidered frequently during the course of remediation; and as the evaluation report presented at the end of the chapter shows, the evaluation process continues during remedial sessions.

The evaluation report is of especial use to the clinician who will work with a client. However, it is also used to convey information to other professionals. Sometimes a separate report is prepared to communicate as concisely as possible with other professional workers (Pannbacker, 1975). The clinician must also communicate findings and recommendations to the client, the parents, or both. This is usually done orally, and the skilled clinician is cognizant of the conditions and time required to communicate clinical information effectively.

Remediation

The term "speech therapy" has no single meaning. Therapy for misarticulation involves a diversity of procedures. Persons who hold to different theoretical viewpoints may approach management of a given articulation problem in quite different ways. At one time, persons who taught courses about disordered articulation left it to their students to devise methods of treatment congruent with information about the nature of the disorder and its etiology. This approach to treatment was based on the assumption that the practitioner would apply knowledge learned from the study in various fields, including child development, mental hygiene, and the psychology of learning. Later, some writers began to outline treatment plans in great detail. Sometimes those plans were compatible with one or another theoretical viewpoint. Other writers presented barrages of treatments, presumably on the assumption that one or another should work and that the clinician would eventually find the right one. Often the same treatments are used whether the articulation disorder is organic or functional. The clinician's efforts may be directed to the elimination or correction of problems that are thought to cause or maintain the articulation disorder, or the clinician may undertake direct modification of articulation behavior. Combinations of these two treatment approaches may also be used.

Treatment of Conditions Underlying Disordered Articulation

If a physical deficit is maintaining an articulation disorder, it should be corrected if possible. In the management of persons with cleft palate, there is essentially universal agreement that development of good speech is dependent on treatment of the palatal defect. Speech will be less than normal until the individual is provided with a speech mechanism that can prevent unwanted escape of air through the nose, and articulation correction will be more efficient if it follows physical treatment of the palate defect.

If a physical condition exists that is not correctable, the speech pathologist must select training goals that are within the potential of the client. A physical condition may so restrict prognosis for speech remediation that treatment is not warranted. If a trial period of treatment is instituted, the time may arrive when the clinician must terminate treatment because of lack of progress. It should be noted, however, that a trial period is structured as a search for information and can end on a note of success even if the target behavior is not achieved.

Some treatments are directed to underlying causes that cannot be observed or measured, but which are inferred on the basis of a hypothesis accepted by the clinician. For example, some clinicians use tongue exercises with articulation clients on the assumption that those exercises will correct possible muscular problems or will increase readiness for learning articulation skills. Such procedures should not be used in the absence of evidence that they increase the efficiency or effectiveness of articulation remediation. Attempts have been made to increase the adequacy of velopharyngeal closure through therapeutic exercise. This work has included movement of muscles against resistance to develop strength (Cole, 1971). Unfortunately, research has not demonstrated that these methods result in appropriate closure during connected speech. As was mentioned earlier, it should be possible to improve the skill with which velopharyngeal muscles are used, and research directed to that goal is continuing.

Therapeutic exercise may be of value to some persons with neurologically based articulation disorders. We observed a patient who suffered brain damage that interfered with his respiratory movements. Physical therapy that improved his respiratory function appeared to contribute directly to his speech. Mysak's (1963) program for speech habilitation in children with cerebral palsy emphasizes procedures directed to posture, reflexes, and other variables important to speech.

Some clinicians seek to identify deficits in psycholinguistic skills that may underlie articulation defects. Deficient speech-sound discrimination may be classified as such a defect. Auditory perceptual training is often applied in treatment of disordered articulation. In Van Riper's (1963) system of articulation remediation, ear training precedes any attempt at sound production. The ear training is intended to teach speakers to listen to speech sounds, discriminate among those sounds, and differentiate between correct and incorrect sound productions. The explicitness with which Van Riper's treatments were described anticipated the development of step-by-step treatment programs that have been developed in recent years.

The popularity of ear training may have resulted in part because it is readily adaptable to training directed to groups of clients. Listening activities are convenient in group work because all children present can be involved in the activity. If emphasis is placed on sound-production work for groups of children, only one person can respond at a time, or the clinician cannot evaluate the responses and inform the speakers about the adequacy of their responses. Successful use of ear training probably requires active listening on the part of the client. Clinician manipulation of auditory and visual cues may be of no value unless the client's attention is directed to those cues; that is, the learner probably should respond to the stimuli with problem-solving behavior (Winitz, 1975).

Ear-training emphasis has been criticized because it led to the practice of bombarding children with speech in a situation emphasizing participation in games rather than working directly on the speech problem (Mowrer, 1970). Clinicians who teach clients to discriminate between grossly different sounds (perhaps vacuum cleaners and barking dogs) or even between correctly and incorrectly articulated words (as produced by the clinician) should be careful that they are not spending their time in teaching discriminations already available to the client. Poor performance on a discrimination task may reflect failure to understand the task rather than failure of discrimination. Backus and Beasley (1951) observed that the important discriminations are those wherein the client discriminates between his or her own correct and incorrect responses, and they also observed that those self-discriminations are dependent on production. Williams and McReynolds (1975) showed that under some circumstances discrimination training does not influence articulation.

In recent years, speech clinicians have reduced use of ear training in favor of articulation training methods that stress speech production. However, perceptual processes involved in acquisition of language by the infant is a topic of current research and may influence speech training in the future. Although we do not consider ear training to be a prerequisite to production training, we do at times consider its use as a supplement to production procedures.

Direct Articulation Training

At some point in therapy, the clinician is likely to attempt direct change of a client's articulation. This may follow attention to causative and maintaining factors, including auditory perceptual deficits, or it may be the first step in therapy.

McDonald's (1964) sensory-motor approach to articulation remediation contributed to a shift in emphasis from ear training to sound-production training. The sensory aspect of this work utilizes kinesthetic and **touch-pressure** sensations as well as audition. Use of kinesthetic and touch-pressure feedback requires the client to sense the movements, positions, and contacts of his or her articulators while producing sounds. Work on the motor level is intended to facilitate correct use of the target sound in a variety of phonetic contexts. Treatment is planned with consideration of the overlapping movements that are involved in speech production.

The term "overlapping" refers to the fact that neighboring sounds that we think of as occurring sequentially actually involve movements of the articulators that occur simultaneously. The term **coarticulation** is now used rather than "overlapping," and coarticulation has been studied extensively. For example, in studying the effect of sounds on preceding and succeeding sounds, investigators have found that the articulation of one sound may be influenced by neighboring sounds even when they are separated by syllable and word boundaries (see Chapter 3). If an individual is to practice a target sound in word and sentence units, units should be chosen so that the child learns to blend or coarticulate the target sound with a variety of neighboring sounds (Shriner, Holloway, and Daniloff, 1969; Winitz, 1975). Choice of facilitating contexts early in training may make a small contribution to the generalization process.

The shift in emphasis from listening training to sound-production training has also been influenced by the work of psychologists concerned with the modification of behavior through operant conditioning (McReynolds, 1970; Bankson, 1974). The procedures used require careful manipulation of **reinforcement** techniques and of stimuli which serve to elicit the behavior of interest. Research has demonstrated the efficacy of this methodology in modifying many kinds of behavior, and the methodology is readily adapted to articulation treatment because articulation behavior is fairly easily observed.* As a result of operant conditioning research, many speech pathologists contend that articulation remediation requires a high rate of speech-production practice and that during practice most of the utterances the child produces should involve correct articulation of the sound being learned.

---

* Speech clinicians do make errors in evaluating articulation responses, and there is some evidence that listening to repetitions of the same sound is associated with shifts in the clinician's perception of the adequacy of the sounds produced (Shelton, Johnson, and Arndt, 1974).

The operant influence on articulation training has led to the development of programs to guide articulation remediation step by step. Persons advocating the use of programed materials (Costello, 1977) report that carefully programed sequences of speech production can result in articulation correction in much shorter periods of time than are required by more traditional methods. Treatment claims must be assessed (Gerber, 1977), but some data supportive of the use of some articulation programs are available. One of the first articulation programs written, the /s/ Pac, was developed by Mowrer, Baker, and Schutz (1968) to correct interdental lisps. Another program example is provided by Irwin and Griffith (1973), who tested a procedure to encourage generalization from key words in which the target sound is produced correctly to other words in which the sound is misarticulated. This procedure, which is termed "paired stimulus training," requires the client to name a key word, then a training word, key word, training word until ten training words have been produced. Each correct response is rewarded by administration of a token that has redemption value known to the learner.

Other programs have been developed, including those by Gerber (1973), Carrier (1970), and Shriberg (1975). A program described by McLean (1970) further illustrates the importance of effective use of stimuli in articulation remediation. In McLean's stimulus-shift procedure, children are taught to produce the target sound correctly in a set of words under different stimulus conditions. The children are shifted from one stimulus condition to another, contingent on achievement of a performance criterion. In work of this kind words containing a target sound are first presented under stimulus conditions most likely to result in correct responses. For example, a child might be asked to watch and listen as the clinician produces a word to be imitated. As the child is successful in imitation, the clinician shifts to use of stimuli that initially would have had a lower likelihood of resulting in correct articulations. A written passage containing the target words is an example of a stimulus condition that might be used later in training. The clinician gradually shifts to stimuli resembling conditions of spontaneous speech.

This section was introduced in terms of a change in clinical emphasis from auditory discrimination training to sound-production training. However, it may now be evident that discrimination between correct and incorrect responses is taught simultaneously with sound production. If a person is asked to produce responses under different stimulus conditions and if he or she is rewarded for correct responses but not for incorrect responses, discrimination is taught as well as production.

Clinical procedures based on operant conditioning are not universally accepted, and they have not solved all clinical problems that arise in articulation remediation. Operant conditioning involves clinician control of the client's behavior through manipulation of stimuli and administration of rewards for correct responses; the child's role in the process is relatively passive. Recently,

198

Winitz (1975) has advocated use of listening procedures in articulation training, at least when the production of a target sound is available to the child. Although Winitz utilized conditioning procedures in the training he recommends, he also places emphasis on involving the child in active conceptual and problem-solving tasks. This viewpoint appears to move the clinician full circle to use of activities that were set aside with operant emphasis on production. However, perhaps the result will be a better amalgam of listening and production training.

Much articulation training is conducted on a group-therapy basis, yet relatively little research has been conducted investigating techniques useful in group research. McDonald (1964a) has discussed means whereby his sensory-motor procedures can be used in group remedial work, and Sommers (1976) has pointed out that group dynamics can be employed to assist groups in solving their articulation problems. Group work should not involve individuals' taking turns, but rather establishment of camaraderie and skilled direction of that good fellowship to the resolution of group members' articulation problems. The use of group dynamics and operant conditioning may be divergent practices.

Articulation remediation can be viewed as involving several steps which are compatible with knowledge concerning acquisition and **automatization** of motor behaviors (Wright, Shelton, and Arndt, 1969). If the individual misarticulates sounds from many phonemes, the distinctive features of the sounds misarticulated should be considered in treatment plans in order to facilitate generalization from the sound or sounds taught to untaught sounds (McReynolds and Engmann, 1975). If an analysis of the client's speech indicates that he or she cannot produce a target sound correctly, a decision may be made to teach production of the sound in isolation from context. If so, the clinician has access to numerous textbook descriptions of how the articulators are used in the production of various sounds. Auditory stimulation may be combined with visual cues and directions concerning proper articulatory placements, close approximations of a target sound may be accepted for a period of time, and satisfactory responses will be rewarded. Or, a first goal may be to teach the client to produce the sound correctly in a set of words. If the client already uses the sound correctly in some words, the number of those words may be extended with training.

After the client has been taught to produce the sound in selected words under one set of stimulus conditions, different stimulus conditions will be employed (imitation, picture naming, conversation, and others). The clinician may give the client information about the correctness of target sounds produced in connected speech as the client reads or talks. A conversation may be recorded and the tape recording stopped and played back when a sound of particular interest is articulated. These techniques are intended to facilitate the automatization of correct responses. The goal of remediation is to establish consistently correct use of phones from all phonemes in spontaneous speech. A method that teaches the client to produce a sound correctly in a set of words cannot stand by itself unless it results in correct use of the sound in the client's spontaneous conversation.

At some point in therapy, perhaps before many correct responses have been elicited, techniques will be used to encourage correct use of the target sound in conversation outside the clinic setting. The parents may be asked to aid the clinician's work by monitoring the child's conversation at home. Parents who appear able to work positively with their children can be given training in the recognition of speech sounds and in judging the correctness of their articulation. They can be asked to keep track of a given number of productions of the target sound each day and to indicate how many were correctly articulated. They would give a reward for correct responses, but ask the child to repeat misarticulated sounds correctly from imitation. All parents aren't prepared to participate in this work, and the clinician may choose to train an aide to serve as an assistant. Sometimes children's classmates have been trained to help. Also, a clinician can conduct work of this kind with groups of misarticulating children. Increasing use is now being made of parents, volunteers, or paid aides in the conduct of corrective procedures planned and supervised by the speech pathologist.

Many clinicians make detailed assessment of articulation learning of at least some of their clients. This helps clinicians to evaluate the services they provide. They may do this by tabulating and plotting the number of practice items that are produced correctly from day to day. They may also sample untaught items for evidence of generalization from training. To determine whether the client is establishing automatic use of the target sound, the clinician will sample use of that sound in spontaneous conversation and in reading. Again, the results will be plotted (Diedrich, 1973). Figure 8.4 illustrates generalization and automatization plots.

Whatever services are provided, the client's active cooperation is required. Johnson's (1956) discussion of the clinical point of view in education is pertinent here. That viewpoint emphasizes that each child is a worthy individual deserving of respect and treatment that is courteous and suitable to his or her needs. Hahn (1961) recommended that the nature of the services provided be related to the child's adjustment and communicative behaviors. Thus the well-adjusted child who misarticulates would be given direct articulation training. A noncommunicative child would be given indirect articulation help; for example, communication would be encouraged through play with toys, and attention to articulation would be worked into the play. A child with psychological problems would be referred for suitable evaluation and treatment. Whatever techniques of treatment are used, a good relationship between clinician and client will be satisfying to each.

Conclusion

Speech pathologists have learned a great deal about articulation disorders. The disorders are well described, and they are reasonably well understood in terms of related variables. Articulation behaviors can be classified with some accuracy,

Figure 8.4

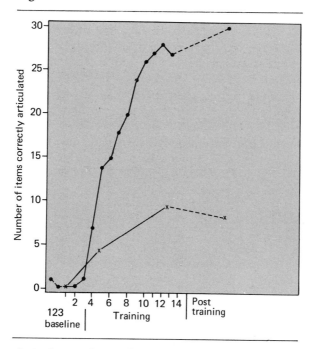

Articulation data collected from a child undergoing correction of the /r/ sound. Data are reported from a sound-production task (SPT) that
sampled /r/ in 30 items imitated after an examiner and also from assessment of 30 /r/ phones as
they appeared in the child's connected speech.
None of the SPT items were directly taught in
training; consequently, improved performance on
that measure presumably reflects generalization
from the training that was provided. These data
indicate that SPT performance improved dramatically during a few lessons that followed pretreat-
ment, baseline testing. Less marked improvement
was observed in the connected speech measure.
Future training for this child would be directed to
activities that would increase correct use of the
target sound in conversation. (Adapted from
V. A. Wright, "Comparison of Imitative and
Spontaneous Speech Samples in the Evaluation of
Articulation Change with Therapy," M.A. thesis,
1969. Data reprinted by permission of the author.)

and treatment methods are very effective with several classes of clients, especially those with palatal defects and those free from serious physical disability. Since articulation errors are often overcome, some persons have a tendency to deprecate the importance of articulation remediation. Nevertheless, most people prefer to speak without articulation errors, and investigators are continuing to strive for improved understanding and control of articulation disorders. Speech pathologists use findings from physical, physiological, and behavioral specialists in their clinical and research endeavors. Currently, interest is especially strong in the application of linguistic information to the study of articulation disorders. Clinical advancements continue to be dependent on speech-pathology research directed to the observation, description, and manipulation of articulation.

Evaluation Report

The following report, taken from a speech clinic file, reflects the collection and use of information in the speech evaluation.

Speech Evaluation Report

Name: Abe	Date of evaluation:
Address:	Date of birth:
Telephone:	Age at evaluation: 4 years, 7 months
Parents:	Referred by: Parent

Statement of the problem   Abe's mother stated that Abe's speech was often unintelligible to her and neighborhood children and he did not use certain sounds including /r/, /l/, /θ/, and /ð/. She was also concerned about his sentence structure.

History   Abe sat at six months and walked at twelve months; however, he did not produce his first word until he was sixteen months of age. The family physician reported that the boy was free from organic abnormality. The boy's father is a professional man, and the mother has a graduate degree. An older brother received articulation remediation between the ages of 4½ and 5½ years.

Behavioral observations   Abe was an attractive and energetic youngster. He stayed alone with the clinician in the clinic room and eagerly attempted all tasks. He was curious about the toys and objects in the room and cooperated well with the clinician.

Tests   Several types of tests were used to evaluate Abe's speech.

Language. On the Peabody Picture Vocabulary Test, Abe received a **standard score** of 119. The norm for this test is 100, with a standard deviation of 15. Abe's conversational language was characterized by sentences seven to ten words in length. He made 20 correct responses on the receptive portion of the Northwestern Syntax Screening Test and 25 correct responses on the expressive portion. He was in the 10th percentile receptively and the 50th percentile expressively. Disagreement between pronouns and verbs and other syntactical errors were evident in the boy's spontaneous speech. He understood and responded appropriately to speech directed to him. His grammar was sufficient to convey his meaning to a listener; however, poor intelligibility sometimes prevented the clinician from understanding Abe's speech.

Hearing. Pure-tone screening was done at 20 dB for the frequencies 250, 500, 1000, 2000, 4000, and 8000 Hz bilaterally. Functional hearing sensitivity was within normal limits bilaterally, but Abe failed to respond to the 4000 Hz tone at 20 dB in the right ear.*

Articulation. Abe's score on the Templin-Darley Screening Test of Articulation was 20. The norm for boys his age is 37, with a standard deviation of 10. Most of his errors were substitutions: ʌ/ɝ, f/θ, w/r, w/l, ʃ/tʃ, b/v, s/z, and d/ð. Abe was stimulable for the /θ/ and /ð/ sounds in isolation and initial and final positions of nonsense syllables.

Summary and recommendations Abe's articulation development was inadequate for a person his age, and his conversational speech was often unintelligible. His scores on the receptive syntax screening indicated he was below the norm for boys his age. Because of these problems, it was recommended that Abe begin articulation and language remediation. His mother stated that she wanted to attempt to get Abe's speech difficulties corrected before he started school the following year.†

---

* Later testing by an audiologist indicated that the boy had a 10–15 dB air-bone gap in his right ear (see Chapter 13). He was referred to an otologist for further evaluation and any treatment needed. The nature of the hearing loss did not explain the articulation and syntax differences described in the report.
† During the early clinic sessions, the boy's articulation was tested in greater depth. It was learned that most of his errors were consistent. Correct production of /ɝ/ (errr) was not achieved even when the sound was presented repeatedly to the boy. He was able to imitate /l/ and /v/ after an examiner. Additional information indicated that the boy was well above average in intelligence and that his language problem was restricted to a small set of syntactical errors. A treatment program was planned and conducted, and Abe's articulation and syntactical problems were cleared with training that was administered over a period of about one year.

Glossary

Apraxia of speech: Inability to make voluntary speech movements even though involuntary movements of the articulators may occur normally. The disorder reflects neurological impairment of the portion of the brain that programs sequences of speech movement, but muscle weakness and spasticity are not involved. Dyspraxia is a less severe form of the same disorder.

Automatization: Development of a learned motor performance to the point where it is skillfully executed without conscious effort.

Cerebral palsy: A neuromuscular disability including weakness, paralysis, or incoordination. This disorder, which results from brain damage prior to, during, or shortly after birth, may involve different portions of the body, including the speech mechanism. Varieties of cerebral palsy marked by distinctive motor impairments are athetosis, spasticity, and rigidity.

Cleft palate: A fissure, or opening, in the roof of the mouth. The opening may involve the soft palate, the hard palate, or both. It may be accompanied by a cleft of the lip.

Coarticulation: The phenomenon whereby the speech mechanism moves simultaneously in the production of speech sounds that are perceived sequentially. For example, in the word "construe," the lips may begin to move toward the /u/ configuration at the same time that other articulators are producing the /n/ sound (Daniloff and Moll, 1968).

Continuant consonants: Phones that are relatively long in duration. Included are fricatives, such as /s/ and /ʃ/, which are produced by the friction of the airstream passing through a narrow orifice, and resonants, such as /n/ and /r/, which involve modification of the laryngeal tone by placement of the articulators.

Dialect: A language usage employed by a group of speakers who are separated from the larger community. A dialect may be characterized by nonstandard articulation, grammar, vocabulary, and rhythm or prosody.

Distinctive features: Physiological and associated acoustical events that distinguish phones of one phoneme from those of another.

Dysarthria: Neurologically based disorder of articulation and sometimes also phonation, prosody, and respiratory function for speech. Performance of both voluntary and involuntary movements is consistently impaired.

Endoscope: An optical instrument equipped with a light and lens. It is used for visual examination of interior portions of the body, including the velopharyngeal closure mechanism and the larynx.

204

Etiology: The cause of a condition or behavior.

Glossectomy: Surgical removal of the tongue. Partial glossectomy is the removal of a portion of the tongue.

Intelligibility: Being understandable to a listener. Intelligibility may be measured by presenting a sample of a person's speech to a panel of listeners.

Kinesthesis: Sense of the position and movement of bodily structures, including the articulators.

Normative data: Quantitative information about the performance of a group of persons on a given measure. Typically data are gathered for groups of normal children of different ages.

Phone: A speech sound; any consonant or vowel. Any sound produced with the speech mechanism may be classified as a phone, even if it is not used to differentiate between words in a given language.

Phoneme: A set or class of speech sounds or phones. Phones may differ from one another moderately and still be members of the same phoneme. However, use of a phone from one phoneme, such as /ʃ/, in place of a member of another phoneme such as /s/ will constitute an articulation error and may change the meaning of an utterance. Sometimes "phoneme" is used synonymously with "speech sound" or "phone."

Prosody: Intonation and stress patterns of an utterance.

Prosthetic speech appliance: An acrylic device fitted to the patient to fill or obturate a palatal cleft, to support a soft palate that moves little or not at all, or to fill space between a short or immobile palate and the pharyngeal walls.

Prosthodontist: A dentist who provides prosthetic aids including dentures, prosthetic speech appliances, and appliances to replace oral-facial tissue removed in the treatment of cancer.

Reinforcement: Influencing the frequency of occurrence of a response by dispensing something valued by the learner.

Secondary palatal surgery: Initial palatal surgery brings tissue together to close a cleft. The palate may also be moved surgically to position it closer to the pharyngeal wall. If initial surgery does not provide adequate velopharyngeal closure for speech, a secondary procedure may be performed. One such procedure is the pharyngeal flap, wherein tissue from the posterior wall of the pharynx is attached to the middle portion of the soft palate.

Standard score: A test score that may be interpreted in terms of location within a normal distribution. For a distribution with a mean of 100 and a standard deviation of 15, standard scores of 85 and 115 would fall as shown on the bell-shaped curve below.

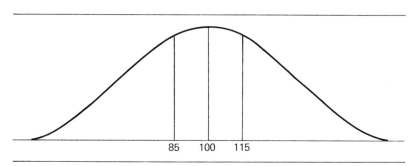

Stimulability: A client's ability to articulate correctly through imitation of a model sounds that he or she usually misarticulates in spontaneous speech.

Stop consonants: Phones produced by the interruption and release of the breath stream, e.g., /p/ and /g/.

Tactile: Feedback process involving contact of bodily structures. Tactile neural signals do not reach conscious awareness and should be contrasted with touch-pressure feedback.

Tongue thrust: One or more of the following performances: (1) displacement of the tongue between the anterior teeth and against the lower lip during the initiation phase of swallow; (2) depression of the mandible and fronting the tongue between or against the anterior teeth during speech; and (3) depression of the mandible and forward tongue position so that the tongue tip is between or against the anterior teeth at rest (Mason and Proffit, 1974).

Touch-pressure: Contact involving bodily structures; it stimulates conscious awareness (Hardy, 1970).

Velum: Soft palate.

Study Questions

1. Articulation errors may be classified as substitutions, omissions, distortions, and additions. Describe each type of error.
2. Articulation disorders associated with organic conditions were discussed in terms of two categories. What are they?
3. When is an organic condition thought to have caused an articulation problem?
4. In what ways does poor velopharyngeal closure interfere with articulation?
5. List professional specialties likely to be represented on the team for a person with cleft palate.

6. What speech parameters may be involved in dysarthria?
7. What is a functional articulation problem?
8. Children who misarticulate are thought to present a high incidence of language disorders. What theoretical viewpoint postulates this relationship?
9. If unable to identify the cause of an articulation problem, what course of action is a speech pathologist likely to follow?
10. Why do we think that no one phenomenon causes all articulation problems?
11. What is the purpose of an articulation screening test?
12. List the aspects of articulation testing.
13. What purpose is served by articulation deep tests?
14. Discuss the examination of the speech mechanism as a part of an articulation evaluation.
15. In what way may distinctive features be used to encourage generalization in articulation treatment?
16. If articulation is better under some stimulus conditions than others, the prognosis for articulation improvement is probably good. What stimulus conditions are used in articulation testing to establish prognosis?
17. A child with a favorable prognosis for spontaneous correction of an articulation problem may not be scheduled for remediation, but rather retested from time to time. What is gained by this process?
18. Articulation remediation focusing on motor speech responses was described as involving several steps. What are they?
19. In articulation treatment what arrangement of stimulus conditions may be used to establish correct articulation in spontaneous conversation?
20. What purpose is served when a clinician utilizes articulation tests and observations to evaluate a client's response to treatment?

Bibliography

ARNDT, W. B., R. L. SHELTON, AND M. ELBERT, "Prediction of Articulation Improvement with Therapy from Early Lesson Sound Production Task Scores," *J. Speech Hearing Res.* 14 (1971):149–153.

ARNDT, W. B., R. L. SHELTON, A. F. JOHNSON, AND M. L. FURR, "Identification and Description of Homogeneous Subgroups within a Sample of Misarticulating Children," *J. Speech Hearing Res.* (1977).

BACKUS, O., AND J. BEASLEY, *Speech Therapy with Children*, Boston: Houghton Mifflin, 1951.

BANKSON, N. W., "Assessment of the Effectiveness of Articulation Therapy," *J. National Student Speech Hearing Assoc.* 2 (1974):13–21.

BOSMA, J. F., ed., *A Second Symposium on Oral Sensation and Perception*, Springfield, Ill.: Charles C Thomas, 1970.

CARRIER, J. K., "A Program of Articulation Therapy Administered by Mothers," *J. Speech Hearing Dis.* **35** (1970):344–353.

COLE, R. M., "Direct Muscle Training for the Improvement of Velopharyngeal Function," in W. C. Grabb, S. W. Rosenstein, and K. R. Bzoch, eds., *Cleft Lip and Palate*, Boston: Little, Brown, 1971.

COSTELLO, J., "Programmed Instruction," *J. Speech Hearing Dis.* **42** (1977):3–28.

CUTTING, J. E., AND J. F. KAVANAGH, "On the Relationship of Speech to Language," *Asha* **17** (1975):500–506.

DANILOFF, R. G., AND K. L. MOLL, "Coarticulation of Lip Rounding," *J. Speech Hearing Res.* **11** (1968):707–721.

DARLEY, F. L., A. E. ARONSON, AND J. R. BROWN, "Differential Patterns of Dysarthria," *J. Speech Hearing Res.* **12** (1969):246–269.

———, *Motor Speech Disorders*, Philadelphia: Saunders, 1975.

DIEDRICH, W. M., *Charting Speech Behavior*, Lawrence: University of Kansas, Extramural Independent Study Center, 1973.

FISHER, H. B., AND M. A. LOGEMANN, *The Fisher-Logemann Test of Articulation Competence*, Boston: Houghton Mifflin, 1971.

FLETCHER, S. G., "Time-by-Count Measurement of Diadochokinetic Syllable Rate," *J. Speech Hearing Res.* **15** (1972):763–770.

GERBER, A., *Goal: Carryover*, Philadelphia: Temple University Press, 1973.

———, "Programming for Articulation Modification," *J. Speech Hearing Dis.* **42** (1977):29–43.

GOLDMAN, R., AND M. FRISTOE, *Test of Articulation*, Circle Pines, Minn.: American Guidance Service, 1969.

HAHN, E., "Indications for Direct, Nondirect, and Indirect Methods in Speech Correction," *J. Speech Hearing Dis.* **26** (1961):230–236.

HANSON, M. L., "Tongue Thrust: Another Point of View," *J. Speech Hearing Dis.* **41** (1976):172–184.

HARDY, J. C., "Development of Neuromuscular Systems underlying Speech Production," in J. E. Fricke and R. T. Wertz, eds., *ASHA Report*, Number 5, Washington, D.C.: American Speech and Hearing Association, 1970.

IRWIN, J. V., "Speech Pathology and Behavior Modification," *Acta Symbolica* **1** (1970):15–23.

———, "The Triota: A Computerized Screening Battery," *Acta Symbolica* **3** (1972):26–38.

IRWIN, J. V., AND F. A. GRIFFITH, "A Theoretical and Operational Analysis of the Paired-Stimuli Technique," in W. D. Wolfe, and D. Goulding, eds., *Learning and Articulation: A Symposium*, Springfield, Ill.: Charles C Thomas, 1973.

JOHNS, D. F., AND F. L. DARLEY, "Phonemic Variability in Apraxia of Speech," *J. Speech Hearing Res.* **13** (1970):556–583.

208

JOHNSON, W., "The Clinical Point of View in Education," in W. Johnson, *et al.*, eds., *Speech Handicapped School Children*, rev. ed., New York: Harper and Brothers, 1956.

JOINT COMMITTEE ON DENTISTRY AND SPEECH PATHOLOGY-AUDIOLOGY, "Position Statement of Tongue Thrust," *Asha* **17** (1975):331–337.

LAPOINTE, L. L., "Neurologic Abnormalities Affecting Speech," in D. B. Tower, Editor-in-Chief, *The Nervous System*, Vol. 3, ed. E. L. Eagles, *Human Communication and Its Disorders*, New York: Raven Press, 1975.

LENNEBERG, E. H., *Biological Foundations of Language*, New York: Wiley, 1967.

MCDONALD, E. T., *Articulation Testing and Treatment: A Sensory-Motor Approach*, Pittsburgh: Stanwix House, 1964a.

————, *A Deep Test of Articulation*, Pittsburgh: Stanwix House, 1964b.

MCGLONE, R. E., AND W. R. PROFFIT, "Patterns of Tongue Contact in Normal and Lisping Speakers," *J. Speech Hearing Res.* **16** (1973):456–473.

MCLEAN, J. E., "Extending Stimulus Control of Phoneme Articulation by Operant Techniques," in F. L. Girardeau and J. E. Spradlin, eds., *A Functional Analysis Approach to Speech and Language*, Washington, D.C.: ASHA Monographs, Number 14, American Speech and Hearing Association, 1970.

MCREYNOLDS, L. V., "Contingencies and Consequences in Speech Therapy," *J. Speech Hearing Dis.* **35** (1970):12–24.

MCREYNOLDS, L. V., AND D. L. ENGMANN, *Distinctive Feature Analysis of Misarticulations*, Baltimore: University Park Press, 1975.

MCREYNOLDS, L. V., J. KOHN, AND G. C. WILLIAMS, "Articulatory-Defective Children's Discrimination of their Production Errors," *J. Speech Hearing Dis.* **40** (1975):327–338.

MCWILLIAMS, B. J., AND R. T. WERTZ, "Speech, Language, and Psychosocial Aspects of Cleft Lip and Cleft Palate: The State of the Art," *ASHA Report*, Number 9, Washington, D.C.: American Speech and Hearing Association, 1973.

MARTIN, A. D., "Some Objections to the Term *Apraxia of Speech*," *J. Speech Hearing Dis.* **39** (1974):53–64.

MASON, R. H., AND W. R. PROFFIT, "The Tongue Thrust Controversy: Background and Recommendations," *J. Speech Hearing Dis.* **39** (1974):115–132.

MOWRER, D. E., "An Analysis of Motivational Techniques used in Speech Therapy," *Asha* **12** (1970):491–493.

MOWRER, D. E., R. L. BAKER, AND R. E. SCHUTZ, *Modification of the Frontal Lisp Programmed Articulation Control Kit S-Pack*, Tempe, Ariz.: Ideas, 1968.

MYSAK, E. D., "Dysarthria and Oropharyngeal Reflexology," *J. Speech Hearing Dis.* **28** (1963):252–260.

NETSELL, R., AND C. S. CLEELAND, "Modification of Lip Hypertonia in Dysarthria using EMG Feedback," *J. Speech Hearing Dis.* **38** (1973):131–140.

PANAGOS, J. M., "Persistence of the Open Syllable Reinterpreted as a Symptom of Language Disorder," *J. Speech Hearing Dis.* **39** (1974):23–31.

PANNBACKER, M., "Diagnostic Report Writing," *J. Speech Hearing Dis.* **40** (1975):367–379.

PHILIPS, B. J. W., AND K. R. BZOCH, "Reliability of Judgments of Articulation of Cleft Palate Speakers," *Cleft Palate J.* **6** (1969):24–34.

POWERS, M. H., "Functional Disorders of Articulation: Symptomatology and Etiology," in L. E. Travis, ed., *The Handbook of Speech Pathology and Audiology,* New York: Appleton-Century-Crofts, 1971.

PRATHER, E. M., D. L. HEDRICK, AND C. A. KERN, "Articulation Development in Children Aged Two to Four Years," *J. Speech Hearing Dis.* **40** (1975):179–191.

RAMPP, D. L., ed., *Proceedings of the Memphis State University's First Annual Symposium on Auditory Processing and Learning Disabilities,* Memphis: Memphis State University Press, 1972.

REES, N. S., "Auditory Processing Factors in Language Disorders: The View from Procrustes' Bed," *J. Speech Hearing Dis.* **38** (1973):304–315.

ROSENBEK, J. C., *et al.,* "A Treatment for Apraxia of Speech in Adults," *J. Speech Hearing Dis.* **38** (1973):462–472.

SANDER, E. K., "When Are Speech Sounds Learned?" *J. Speech Hearing Dis.* **37** (1972):55–63.

SHELTON, R. L., A. JOHNSON, AND W. B. ARNDT, "Variability in Judgments of Articulation when Observer Listens Repeatedly to the Same Phone," *Perceptual Motor Skills* **39** (1974):327–332.

SHRIBERG, L. D., "A Response Evocation Program for /ɝ/," *J. Speech Hearing Dis.* **40** (1975):92–105.

SHRINER, T. H., M. S. HOLLOWAY, AND R. G. DANILOFF, "The Relationship between Articulatory Deficits and Syntax in Speech Defective Children," *J. Speech Hearing Res.* **11** (1969):319–325.

SOMMERS, R. K., "Group Dynamics and Articulation Therapy." Paper presented at the Modern Methods for Articulation Therapy Workshop, Speech and Hearing Clinic, School of Speech, and the Division of Continuing Education, Kent, Ohio: Kent State University, 1976.

TEMPLIN, M. C., AND F. L. DARLEY, *The Templin-Darley Tests of Articulation,* 2d ed., Iowa City: Bureau of Educational Research and Service, Division of Extension and University Services, University of Iowa, 1969.

VAN DEMARK, D. R., "A Factor Analysis of the Speech of Children with Cleft Palate," *Cleft Palate J.* **3** (1966):159–170.

VAN RIPER, C., *Speech Correction Principles and Methods,* 4th ed., Englewood Cliffs, N.J.: Prentice-Hall, 1963.

VAN RIPER, C., AND R. L. ERICKSON, *Predictive Screening Test of Articulation,* 4th ed., Kalamazoo: Continuing Education Office, Western Michigan University, 1975.

WILLIAMS, G. C., AND L. V. MCREYNOLDS, "The Relationship between Discrimination and Articulation Training in Children with Misarticulation," *J. Speech Hearing Res.* **18** (1975):401–412.

WINITZ, H., *Articulatory Acquisition and Behavior*, New York: Appleton-Century-Crofts, 1969.

————, *From Syllable to Conversation*, Baltimore: University Park Press, 1975.

WRIGHT, V. A., "Comparison of Imitative and Spontaneous Speech Samples in the Evaluation of Articulation Change with Therapy," M.A. thesis, University of Kansas, 1969.

YOSS, K. A., AND F. L. DARLEY, "Therapy in Developmental Apraxia of Speech," *Language, Speech, and Hearing Services in Schools* 5 (1974):23–31.

CHAPTER 9
Overview

Disorders of voice include use of inappropriate pitch or loudness, unsatisfactory voice quality, and loss of voice. Disorders of voice quality include breathiness similar to that used by an occasional actress and also hoarseness which is unpleasant and rough-sounding. Vocal pitch, loudness, or quality may differ from the acceptable only slightly or severely, or an individual may be without voice. Voice disorders are especially likely to result from misuse or abuse of the larynx or from laryngeal disease, injury, or malformation. Perhaps the most dramatic voice difference is the loss of voice that coincides with the surgical removal of the larynx in treatment of laryngeal cancer.

This chapter is concerned with the nature of different classes of voice disorders and with their evaluation and treatment through training. Clinical voice training is usually effective in teaching an individual to use the vocal mechanism efficiently and to produce a good voice in the process. This service can result in the reduction or elimination of nodules that sometimes form on the vocal folds when an individual misuses the larynx. Even the individual who loses the larynx to cancer has an excellent chance of reacquiring "voice" and intelligible speech.

Ralph L. Shelton, Ph.D.
University of Arizona

Disorders of Phonation

Introduction

The human voice is produced by the respiratory system and larynx, and articulators above the larynx influence the voice by changing the configuration of resonating cavities of the vocal tract. Misuse of or damage to the larynx may cause voice disorders which may involve pitch, loudness, quality, combinations of those variables, or loss of voice. Surgical removal of the larynx eliminates the capacity to produce normal voice and necessitates voice production by use of either the esophagus or a mechanical aid. Excessive nasality, which is usually associated with poor velopharyngeal closure (Chapter 8), may also make a voice unacceptable to listeners. This chapter will introduce voice disorders from the viewpoint of the speech pathologist who is interested in evaluation and treatment.

Description

Pitch, loudness, and quality, which are involved in disordered phonation, may be understood in terms of how they are measured. Pitch and loudness are psychological perceptions generally corresponding to the acoustic parameters (see Chapters 4 and 6) of fundamental frequency (F_0) and sound pressure (SP). To measure vocal pitch, speech clinicians often match a sample of sustained phonation with standard notes of known frequency. These notes may be generated by a piano, pitch pipe, or electrical **oscillators.** Similar procedures may be used to measure loudness. However, reference tones must be generated electronically to provide the precise sound pressures desired. Frequency and sound pressure may be measured directly by use of electronic instruments. Fundamental frequency, the lowest frequency in a complex sound, may be measured by filtering out harmonic frequencies, leaving only the fundamental, which is then fed into an electronic frequency counter. Intensity can be measured by use of sound-level meters, devices that can indicate sound pressure in decibels (dB). Voices may be too high or low in frequency, too intense, or not intense enough. Laryngeal control of frequency (and pitch), respiratory-system control of intensity (and loudness) and other physiological aspects of voice were introduced in Chapter 3.

Pitch and loudness, as described above, are unidimensional variables based primarily on frequency and sound pressure, respectively. Voice quality, however, is more complicated. It is a multidimensional phenomenon composed of several components, each of which may vary somewhat independently of the others. Perkins (1971, p. 489) wrote that voice quality can be defined acoustically "as the distribution of energy among the various frequencies within the acoustic spectrum." Voices that are perceived as disordered in quality often involve variability in duration from one period of the acoustical wave to the next (Chapter 4), and amplitude variability from period to acoustical period has also been observed in disordered voices. Each form of aperiodicity appears to be related to

214

perception of vocal roughness (Michel and Wendahl, 1971).* If the vocal folds are not adequately closed, air passing through the folds may create noise. Thus voice-quality disorders may involve small deviations in acoustic periodicity, production of noise, or combinations.

Perception of voice quality is more difficult to study than perception of pitch and loudness. There is no single measure of perceived voice quality. Perkins (1971) discussed voice quality as a part of perceived sound other than pitch or loudness, and he stated that quality is essential to identification of a speaker and to other discriminations that may be made.

Numerous terms have been used to describe various deviations from normal vocal quality: rough, harsh, hoarse, breathy, strident, nasal, and others. However, these terms mean different things to different people, and research has shown that individuals often do not use the terms consistently or reliably. That is, a recorded voice sample that is categorized as "harsh" at one listening may be labeled differently by the same judge at a later listening session. To avoid problems of reliability in evaluating voice, Michel and Wendahl (1971) advocate study of voice disorders through use of physiological and acoustical measures that do not require listener judgments. These measures reflect operation of the respiratory system and larynx in voice production. Wilson (undated) devised training procedures to increase the reliability of voice ratings, and many clinicians now use instrumental measures and voice ratings to supplement each other. Indeed, both must be used if we are to establish that the instrumental measures are related to listeners' perception of voice. That perception is fundamental to the concept of a voice disorder. Panels of clinicians trained to use rating scales do produce reliable ratings that may be used for this purpose.

The incidence of voice disorders appears to be rather high. Although Senturia and Wilson (1968) estimated the incidence in school children to be 6 percent, Yairi, Currin, and Bulian (1974) screened approximately 1500 school children and identified hoarseness in about 13 percent. However, only approximately 3 percent presented problems that were clinically significant. Approximately 50 percent of a subset of 251 children continued to be hoarse when reexamined a year later. Silverman and Zimmer (1975) reported that 23 percent of 162 children in a Hebrew day school presented chronic hoarseness and that many of them presented **vocal nodules,** which are described below. Deal, McClain, and Sudderth (1976) established a screening program for voice disorders in a Texas school district of about 15,000 students. One hundred and twenty-four children were referred to the school speech pathologists, who in turn referred 77 of the children for examination by physicians specializing in disorders of the ear, nose, and

---

* Aperiodicity in the form of the two vocal folds vibrating at different rates may give the perception of two voices, or diplophonia (Frank Wilson, personal communication). Diplophonia has also been attributed to simultaneous vibration of both true and false vocal folds.

throat **(otolaryngologists).** Thirty-four children were found to have nodules, seven presented edematous (containing fluid) vocal folds, seven presented allergy problems, and four could not be examined. The remainder were medically normal. Information about the incidence of voice disorders in teachers is presented later.

The goal of speech-pathology services for individuals with disordered voice is to help the speakers produce a voice that is satisfactory to themselves and their listeners. The speakers must be comfortable in their production of that voice, and their voice productions should not be abusive to the vocal mechanism. In the next section, voice disorders will be described and discussed in etiological terms.

Etiology and Related Variables

Problems Associated with Speaker Misuse and Abuse of the Larynx

Improper use of the larynx may result in physical damage to the larynx, change in the voice, or both. Thus misuse of the larynx during phonation or other acts such as throat clearing may abuse both the larynx and the voice.

Misuse of the larynx in voice production often involves faulty approximation of the vocal folds. Brackett (1971) described a continuum of vocal-fold closure from abducted **aphonia,** where the folds are completely open (see Fig. 9.1), through normal vocal-fold closure for phonation to **hypervalvular phonation,** where the folds are brought together (adducted) with excessive force. He pointed out that if the vocal folds are completely open, there is low laryngeal resistance to air flow, and no voice is produced. If the folds are partially closed, a whisper may be produced. Closer approximation of the vocal folds may result in moderate vocal-fold vibration, but the voice is breathy. In vocal-fold closure satisfactory for normal phonation, the folds are so approximated that there is little variation in the opening and closing of the vocal folds from cycle to cycle.

In hypervalvular phonation, the vocal folds are moved together too tightly, and the portion of the vibratory cycle when the folds are closed is given an increased amount of time. Brodnitz (1965) stated that hypertense vocal-fold closure necessitates an increase in the subglottal air pressure required to produce voice. That is, when the folds are held tightly closed, it takes greater air pressure to blow them open. **Dysphonia,** or partial loss of voice, is associated with abuse of this kind, but may result from other causes as well. The term **hard glottal attack** is used to describe the forceful closure of the vocal folds that may be part of hypervalvular phonation. The vocal folds may strike each other with sufficient force to cause irritation. With continued abuse, tissue thickening and then vocal nodules may develop within the larynx. Other patterns of abuse may cause **vocal polyps,** which may result from a single episode of vocal abuse, perhaps in con-

Figure 9.1

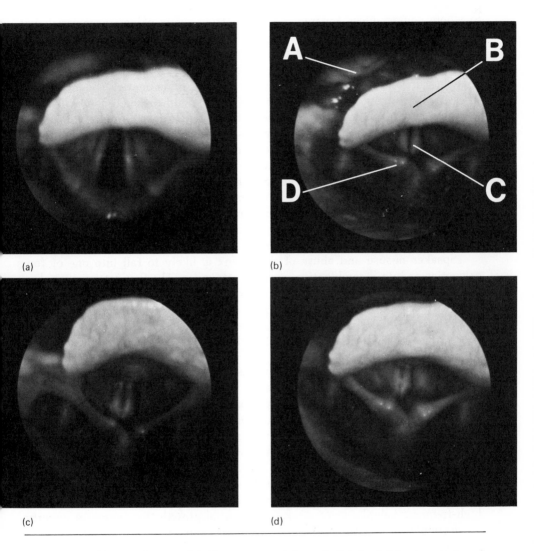

The vocal folds: (a) the vocal folds open, or abducted; (b) the folds almost closed, or adducted, during a breathy phonation; (c) the folds during normal phonation; and (d) an attempted hyperfunctional adduction of the folds. In (b), A represents the base of the tongue, B the epiglottis, C a true vocal fold, and D an arytenoid cartilage. (Photos by Dennis Ruscello and Ralph Shelton, University of Arizona.)

junction with a respiratory illness, or contact ulcers, which may result from forced use of a low pitch. Cherry and Margulies (1968) described three patients in whom contact ulcer apparently resulted from reflux of gastric material that served as an acidic bath for portions of the larynx. Treatment of peptic esophagitis restored larynx and the voice in these patients.

A nodule is a buildup of a layer of tissue similar to a callus, and a polyp is an enlargement that may be filled with fluid or other matter (Boone, 1971). These changes may appear on one or both folds, and their site is usually one-third the length of the folds from their attachment to the thyroid cartilage (see Fig. 3.4). Boone stated that these changes influence the mass of the vocal folds and result in dysphonia involving breathiness and lowered pitch. Contact ulcers develop where the vocal fold attaches to the arytenoid cartilage. These ulcers usually develop on both folds. The patient with contact ulcers may state that his or her voice tires easily and may also report laryngeal pain. A speaker may be more concerned with laryngeal fatigue or pain associated with poor use of the larynx than with poor voice quality. Obviously, gentle initiation and use of voice are frequent goals in voice rehabilitation.

Speaker misuse and abuse of the larynx is likely to fall into one of four categories or into a combination of those categories. The first category involves persons who use poor vocal skills. The second involves excessive shouting, which is often observed in children. The third category involves chronic respiratory conditions or other irritations that cause individuals to clear the throat and cough, thus abusing the larynx. The fourth category is nonorganic loss of voice.

Unskilled use of the larynx and respiratory mechanism Laryngeal abuse may involve use of inappropriate fundamental frequency levels or excessive vocal intensity as well as the inadequate approximation of the vocal folds described earlier. Frequency problems include use of a frequency level that is inappropriate for the size of the speaker's larynx. Frequency range may be defined as the difference between the lowest and highest fundamental frequencies that a person can produce, and the frequency that is used most often (modal frequency) should be approximately one-third of the speaker's range from lowest F_0. Another frequency problem which sometimes exists involves continued use of a high-frequency child's voice after the laryngeal growth that occurs at puberty.

Examples of individuals using inappropriate pitch level include a prepubertal child belting out pop-tunes in a low voice during a local television amateur program. We don't know what happened to the lad's voice, but a young woman singer whom we met professionally and who used a style similar to that of the child developed marked vocal nodules. A politician insisted on using a low-pitch voice to convey an authoritative image, despite the fact that he ended his speaking day with a painful throat. He persisted in low-pitch usage even though his larynx was chronically inflamed.

Improper breathing patterns may also influence voice adversely. Many voice texts say that proper inspiration for speech involves elevation and expansion of the lower rib cage simultaneously with expansion of the abdomen. An individual who elevates the shoulders or markedly contracts muscles in the neck or shoulder areas when breathing for speech is using a pattern that is potentially abusive to the larynx. That is, the breathing pattern described is likely to be accompanied by laryngeal tension and hypervalvular phonation. Respiration for phonation requires prolongation of expiration. Boone (1971) reported that some persons exhale a good deal of air before beginning phonation, which of course is not compatible with efficient phonation. Speakers may also attempt to continue an utterance after they have run out of breath. Such effort is likely to involve production of undesirable laryngeal muscle activity.

Persons who use their voices professionally or who speak under conditions of stress or in noisy environments are especially likely to present voice pathology associated with poor speaking skills. We've cited performers and politicans. European literature abstracted in *dsh Abstracts* also cites teachers as presenting a high risk for voice disorders. Vasilenko (1972) reported that teachers of young children were especially vulnerable to voice disorders. Thirty-six percent of a group of nursery and kindergarten teachers presented functional and organic diseases of the larynx. Apparently much of this problem can be attributed to poor speaking behaviors, and Vasilenko recommended that teachers be taught (1) information about the voice and speech mechanism; (2) means of voice and speech production that are not abusive to the vocal mechanism; and (3) the ability to recognize work conditions that might contribute to development of voice disorders. They should also receive suitable otolaryngological medical service. Seidner and Loewe (1972) commented that a widely held viewpoint is that persons with allergic diseases of the upper respiratory tract should not be accepted into teacher training. (They differentiated between classes of allergic disease that would and would not interfere with teaching.) Perhaps danger to the voice is low in American elementary schools, where teachers may work with small groups rather than lecturing to entire classes. Nevertheless, we would recommend that the school speech pathologist's knowledge of voice disorders and their management be considered as a resource for school faculty as well as for students. Indeed, in-service voice training conducted by the speech pathologist could be part of continuing education for teachers.

Anyone speaking in noise for long periods is likely to suffer vocal abuse by speaking loudly in order to be heard over the noise. Children may yell for the joy of it. Shouting as a form of vocal abuse is sufficiently prevalent to warrant its own category.

Excessive shouting   Prolonged shouting is a source of laryngeal abuse often associated with nodules in children. Spirited yelling at ballgames has resulted in temporary dysphonia in many persons, and children who yell frequently and vigorously may develop nodules. Forms of vocal play used by children—for example imitating car and airplane engines—can have the same effect as shouting. Fortunately, many children respond quickly to training techniques intended to remind them to stop yelling.

Loud speech is especially likely to be harmful if it is produced by increasing laryngeal constriction or tension. Loudness should be generated by increasing subglottal air pressure with the respiratory mechanism, not by use of excessive laryngeal muscle contraction. Novice drill instructors who tense the neck to shout commands may well abuse themselves as well as their charges (see Fig. 9.2). Consulting with a colleague over a background of factory noise, visiting with a friend next to a noisy air conditioner, conversing in a fast-moving car

Figure 9.2

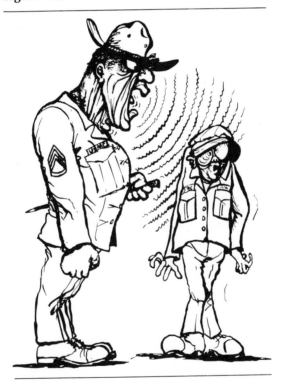

Shouting may abuse the larynx by causing excessive tension within the larynx and nearby muscles. (Cartoon by David O'Day, University of Arizona.)

with the windows open, or other common speaking situations may lead to shouting and abuse of the larynx and voice.

Chronic respiratory conditions An individual may also abuse the larynx through acts not associated with speech, notably through use of excessive coughing and throat clearing which may be associated with respiratory disorders, such as allergy and post-nasal drip. The vocal mechanism may suffer from allergy in two ways: (1) inflammation as a direct response to allergens; and (2) irritation caused by coughing that results from the allergens. It seems inappropriate to classify all respiratory discomfort as ailment on the part of the sufferer. Rather, the **pathology** would seem to be in the air pollution itself and perhaps in the heads of the people who created it. Smoking and use of alcohol may irritate the larynx and influence the voice adversely. However, those two pollutants are self-inflicted except when the smoke inhaled is from someone else's cigarette.

Nonorganic loss of voice Sometimes the voice is completely lost even though pathology is not present. This loss may follow a period of acute psychological stress or a period of temporary laryngeal pathology. Sometimes this loss is called *hysterical aphonia* (Murphy, 1964) and sometimes *functional aphonia* (Boone, 1971). The term "hysterical" implies a psychoneurotic causation and a need for psychotherapy as a treatment. "Functional" is a more neutral label so far as causation is concerned, and Boone reports that functional aphonia has often been corrected successfully through clinical voice-training procedures. The clinician may attempt to elicit reflexive phonation, perhaps by having the patient cough, and to help the client use that phonation in a sequence of acts progressively approximating running speech.

Voice Problems Associated with Laryngeal Disease, Injury, or Malformation

As indicated above, laryngeal abuse may influence the voice and lead to laryngeal changes which in turn may adversely influence the function of the larynx further. However, there are many physical conditions that influence the larynx and often the voice as well that are not the result of abusive behaviors produced by the speaker. Voice disorders associated with these conditions often resemble those resulting from misuse and abuse of the larynx.

One category of laryngeal disorders is unilateral or bilateral vocal-fold paralysis, caused by illness or injury. One or both folds may be maintained in either an open or closed position. A patient who cannot bring the folds together will not be able to generate a normal voice. Some individuals learn to move a normal fold past midline to compensate for inadequate movement of the other fold. If the folds are maintained near a midline position, the individual will not be able to breathe properly. The conditions described usually result

221

from damage to the nerve that directly connects with the involved muscle.* However, neurological damage higher in the nervous system can interfere with the extent or coordination of vocal-fold movements. Various diseases may result in weakness or malfunction of the laryngeal muscles. For example, increase in breathiness, nasality, and imprecise articulation with prolonged speaking are observed in myasthenia gravis, a neurological illness involving muscle weakness (Aronson, 1971).

A second major class of laryngeal problems involves tumors. Tumors may be malignant (cancerous) or benign (noncancerous). Benign tumors may become malignant, and either class of tumor can cause voice disorders. Cancer of the larynx requires medical treatment if the patient's life is to be saved. A frequently used treatment, partial or total removal of the larynx, is called a **laryngectomy.** About 25 percent of patients with laryngeal cancer receive partial laryngectomy (Moore, 1975). According to Moore, the portion of the larynx above the vocal folds may be removed with little effect on voice; however, removal of one side of the larynx may cause hoarseness and reduction in vocal intensity.

Total laryngectomy leaves the patient voiceless. In later sections, some emphasis will be given to the matter of teaching esophageal speech to the person with no larynx **(laryngectomee).** Laryngectomized persons may also speak through use of a vibrator called an artificial larynx. Esophageal speech and speech produced with the artificial larynx can be suitably intelligible (Fig. 9.3).

Persons with laryngeal cancer are sometimes treated by **radiation therapy.** Murray, Bone, and Von Essen (1974) studied a 49-year-old male musician just prior to, during, and eight weeks following cobalt radiation for treatment of a vocal-fold cancer. Prior to treatment, the patient reported that his voice had become strained, and medical diagnosis showed a **lesion** which impaired motion of the affected vocal fold. Thirty-nine days of cobalt treatment eliminated the lesion, and eight weeks after treatment, visual examination showed only slight redness of the folds. Instrumental measures of frequency and airflow rate indicated that with treatment, the patient's frequency range had increased, and excessive air-flow† rate was dramatically reduced. Nevertheless, the patient's voice continued to be hoarse eight weeks after treatment. The authors concluded that vocal rehabilitation may be needed by persons who undergo radiation for vocal-fold cancer.

---

* Haglund, Knutsson, and Martensson (1974) studied electrical activity associated with the vocal or cricothyroid muscles or both in 18 persons thought to have dysphonia of functional origin. Ten of these patients presented evidence of neurogenic lesions. The authors conclude that neurogenic lesions in laryngeal muscles may be responsible for some voice disorders thought to reflect habitual or psychogenic origin.
† A tumor or a nodule may obstruct complete closure of the vocal folds. Any resulting opening allows air leakage during phonation.

Figure 9.3

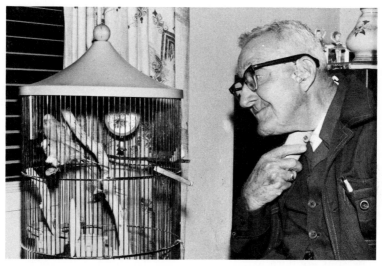

This gentleman lives alone at 87 years of age—seven years following the surgical removal of his larynx. He uses both esophageal speech and an electrolarynx to talk with his many friends and to his pets. He also has a hearing loss of a type that is not overcome by amplification, and he often wears his glasses without bothering to insert the earmolds of his bilateral, glasses-type hearing aids. (Photo by Nate Shelton, University of Arizona.)

Papillomas are one category of benign tumor that occur in the larynx—usually in children before the age of puberty. These wartlike growths are believed to result from viral infection. Although papillomas tend to disappear at puberty, it may be necessary to treat them medically or remove them surgically, and then they may grow back. Indeed, airway obstruction caused by papillomas may necessitate **tracheotomy** to provide an airway for respiration. This means that surgery is performed to create an opening in the neck below the larynx to permit breathing.*

A tracheotomy prevents a person from using the larynx for voice—unless it is plugged temporarily, perhaps with a finger—because it allows the subglottal air pressure to escape below the vocal folds. Complete airway obstruction above the tracheotomy opening would prevent phonation even during momentary closure of the tracheotomy. Weinberg and Westerhouse (1973) described a

---

* A tracheotomy opening may close spontaneously over time, but the opening can be maintained by use of a special tube.

223

child who underwent tracheotomy at age two because of papillomatosis and who was still tracheotomized when she was studied at age 12. She received no speech instruction, but on her own acquired pharyngeal speech. That is, she learned to produce sound by taking air into the pharynx and then directing it between the approximated tongue and palate to make a noise that could be used as a voice. The speech produced was of poor intelligibility, and the authors hoped to help the girl to develop a different, more effective way of speaking.

Patients may suffer other diseases that influence laryngeal function. For example, impairment of laryngeal joint function by disease or metabolic disturbance will impair vocal-fold **adduction** and **abduction. Endocrine** gland problems that retard laryngeal growth in the male will cause vocal pitch inappropriate to the sex of the speaker. **Virilization,** or the acquisition of masculine body characteristics by a female, may include laryngeal growth and development of a low-pitched voice. Women who take ovulation inhibitors are subject to this danger (Wendler, 1972) as are girls or women who take anabolic (promoting the assimilation of food) medication in treatment of loss of appetite (Pruszewicz *et al.*, 1973).

Some persons are born with webs of tissue that connect the vocal folds, usually in their front portion. One boy we knew was born with cleft palate and a laryngeal web, and he presented a combination of vocal roughness, or hoarseness, and **hypernasality.** The web was cut surgically, but some vocal aperiodicity remained. We also met a woman who created a laryngeal web and other defects of the speaking and swallowing mechanisms when she swallowed lye in a suicide attempt. Both voice and articulation were adversely influenced.

Finally, the larynx may be fractured or otherwise damaged in accidents. A danger here is that the damage will obstruct the airway, thus endangering or taking the victim's life. Accidents and other laryngeal conditions are discussed in voice-disorders texts (Boone, 1971; Moore, 1971).

Voice quality may also be influenced by defects above the larynx. Hypernasality provides a frequently observed example of this kind of problem. If an individual fails to close the velopharyngeal port during speech, the oropharynx and nasopharynx are coupled, and the nasopharynx may then greatly influence the voice through the resonance process described in Chapter 4. The result is an excessively nasal voice. Like articulation, hypernasality involves the movement of structures above the larynx, and it serves to remind us that phonation and articulation are not independent of each other. Laryngeal function is thought to be influenced by the position of the articulators, and it seems likely that hypernasality involves interaction between the vocal tract and the larynx.* Cleft pal-

---

* Spectrographic displays (Chapter 4) of hypernasal voices show certain characteristics, including a loss of energy in the first formant and a shift in formant frequencies. Schwartz (1971) pointed out that these characteristics can be produced at the larynx as well as through defects of velopharyngeal closure.

ate persons who present hypernasality are especially likely to do so on vowels produced with the tongue high (Table 3.1) in the mouth (Carney and Sherman, 1971). Presumably the high tongue position partially blocks the oral passage, thus directing sound through the velopharyngeal passage into the nasopharynx.

Perceptually extreme hypernasality is easily identified. However, changes in nasal resonance within individuals and small differences in nasal resonance among individuals are difficult to judge reliably. Anyone demonstrating hypernasality should be studied for adequacy of velopharyngeal closure, and hypernasality should be differentiated from denasality, which results from obstruction of the nasal passages. The person presenting denasality has difficulty articulating nasal consonants (/m, n/ and /ŋ/) clearly and is sometimes said to sound like an individual with a head cold.

Other Variables Related to Voice

For many years, the viewpoint was widely accepted that nonorganic voice problems are symptoms of neurosis. Murphy (1964), who discussed variables that may influence a speaker's vocal characteristics, stated that in a child free from organic defects, voice disorders must be understood in terms of conflicts or confusions the child experiences. Murphy wrote that imitation influences voice, as do parent-child relationships and identification with loved or admired persons. Many people tend to associate voice characteristics with personality type, and voice may reflect one's self-image. As a symptom of neurosis, a voice disorder could serve as a defense against emotional discomfort. The disorder could provide the speaker with secondary gain—with an excuse for failure to achieve.

Despite the long-standing interest in the relationship between voice and personality, relatively few data are available. There is little research to support the clinical theory that voice disorders may reflect personality problems. Bloch and Goodstein (1971) summarized a review of ten years of research as follows: "The number of studies in this area is very few, and little remains known about personality as an etiological, consequential, or therapeutic factor in voice disorders." Much current clinical speech practice is based on the viewpoint that nonorganic voice disorders are observed in persons who make poor use of the larynx but who are free from neurosis.

Perkins (1971) noted that relatively little research has been done on behavioral aspects of voice production. Acceptance of the viewpoint that nonorganic voice disorders reflect psychoneurotic adjustment may have reduced motivation for research. Also, the clinician has not had reliable voice measures readily available for use in research.

The physiology of voice production and the acoustics of the voice signal have received extensive study in recent years. This research is responsible for our understanding of the vocal phenomena discussed in the previous section. A good deal of information is known about fundamental frequency, periodicity, subglottal air pressure, air flow, and similar phenomena. Investigators have tried to identify components of specific voice disorders. For example, Isshiki and his associates (1969) studied hoarseness perceptually and used statistical procedures to identify its components. Perceptual factors identified were termed roughness, breathiness, and asthenia (weakness). Voice measures have also been studied in relation to age, sex, race, and pathological conditions. For example, Hollien and Shipp (1972) (Hollien, 1972) have collected valuable data about fundamental frequency in adult males. Michel and Wendahl (1971) wrote that investigators are particularly interested in finding readily usable measures of laryngeal function. Such measures would help in the description of vocal phenomena, in the identification of variables correlated with vocal phenomena, and in the management of voice disorders. Measures of frequency, periodicity, and air flow appear to have especial promise for diagnostic use. Clinicians have especial need for measures that enable them to provide their clients with information about the adequacy of responses made in remedial work. That information should be available during a response or immediately after it is made.

Assessment

Because of the strong possibility of organic lesion or disability in patients with laryngeal voice disorders, the speech pathologist usually does not work with these patients until they have undergone examination by an otolaryngologist. The medical examination will include observation of the larynx by mirror and reflected light (Fig. 9.4) or perhaps by use of an optical instrument termed an **endoscope,** or laryngeal telescope. The physician will determine whether any condition is present that requires medical treatment and whether the patient's physical condition contraindicates voice training. Evaluation by additional medical and behavioral specialists may be needed. Hearing should be tested, because hearing loss may account for misuse of the voice; for example, persons with some kinds of hearing loss tend to speak loudly. If a person appears to be a candidate for voice rehabilitation, the speech pathologist will need to make many observations before initiating training.

The voice evaluation will include consideration of the physician's description of the problem and of the condition of the larynx. The patient will be asked to report any concerns about his or her voice. The patient's motivation for voice rehabilitation will be a factor in its effectiveness, and it is the patient's decision whether or not to take remedial voice work. One patient—indeed the first patient—referred to the author by an otolaryngologist stated emphatically that he only wanted to know whether he had tuberculosis and that he was not concerned about his voice: "I don't want to be no damned opera singer." The patient was an employee of the medical center where the examinations were per-

Figure 9.4

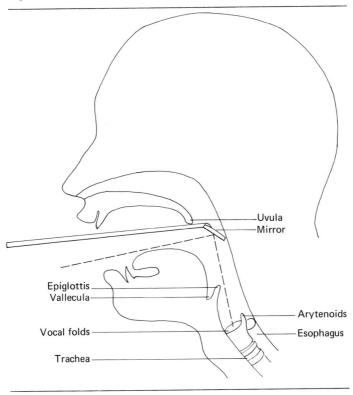

Use of a mirror in examination of the larynx.

formed, and he went about his business for many years, presumably not at all concerned about a raspy voice.

The examiner will be interested in the origin of the voice problem and the duration of its existence. Environmental factors, such as noise and allergens, that may influence voice should be discussed with the patient. Special consideration is given to any history of vocal misuse. A voice sample should be recorded during the evaluation to provide a reference point against which to identify later changes in voice.

The patient's speech organs will be observed for speech function. The examiner will attempt to identify sites in the speaking mechanism that are tense during phonation. Occasionally, excessive muscle activity in the jaw and neck regions can be detected. The individual will be examined to determine whether his or her respiratory patterns are satisfactory for speech. Diaphragmatic-abdominal breathing involves expansion of the abdomen and lower thorax on inhalation and their gradual return during exhalation. This pattern is sometimes taught to voice clients. It can be visualized by use of a kymograph, a device to record expansion and contraction movements sensed through use of an expandable tube placed around the client's ribcage or abdomen. Other respiratory variables that may be measured include **vital capacity,** maximum duration of controlled sustained blowing, maximum duration of controlled sustained phonation, and air flow during phonation of a comfortable /ɑ/. By comparison with norms, information is gained about the individual's respiratory function for phonation. More important, change in these patterns over time can provide information about the individual's learning during voice training.

The voice itself will also be studied in diagnosis. A sound-level meter may be used to measure modal, or most frequently used, sound pressure and also the sound-pressure range that the client can produce. Modal and range measures will also be made for F_0. As was mentioned earlier, F_0 can be measured by filtering out harmonic frequencies, leaving only the fundamental, which is then fed into an electronic frequency counter. Another method of measuring frequency involves use of a storage oscilloscope, which is an instrument that can display and store on a screen various wave forms, including that of the voice. Some oscilloscopes can display two signals simultaneously. To measure F_0, the wave form of the voice is stored on half of the oscillographic screen, and a wave form generated by a frequency oscillator is displayed on the other half of the screen (Shearer, 1972). The frequency of the second sound is adjusted until the duration, or period, of a single cycle matches the period of the voice being measured. The frequency of the voice under study then corresponds to a setting which may be read from the oscillator dial. Many voice samples must be studied to obtain a reliable index to modal frequency. Modal frequency is compared with the frequency located one-third of the distance from the bottom to the top of the frequency range. If there is significant discrepancy, the speaker may be trained to make a slight shift in modal frequency.

Clinicians may also undertake to rate aspects of voice perceptually. In an attempt to provide the clinician with training that will permit reliable judgments of voice, Wilson (undated) collected tapes of persons with various voice problems. These voice samples were scaled for voice phenomena involving pitch, resonance, and varying patterns of glottal closure. Laryngeal function of the patients who produced these voices was observed and described by a laryngologist. Use of such training materials undoubtedly increases the reliability with which voices are placed into different diagnostic categories, such as hypofunctional or hyperfunctional closure of the glottis.

New instrumentation may be developed that will give the clinician information important to the management of voice-quality problems. An example of research that will result ultimately in improved clinical service is a study by Crystal *et al.* (1970) which showed that a laryngeal aperiodicity factor correlates with vocal-fold pathology. This aperiodicity was identified by computer evaluation of waveshape information derived from recorded speech samples.

Our consideration of voice evaluation will be concluded with an introduction to procedures used for the evaluation of velopharyngeal closure. Normal speech requires complete contact between the soft palate (velum) and the posterior wall of the pharynx, and hypernasality may be caused by defects of closure. Therefore, persons observed to produce hypernasality should be tested for adequacy of velopharyngeal closure. Various speech behaviors are indicative of poor closure. Audible nasal escape of air during the production of consonant sounds is a key symptom. To hear this escape, the clinician may employ a listening tube which consists of rubber tubing with an olive-shaped glassed tube in each end (Blakeley, 1972). One end is placed in the client's nose and the other end in the examiner's ear. U-tube water manometers may also be used to measure nasal escape of air (Hess, 1976). Displacement of water in the manometer indicates the amount of pressure that is associated with the air escape. Other manometers may be used to measure the difference in oral pressures during blowing with the nose open and again with the nose pinched closed (Morris, 1966). Given equal blowing effort under the two conditions, poor velopharyngeal closure is indicated if greater blowing pressure is produced with the nose closed. Measurement of air pressure and flow with more elaborate equipment permits accurate estimation of the size of velopharyngeal opening during the production of specific speech sounds (Warren and Devereux, 1966). Facial grimace around the nose may also indicate poor velopharyngeal closure. Velopharyngeal closure may be directly observed by the use of X-ray with the image recorded on motion picture film or videotape. Endoscopes may be placed into the mouth or nose, thus permitting observation of velopharyngeal closure (Willis and Stutz, 1972).

The voice evaluation should lead to specific recommendations. This requires that the clinician be able to predict future voice phenomena. If voice training is needed, the examiner should specify what changes in voice usage need to be made and how they might be accomplished.

Prognosis

The prognosis for voice improvement in individuals presenting laryngeal abuse is thought to be good. However, little research has been done about changes in the voice of individuals with functional voice problems regardless of whether they receive voice training. In contrast to work in articulation, no effort has been made to identify variables that may predict spontaneous improvement. Gundermann, Krone, and Bremer (1968) wrote that infantile hoarseness may lead to dysphonia in adults. Moore (1971) stated that "[voice] therapeutic measures are frequently not subject to predictable results from patient to patient." Both Boone and Brodnitz have commented that voice training should be effective within a relatively short period of time—perhaps two months. Although the prognosis for improvement with training is generally good for individuals presenting vocal abuse, research is needed to identify specific variables indicative of probable success or failure. Perhaps one important variable is the effort the client exerts to incorporate new behaviors into voice production. That is, voice improvement appears to be something that is accomplished by the client with the help of the clinician. A condition called spastic dysphonia has a poor prognosis for improvement, regardless of the treatment used* Spastic dysphonia, which in some ways resembles vocal stuttering, involves excessive activity in the muscles that close or open the vocal folds.

Change in organically based voice disorders is determined in part by the nature of the disability and its course. Voice training will also be influential; however, gains made with training are limited by the condition of the mechanism. For example, in working with an individual with vocal-fold scarring or partial loss of the larynx, the speech pathologist seeks the best, most efficient voice usage that the mechanism will support. Cornut and Pierucci (1969) claim that voice retraining is helpful in persons with problems of laryngeal paralysis. One goal of training may be to help the speaker to accept a voice that is unusual in one or more parameters.

Perhaps more is known about factors that influence the learning of **esophageal speech** by the laryngectomized person than is known about prognosis for recovery from other voice disorders. Diedrich and Youngstrom (1966) measured the **pseudoglottis** from X-ray motion picture frames and did not find their measures to be highly related to speech-skill measures. However, some individuals probably have difficulty learning esophageal speech because of lack of a suitable mechanism. Diedrich and Youngstrom did find esophageal speech skill to be related to hearing acuity and to the amount of time that had passed since surgery. The latter finding suggests that continuation of esophageal speech practice is important to the development of speaking skill.

Wolfe, Olson, and Goldenberg (1971) reported that persons they studied who developed excellent esophageal speech had effective muscle action in closing the stomach from the esophagus. Persons who failed to learn adequate speech, however, suffered inflammation of the esophagus and reflux of fluid from the stomach into the esophagus.† Wolfe *et al.* hope to conduct research that might

---

*   Recently surgeons have alleviated this condition by severing the recurrent laryngeal nerve unilaterally so that the glottis remains partially open at all times; although this results in a breathy voice, it also appears to result in easier phonation and reduction of patient distress.

†   These conclusions are supported by the work of Winans, Reichbach, and Waldrop (1974), who used manometry to study constriction of the cricopharyngeal sphincter, which is located at the top of the esophagus and which must partially open to allow air into and out of the esophagus for esophageal speech to be produced. Cricopharyngeal sphincter pressure at rest was lower in laryngectomees with fluent esophageal speech than in persons who failed to develop esophageal speech.

allow prediction of esophageal speech skill from observations made before surgery. Additional variables may impair esophageal speech learning. For example, alcoholism is thought to detract from such learning, perhaps because it reduces motivation to learn. Research is needed that will enable the speech pathologist to make more precise predictions of the outcome of vocal rehabilitation.

Treatment

Laryngeal Voice Disorders

For some persons with voice disorders, the first treatment is medical in nature. For example, tumors may be removed, or teflon may be injected into the larynx to displace a paralyzed vocal fold toward midline. Teflon is a plastic which because of its inert biological quality is well tolerated by body tissues (Kirchner, Toledo, and Svoboda, 1966), and its injection into the larynx of a person with one paralyzed fold will displace that fold toward midline, where it may be contacted by the normally moving fold. Other medical treatments, e.g., management of allergic conditions, may be directed to conditions that influence the function of the vocal mechanism.

Psychotherapy may be needed by some patients. However, Boone (1971) wrote that training techniques directed to proper use of the voice mechanism can result in satisfactory solution of most functional voice disorders. As was mentioned earlier, he stated that even functional aphonia can often be corrected by training procedures.

Attention may also be given to environmental factors that influence voice. A person who must work in a noisy environment may be taught means of conserving voice in noise, and repetition of treatment may be required with periodic exposure to an adverse environment. Moore (1971) pointed out that use of air conditioners and other devices may control allergens or other pollutants in the air, thereby reducing irritation to the larynx.

With regard to voice remediation itself, training techniques will be chosen that can be expected to bring about voice-behavior changes needed by the individual. Usually the clinician's goal is to teach behaviors that will correct the voice problem permanently. Boone (1971) has described a number of procedures used in voice training, including many which are appropriate for individuals with either functional or organic voice disorders. Boone emphasized the search for behaviors that the patient can accomplish and that will improve his or her use of voice. Early in training, the clinician will ask the patient to experiment with different manners of voice production in order to identify the most satisfactory voice or manner of voice production that the individual can use. In this exploratory process the patient will be asked to vary pitch, loudness, air flow, effort, posture, and other variables. Moore (1971) emphasized that early in training, exercises should be restricted to short periods, and minimum loudness generally should be used. That is, the clinician should avoid behaviors that may contribute to laryngeal abuse.

For persons who do not bring their vocal folds together, remediation will be directed to increase in fold approximation. For example, pushing exercises may be used to increase adduction. In pushing exercises, the patient raises the arms so that the fists are close to the chest and then lowers the arms in a forceful manner (Brodnitz, 1965). Reflexive glottal closure is likely to accompany this act. Pushing may be practiced simultaneously with attempts at phonation; however, pushing exercises are contraindicated in an individual with a hyperfunctional voice problem.

Individuals presenting hyperfunctional use of the larynx will be taught to use less forceful fold approximation, especially during initiation of phonation. Several authors have described the use of chewing movements in voice remediation, because use of these movements is thought to contribute to relaxation of the speaking mechanism. Apparently tension is less likely to occur in muscles when they are moving a structure. Moore (1971) pointed out that relaxation may be accomplished by deliberately turning off tensed muscles. Quiet speech may possibly contribute to reduction in laryngeal muscle activity, and a sound-level meter may be used to monitor vocal intensity and to teach use of a less intense voice.

Breathy voice production is sometimes deliberately used in treatment of hyperfunctional voice usage. However, it is possible to produce a breathy voice and excessive laryngeal muscle activity simultaneously. Basmajian (1972) has reported that muscle relaxation may be efficiently accomplished by giving the subject visual or auditory **biofeedback** of electrical activity in the muscles of interest. In the future, this procedure may be tested for utility in the treatment of voice disorders. There is some evidence that relaxation learned under these feedback conditions can be used in the absence of the biofeedback instrumentation. Moore (1971) noted that relaxation can be described in terms of well-coordinated activity of muscles that oppose one another.

Many other procedures may also be used to relieve hyperfunctional phonation. Clinicians frequently use techniques to decrease any shouting a patient does; indeed, work may be done to decrease the patient's amount of speaking. Singing may also be discouraged, in that vocal abuse during singing is a key behavioral fault in some voice patients. Improvement of articulation and diction may increase intelligibility and thereby alleviate apparent need for loud speech. Attention may be paid to posture, because upright posture may facilitate easy voice production. Attention to mental hygiene may also be helpful; Moore stated that loud responses to emotional stimuli may be amenable to training and that the patient may need to learn to manage emotional states as a prerequisite to relaxed voice production.

Laryngeal abuse may involve nonspeech acts, such as coughing and clearing the throat. Since these acts involve forceful closure of the vocal folds, they are discouraged by the voice clinician. Boone (1971) suggested that a person be taught to clear the throat by sniffing and swallowing. Zwitman and Calcaterra (1973b) recommended a "silent" cough wherein the individual inhales and then expels air forcefully through the larynx without producing voiced sound. Perhaps a combination of sniffing and unvoiced cough will provide the relief the patient seeks from irritation of the larynx by accumulation of mucus.

At present, the speech pathologist must infer hyperfunctional approximation of the vocal folds from visual identification of muscle activity in the speaking mechanism and from auditory cues in the voice. The client may be able to introspect laryngeal muscle tension during voice phonation. With study and experience, the clinician can work with these phenomena.

Depending on the problem the patient presents, techniques may be used to teach respiratory patterns that make efficient use of the available air supply. The individual can be taught to produce loudness when it is needed by increasing subglottal air pressure through respiratory effort rather than by increasing laryngeal muscle activity.

Some texts emphasize the importance of ear training to make the patient aware of auditory cues important to voice production. Tapes such as those prepared by Wilson (undated) for training clinicians to judge voice qualities may also be helpful in teaching an individual to evaluate and monitor his or her own voice. Video-tape equipment may be helpful for orienting the patient to his or her breathing patterns, posture, and use of excessive muscle activity in the speaking mechanism.

If the voice clinician is to utilize the ear in evaluating responses a client produces during remediation, he or she must be able to evaluate small changes in voice reliably and accurately. That is, if a clinician cannot reliably identify changes in a given parameter of voice as they occur, that parameter cannot be manipulated efficiently in voice training, because the clinician's advice to the patient will be contradictory. When judgments of small differences in voice quality are difficult to make, the clinician must rely on other observations to guide the remediation process (Chapter 7). Fortunately, as the paragraphs above indicate, there are many phenomena that the voice clinician can appropriately manipulate in this clinical work. However, new instrumental measures that will supplement the senses of the clinician and the client need to be developed and tested.* An instrument that is capable of providing an index to laryngeal muscle activity would enhance the efficiency of voice evaluation and remediation.

---

* Daly and Johnson (1974) used a biofeedback device called TONAR to train out hypernasality in mentally retarded individuals. The device picked up sound energy at the nose and mouth, processed the information by computer analysis, and displayed

Studies are needed that measure changes in voice and voice production under conditions of well-controlled treatment, and the development of step-by-step treatment programs can contribute to the accomplishment of that goal. Drudge and Philips (1976) described a 31-step program developed for use with patients presenting hoarse voice quality resulting from vocal abuse, and they described the use of the program with three persons who had vocal nodules. Nodules disappeared from two of the patients, and the third had a reduction of nodule size during the course of 16 half-hour sessions.

The data pool regarding effectiveness of vocal rehabilitation is small, but other authors have also reported that voice training is highly effective in modifying vocal abuse and eliminating or reducing vocal nodules (Deal et al., 1976). Fisher and Logemann (1970) used a high-speed motion picture camera and a laryngeal mirror to document change in laryngeal function of a 19-year-old actress as she underwent vocal rehabilitation involving a moderate increase in F_0. The patient's bilateral vocal nodules were reduced, and she was able to resume her acting career.

Alaryngeal Speech

To produce esophageal speech, the laryngectomized person must inject air into the esophagus and then must set tissue at the top of the esophagus into vibration by expelling the air from the esophagus. This process was described above briefly. An early step in esophageal speech training involves teaching the client to inject air into the esophagus. Swallowing was once emphasized for this purpose, but it is not often used now, because much of the air swallowed goes into the stomach. More efficient injection is accomplished by pressing the tongue against the roof of the mouth so that contact is made between the front of the tongue and the tissue behind the upper, central teeth. The palate elevates reflexively. As tongue contact is then extended backwards, air is compressed in the mouth and forced into the esophagus. This process is facilitated as the speaker learns to relax the tissue at the top of the esophagus. A related method of forcing air into the esophagus involves production of consonants that require oral pressure. With little or no training, laryngectomized persons are able to produce voiceless consonants with air that is in the mouth. Production of sounds such as /p/, /t/, and /k/ tends to compress air and to direct it into the esophagus, thus preparing the speaker for voiced sounds that follow the voiceless plo-

---

the information to the learner. The learner was then given the opportunity to improve performance, and reinforcement was provided in response to success. Stevens, Kalikow, and Willemain (1975) conducted similar work with deaf speakers. However, they used an accelerometer to pick up sound energy at the nose. Presumably the training conducted in each study influenced velopharyngeal closure movements.

sives. This so-called plosive injection contributes to the fluency of esophageal speech in that it helps the speaker to add to the esophageal air supply during conversational speech. Some speakers find that air injection is helped by a sniffing action or inhalation, and injection and inhalation may be used in combination. Early lessons will concentrate on getting air into the esophagus and on the utterance of consonant-vowel combinations or vowels by themselves. Consonants that require buildup of oral air pressure are emphasized in the early work. With progress, longer units involving greater phonetic diversity are worked into the lessons. Specialists in this area emphasize that the speaker should master the first steps before attempting conversation.

The artificial larynx provides an alternative method of speaking for the person who has undergone a laryngectomy (Zwitman and Disinger, 1975). Some of these devices use batteries to set a diaphragm into vibration. If the diaphragm is placed in contact with soft tissue under the chin, it provides a sound source, or alaryngeal voice. Other of these devices consist of tubing and a reed. The tubing is used to direct air from the tracheal stoma past the reed, which is set into vibration, and into the mouth. The vibration provides an alaryngeal voice. Many persons learn to use these devices quickly; however, they do require close attention to articulation and phrasing.

At one time, laryngectomized persons were discouraged from using the artificial larynx unless they had failed to learn esophageal speech. Indeed, it continues to be a common practice to discourage use of the artificial larynx for fear that success will decrease motivation for learning esophageal speech. However, Diedrich and Youngstrom (1966) and others have argued that the artificial larynx should be made available to the patient early. It provides the patient with a method of communication and encourages articulation practice. Many persons have used the artificial larynx while successfully learning esophageal speech.

We often think of laryngeal cancer as a disease that occurs late in life. However, Peterson (1973) described a child who was laryngectomized at 20 months of age because of cancer. Engineers from the Western Electric Bell System in Indianapolis remodeled an electrolarynx to provide a vibrating diaphragm that would fit the child, and Peterson provided the child with esophageal speech training and with training intended to facilitate articulation and expressive language. At the time the patient report was written, the child used a combination of esophageal, electrolaryngeal, and buccal speech to communicate with family and friends. The child had acquired the buccal speech, which does not provide good intelligibility, on his own. It involves trapping air in a cheek and using that air to produce sound "Donald Duck" style.

Surgeons have developed operations that enable laryngectomized persons to use their own pulmonary air to produce voice. This requires either surgical creation of a passageway from the trachea to the pharynx (Zwitman and Calcaterra, 1973a) or coupling a prosthetic device to the trachea and pharynx. These procedures have not been used a great deal and should be considered as experimental.

235

Conclusion

Research directed to the structure and function of the larynx, laryngeal diseases, the voice, and application of behavioral principles to the treatment of voice phenomena has greatly increased our understanding of voice disorders. Much greater use is being made of operational terminology in the consideration of voice phenomena. This in turn makes the assessment of behavioral treatments for voice disorders more manageable. As voice treatments are submitted to scientific tests, the clinician can become increasingly confident in the clinical tools. The clinician can also eliminate the use of practices that prove to have no beneficial effect. The combination of research and careful application of research findings ultimately results in a more precise and hence more effective voice remediation.

This chapter has been introductory in nature. The reader who qualifies for career in speech pathology will, of course, study voice disorders intensively in intermediate and advanced texts and in periodical literature. Recently various instruments have been placed on the market that should help the clinician provide biofeedback to patients about frequency, sound pressure, nasality, and other phenomena. Study of communication disorders is a continuing process both for the student in training and for professionals in the field.

Glossary

Abduction: When used in reference to the larynx, this term pertains to movement of the vocal folds away from midline.

Adduction: When used in reference to the larynx, this term pertains to movement of the vocal folds toward midline.

Aphonia: Loss or absence of voice.

Biofeedback: Use of instrumentation to provide information to a person about ongoing bodily activity.

Dysphonia: A partial loss of voice.

Endocrine: Any of several ductless glands which control growth and other bodily functions.

Endoscope: An instrument for examining the interior of a cavity or canal. The instrument carries light to the structure to be viewed and a lens to send an image back to the eyepiece. Endoscopes may be used with cameras.

Esophageal speech: Production of voice by injecting air into the esophagus and then using it to set tissue at the top of esophagus into vibration.

Hard glottal attack: Forceful approximation of the vocal folds during the initiation of phonation. Hard glottal attack may be one portion of a pattern of hypervalvular phonations.

Hypernasality: Excessive nasal resonance.

Hypervalvular phonation: Use of excessive tension in the larynx during vocal-fold approximation. The closed portion of the vibratory cycle is given an increased amount of time.

Laryngectomee: Colloquial term used to refer to an individual who has had the larynx removed.

Laryngectomy: Surgical removal of the larynx.

Lesion: An alteration of structure or function resulting from disease or injury.

Oscillator: A device for producing sound vibrations.

Otolaryngologist: Physician specializing in disorders of the ear, nose, and throat.

Papilloma: A noncancerous tumor of the larynx; it occurs most frequently in prepubertal children.

Pathology: Disease, injury, or malfunction of a body part.

Pseudoglottis: The tissue that is placed in vibration to produce esophageal or other alaryngeal speech. In esophageal speech, tissue at the junction of the pharynx and esophagus serves as the pseudoglottis. Also termed neoglottis (new glottis).

Radiation therapy: Use of radium or cobalt rays to destroy cancer cells.

Tracheotomy: Surgical creation of an opening, or stoma, in the trachea below the larynx. This procedure is used to allow a person to breath despite an airway obstruction at a higher level.

Virilization: The acquisition of masculine bodily characteristics by a female.

Vital capacity: The maximum volume of air that can be voluntarily exhaled following a maximum inspiration.

Vocal nodule: A buildup of a calluslike layer of tissue on the vocal fold.

Vocal polyp: A tissue enlargement that may be filled with fluid or other matter.

Study Questions

1. Disorders of voice may involve pitch and what other phenomena?
2. Pitch and loudness correspond to what acoustical phenomena?
3. What is meant by the statement that voice quality is a multidimensional phenomena?
4. Contrast vocal-fold movement in breathy and hypervalvular phonation.
5. List four categories of misuse or abuse of the larynx that can result in voice disorder.

6. Describe proper respiratory movements for voice production.

7. What is the effect on voice of paralysis of one or both vocal folds in open position?

8. In what way may benign tumors influence voice? Malignant tumors?

9. In what way may a lack of velopharyngeal closure influence voice?

10. Why is otolaryngological examination of the voice-disorder patient important?

11. Voice evaluation includes consideration of tension in the speaking mechanism, respiratory patterns, and vocal intensity and frequency. Summarize chapter comments on these evaluation procedures.

12. With what degree of precision may a speech pathologist predict future voice usage in a voice-disorder patient?

13. Pushing and chewing exercises are directed to vocal-fold movement patterns at the opposite ends of a continuum. Explain.

14. How may biofeedback devices be used to teach improved use of the larynx in voice production?

15. What variables in addition to voice training may be useful in helping a patient to overcome a voice disorder?

16. How is air injection involved in learning to use esophageal voice?

17. What means of producing voice are available to the laryngectomized person in addition to esophageal voice?

Bibliography

ARONSON, A. E., "Early Motor Unit Disease Masquerading as Psychogenic Breathy Dysphonia: A Clinical Case Presentation," *J. Speech Hearing Dis.* **36** (1971):115–124.

BASMAJIAN, J. V., "Electromyography Comes of Age," *Science* **176** (1972):603–609.

BLAKELEY, R. W., *The Practice of Speech Pathology*, Springfield, Ill.: Charles C. Thomas, 1972.

BLOCH, E. L., AND L. D. GOODSTEIN, "Functional Speech Disorders and Personality," *J. Speech Hearing Dis.* **36** (1971):295–314.

BOONE, DANIEL R., *The Voice and Voice Therapy*, Englewood Cliffs, N.J.: Prentice-Hall, 1971.

BRACKETT, I. P., "Parameters of Voice Quality," in L. E. Travis, ed., *Handbook of Speech Pathology and Audiology*, New York: Appleton-Century-Crofts, 1971.

BRODNITZ, F. S., *Vocal Rehabilitation*, 3rd ed., American Academy of Ophthalmology and Otolaryngology, 1965.

CARNEY, P. J., AND D. SHERMAN, "Severity of Nasality in Three Selected Speech Tasks," *J. Speech Hearing Res.* **14** (1971):396–407.

CHERRY, J., AND S. J. MARGULIES, "Contact Ulcer of the Larynx," *Laryngoscope* **78** (1968): 1937–1940.

CORNUT, G., AND B. PIERUCCI, "Contribution à l'étude de la Paralysie Récurrentielle du Point de Vue Phoniatrique," *J. Franc. ORL* **17** (1968):665–672. Abstracted in *dsh Abstracts* **9** (1969):284.

CRYSTAL, T. H., W. W. MONTGOMERY, C. L. JACKSON, AND N. JOHNSON, *Final Report: Methodology and Results on Laryngeal Disorder Detection Through Speech Analysis*, Vol. I, 1970. Prepared for Public Health Service, Health Services and Mental Health Administration, Regional Medical Programs Service, 5600 Fishers Lane, Rockville, Maryland 20852.

DALY, D. A., AND H. P. JOHNSON, "Instrumental Modification of Hypernasal Voice Quality in Retarded Children: Case Reports," *J. Speech Hearing Dis.* **39** (1974):500–507.

DEAL, R. E., B. MCCLAIN, AND J. F. SUDDERTH, "Identification, Evaluation, Therapy, and Follow-Up for Children with Vocal Nodules in a Public School Setting," *J. Speech Hearing Dis.* **41** (1976):390–397.

DIEDRICH, W. M., AND K. A. YOUNGSTROM, *Alaryngeal Speech*, Springfield, Ill.: Charles C Thomas, 1966.

DRUDGE, M. K. M., AND B. J. PHILIPS, "Shaping Behavior in Voice Therapy," *J. Speech Hearing Dis.* **41** (1976):398–411.

FISHER, H. B., AND J. A. LOGEMANN, "Objective Evaluation of Therapy for Vocal Nodules: A Case Report," *J. Speech Hearing Dis.* **35** (1970):277–285.

GUNDERMANN, H., U. KRONE, AND C. BREMER, "Die Puerile Dysphonie," *Dtschl. Gesundh.-Wes.* **23**, 34 (1968):1610–1612. Abstracted in *dsh Abstracts* **10** (1970):91.

HAGLUND, S., E. KNUTSSON, AND A. MARTENSSON, "An Electromyographic Study of the Vocal and Cricothyroid Muscles in Functional Dysphonia," *Acta Oto-Laryngol.* **77** (1974):140–149.

HESS, D., "A New Experimental Approach to Assessment of Velopharyngeal Adequacy: Nasal Manometric Bleed Testing," *J. Speech and Hearing Dis.* **41** (1976):427–443.

HOLLIEN, H., AND T. SHIPP, "Speaking Fundamental Frequency and Chronologic Age in Males," *J. Speech Hearing Res.* **15** (1972):155–159.

ISSHIKI, N., H. OKAMURA, H. TANABE, AND M. MORIMOTO, "Differential Diagnosis of Hoarseness," *Folia Phoniat.* **21** (1969):9–19.

KIRCHNER, F. R., P. S. TOLEDO, AND D. J. SVOBODA, "Studies of the Larynx after Teflon Injection," *Arch. Otolaryng.* **83** (1966):350–354.

MICHEL, J. F., AND R. WENDAHL, "Correlates of Voice Production," in L. E. Travis, ed., *Handbook of Speech Pathology and Audiology*, New York: Appleton-Century-Crofts, 1971.

MOORE, G. P., *Organic Voice Disorders*, Englewood Cliffs, N.J.: Prentice-Hall, 1971.

——, "Voice Problems Following Limited Surgical Excision," *The Laryngoscope* **85** (1975):619–625.

239

MORRIS, H. L., "The Oral Manometer as a Diagnostic Tool in Clinical Speech Pathology," *J. Speech Hearing Dis.* **31** (1966):362–369.

MURPHY, A. T., *Functional Voice Disorders*, Englewood Cliffs, N.J.: Prentice-Hall, 1964.

MURRAY, T., R. C. BONE, AND C. VON ESSEN, "Changes in Voice Production During Radiotherapy for Laryngeal Cancer," *J. Speech Hearing Dis.* **39** (1974):195–201.

PERKINS, W. H., "Vocal Function: A Behavioral Analysis," in L. E. Travis, ed., *Handbook of Speech Pathology and Audiology*, New York: Appleton-Century-Crofts, 1971.

PETERSON, H. A., A Case Report of Speech and Language Training for a Two-Year-Old Laryngectomized Child," *J. Speech Hearing Dis.* **38** (1973):275–278.

PRUSZEWICZ, A., A. OBREBOWSKI, W. JASSEM, AND H. KUBZDELA, "Marked Acoustic Characteristics in Girls' Virilized Voices," *Folia Phoniat.* **25** (1973):331–341.

SCHWARTZ, M. F., "Acoustic Measures of Nasalization and Nasality," in W. C. Grabb, S. W. Rosenstein, and K. R. Bzoch, eds., *Cleft Lip and Palate*, Boston: Little, Brown, 1971.

SEIDNER, V. W., AND G. LOEWE, "Fitness for Speaking Professions with Allergic Diseases of the Upper Respiratory Tract," *Dtsch. Gesundheitw.* **27** (1972):1913–1915.

SENTURIA, B. H., AND F. B. WILSON, "Otorhinolaryngic Findings in Children with Voice Deviations," *Annals of Otol. Rhinol. Laryngol.* **77** (1968):1027–1041.

SHEARER, W. H., "Diagnosis and Treatment of Voice Disorders in School Children," *J. Speech Hearing Dis.* **37** (1972):215–221.

SILVERMAN, E. M., AND C. H. ZIMMER, "Incidence of Chronic Hoarseness among School-Age Children," *J. Speech Hearing Dis.* **40** (1975):211–215.

STEVENS, K. N., K. N. KALIKOW, AND T. R. WILLEMAIN, "A Miniature Accelerometer for Detecting Glottal Waveforms and Nasalization," *J. Speech Hearing Res.* **18** (1975):594–599.

VASILENKO, Y. S., "Diseases of the Vocal Apparatus in Educators of Kindergartens and Nurseries," *Zh. Ush. Nos. 8. Gorl. Gol.* **4** (1972):21–25.

WARREN, D. W., AND J. L. DEVEREUX, "An Analog Study of Cleft Palate Speech," *Cleft Palate J.* **3** (1966):103–114.

WEINBERG, B., AND J. WESTERHOUSE, "A Study of Pharyngeal Speech," *J. Speech Hearing Dis.* **38** (1973):111–113.

WENDLER, J., "Effect of Ovulation Inhibitors on Cycle-Dependent Fluctuations of Voice Capacity," *Folia Phoniat.* **24** (1972):259–277.

WILLIS, C. R., AND M. L. STUTZ, "The Clinical Use of the Taub Oral Panendoscope in the Observation of Velopharyngeal Function," *J. Speech Hearing Dis.* **37** (1972):495–502.

WILSON, F. B., "The Voice Disordered Child: A Descriptive Approach," *Language, Speech, and Hearing Services in Schools*, No. 4, Washington, D.C.: American Speech and Hearing Assoc., 9030 Old Georgetown Road 20014, n.d.

WINANS, C. S., E. J. REICHBACH, AND W. F. WALDROP, "Esophageal Determinants of Alaryngeal Speech," *Arch. Otolaryngol.* **99** (1974):10–14.

WOLFE, R. D., J. E. OLSON, AND D. B. GOLDENBERG, "Rehabilitation of the Laryngectomee: The Role of the Distal Esophageal Sphincter," *The Laryngoscope* **81** (1971):1971–1978.

YAIRI, E., L. H. CURRIN, AND N. BULIAN, "Incidence of Hoarseness in School Children over a One Year Period," *J. Commun. Disord.* **7** (1974):321–328.

ZWITMAN, D. H., AND T. C. CALCATERRA, "Phonation Using the Tracheo-Esophageal Shunt after Total Laryngectomy," *J. Speech Hearing Dis.* **38** (1973a):369–373.

———, "The 'Silent Cough' Method for Vocal Hyperfunction," *J. Speech Hearing Dis.* **38** (1973b):119–125.

ZWITMAN, D. H., AND R. R. DISINGER, "Experimental Modification of the Western Electric #5 Electrolarynx to a Mouth-Type Instrument," *J. Speech Hearing Dis.* **40** (1975): 35–39.

241

In a literal sense, "disorders of fluency" could refer to several varieties of anomalous speech. In actual usage, however, this designation is most often implicitly understood to refer to stuttering. There are several reasons for this. First, only two fluency disorders—stuttering and cluttering—are evidently "primary" speech disorders. A "primary" speech disorder is an entity, a condition in itself, rather than an aspect of (and therefore secondary to) some other condition. In comparison, anomalies of fluency associated with conditions such as cerebral palsy or Parkinsonism are evidently partial manifestations of these neurologic disorders, which also have other, more dramatic symptoms. In such conditions the fluency anomalies are secondary in nature. Second, stuttering is the most prevalent fluency disorder; it is reported far more frequently than any other speech anomaly of this kind.

The primary disorders of fluency are likely to impress the listener as quite dramatic. They occur relatively infrequently in the general population and are thus something of a curiosity on this ground alone. Usually they are very noticeable because of their prominent and distinctive characteristics. They are evidenced by individuals who otherwise seem

CHAPTER 10
Overview

Disorders of Fluency

quite normal in appearance and actions. Stuttering, in particular, may appear intermittently, and this seeming on-and-off quality is bemusing. In other respects as well they are unique disorders, and they have held a fascination for very many people over a very long time.

Unlike most other disorders of speech, in which there is either a rather well-known cause or a reasonably good suspicion of etiology, the origin of the fluency disorders remains unknown, despite the fact that investigation has been quite extensive. Although a great deal is known about these disorders, they are still not very well understood.

Marcel Wingate, Ph.D.
Washington State University

Introduction

Two major types or patterns of defective speech are recognized as disorders of fluency—**stuttering** and **cluttering.** Each of these disorders has a distinctive appearance which is well characterized by the word used to name it. This point will be developed later in the chapter, in the appropriate sections giving a description of each disorder.

The disorders of fluency are sometimes referred to as disorders of rhythm. The term **fluency** is preferable for several reasons. First, the word "rhythm" indicates a definite regularity of recurrence, such as that found in the "time" or "beat" of music. As applied to speech, "rhythm" would mean that some feature of the spoken language recurs with a definite regularity. Various languages may be described as having recurring patterns in expression, but they do not recur with the regularity suggested by the word "rhythm." Second, it is not at all clear that the speech disorders of the type considered in this chapter are adequately represented as deviations in the recurring pattern of a language, whatever that pattern might be. In contrast, they are appropriately represented as disturbances in the ordinary flow of oral verbal expression.

The word "fluency" is more descriptive and more accurate as the general term for these speech disorders. In fact, whereas "rhythm" refers to many kinds of events that are in no way related to speech, "fluency" is used almost exclusively to refer to speech performance. A typical dictionary definition of fluency emphasizes ease and smoothness of speech. Fluency in speaking one's native language is pretty much taken for granted, since almost everyone meets the implicit standards of fluency. In common usage the word "fluent" is most often used to describe a person's ability to speak a second language. Someone is said to be fluent in a foreign language when she or he is able to speak it with facility, with the expressive skill of the typical native speaker of that language.

The usual speech of most native speakers of a language does seem to flow continuously and smoothly. However, the seeming smoothness and continuity of normal speech is more appearance than reality (Goldman-Eisler, 1968). Ordinary speaking contains various kinds of interruptions in verbal flow, which sometimes occur quite frequently. First, there are the intermittent brief silences, of varying duration, that help to impart meaning in speech. In the written form of language these silences are represented by commas, semicolons, periods, and dashes. These intervals are a normal part of oral language expression and are completely unnoticed unless their duration extends beyond certain implicit criteria of expected duration, that is, if they are too short or too long.

Other aspects of oral expression are more properly considered irregularities in fluency, since they are not actually part of the "grammar" of verbalization. A very common **disfluency,** or **nonfluency,** of this type is the **filled pause,** a sound used to fill what would otherwise be a silent interval in the flow of words. This sound is most often represented as "uh," but it sometimes occurs as "um" or as "er." Most often it indicates that the speaker is searching for a word or a form of expression.

There are other kinds of disfluency that occur in normal speech. Sometimes speakers repeat words or phrases that may contain several words. Occasionally they may repeat part of a word. Not infrequently speakers may change their minds about what they had started to say and will then revise their oral messages, changing certain words already said or those they were about to say.

These are examples of the kinds of "disfluency" that are present in normal "fluent" speech. They are the kind of irregularity in fluency identified as **normal nonfluencies.** Most of the time they are hardly noticed; ordinarily the listener is either sufficiently attentive to the speaker's message to be largely unaware of the disfluencies or discounts them through an implicit recognition of the circumstances that most likely occasioned their occurrence. For instance, the listener may not notice a protracted silent interval or may not "hear" the speaker say "uh" during a pause, realizing that the disfluency reflects a search for an appropriate word or phrase that the speaker momentarily does not recall. Normal fluent speech, then, contains a variety of disfluencies, and it may contain a fair number of them.

Individuals differ to some extent in the frequency with which disfluencies occur in their speech. Ordinarily we are not particularly aware of these individual differences, probably because on the whole the differences are small. We do note the extremes—the mellifluous speaking of the broadcast commentator versus the stumbling speech of someone who "hems and haws"—but these extremes are unusual, which is why they are noticed.

It is important to keep in mind that for any one individual, the amount of disfluency varies from time to time and particularly from situation to situation. There are certain circumstances in which anyone is likely to be more disfluent than usual, e.g., when temporarily confused or overly excited. For most persons it is only under such special conditions that their speech is noticeably disfluent. It is the rare individual whose characteristic speech contains really notable irregularities in fluency. Even with such individuals, however, we are inclined to notice only the more obvious disfluencies—such as excessive use of "uh"—and to overlook less prominent disfluencies—such as revisions. Moreover, speech can be quite disfluent without being considered to be a disorder of fluency.

This implies that it is possible to make a distinction between normal disfluency and abnormal disfluency; thus abnormal disfluency differs in some special way from what is considered to be normal disfluency. This same point was made earlier, in another fashion, in saying that the words "stuttering" and "cluttering" aptly characterize the respective disorders they name. That is, these words denote speech patterns that are sufficiently unique to be distinguishable from each other *and* from normal speech, with such disfluency as it generally contains.

A qualitative distinction between normal and abnormal disfluency has been accepted for centuries. However, in the past 30 years many individuals in the field of speech pathology (essentially within the United States) have adopted the point of view that there is no essential distinction to be made between "normal" and "abnormal" disfluency (Bloodstein, 1970; Johnson et al., 1959, 1967). The basic point of this belief is that all disfluency is on a continuum, ranging from very little to very much. Those who accept this view argue that all speakers are disfluent at one time or another and that what some people wish to call abnormal disfluency is simply a marked degree of disfluency. Interestingly, this argument has been developed in respect to stuttering, but not in regard to cluttering, where it should be equally applicable.

There are several reasons for this belief, but basically it is an expression of a theoretical viewpoint. This is important to note in the study of fluency disorders, since **theory**, such as it is, makes up a substantial part of the subject matter of stuttering and cluttering, especially stuttering.

Chapter 1 discussed the matter of theory and its relevance and value to the sciences of speech and hearing. Theory was identified as an intellectual formulation developed in an effort to explain phenomena. A theory is constructed by relating available factual information with hypothetical concepts, which are the ideas (really the "guesses") of the person formulating the theory. One must keep in mind the "guess" character of these concepts, particularly in simple theories or those in an early stage of development. As mentioned in Chapter 1, early theories tend to be primitive and may be little more than an idea or two stuck onto a few scattered facts.

Theories are supposed to be valuable in providing a frame of reference and guidelines for the development of understanding. Unfortunately, theories may often stultify understanding. Developers and supporters of theories are much inclined to nurture and protect these creations and, in the effort to prevent the construction from crumbling, concern themselves more with the concepts (the guesses) than with the available facts, especially those contradictory to the theory. Certain facts may be shaped to fit, of course, but others may have to be ignored in order to keep a flimsy structure standing.

The student, then, is well advised that the bulk of what has been written and said about the fluency disorders, particularly stuttering, is likely to be heavily saturated with some favored interpretation. A serious problem in the field is that much of what has come to be accepted as "common knowledge" or as essential truth is actually very questionable. Overgeneralization is a common fault; conjecture often has equal status with fact.

The uncertainty, contradiction, and confusion existing in the field of the fluency disorders are principally manufactured, but the disorders themselves have contributed substantially to this condition. They are perplexing disorders, but in that perplexity lies much of their fascination.

Stuttering

Description

There is little doubt that any lay person, unsophisticated in respect to speech disorders, has a pretty good idea of what is meant by the word "stutter" or its derivative forms. This person, who may not be able to specify in a very articulate manner the criteria by which stuttering can be identified, has little reason to doubt his or her unschooled knowledge. The fact that most lay people do know what is meant by stuttering is attested most clearly by evidence that so many can readily give a very convincing imitation of it. It is not until one becomes more sophisticated in the field of speech pathology, and especially in the fluency disorders, that a person may begin to doubt whether he or she can reliably identify stuttering. This is because many broad claims, and a good deal of quibbling, have developed in regard to what disfluency features are distinctive of stuttering. This situation led one authority to remark that "everyone but the experts knows what stuttering is." The implication in this remark is that certain experts have created a problem that should not exist.

Admittedly there are certain problems involved in the accurate identification of some specific instances of stuttering. Fundamentally this results from a lack of adequately refined criteria. The discussion of normal-abnormal in Chapter 1 explained that the designation of what is abnormal depends essentially on our knowledge of what is normal. However, it was also pointed out that this obvious and seemingly simple basis for distinction can be quite elusive to rigorous description and quantification. And so it is with the identification of stuttering; we do not have a refined, specific set of criteria by which we can invariably distinguish, in every specific instance of doubt, between a stutter and a normal disfluency. Unfortunately, little has been done to isolate the significant criteria. Instead, this limitation has been used as support for the argument that stuttering and normal disfluency are continuous and that whatever difference exists between them is only a matter of degree. This is a specific example of how "theory," or a conceptual viewpoint, has profoundly influenced a very basic consideration in stuttering—the matter of its identification.

The problem of identifying refined criteria for making consistent and valid judgments about every questionable disfluency may eventually be resolved, and certainly efforts must be made in that direction. However, there already exist sufficient criteria by which most instances of stuttering can be identified. There is overwhelming direct and indirect evidence that in the final analysis, both lay person and "expert" are able to identify stuttered speech quite reliably and that in their use of the word "stuttering," both are referring to the same basic set of observations.

We can, then, proceed to talk about stuttering with the understanding that in substance everybody knows what everybody else is talking about and that everybody is referring to the same thing. For the present, we can offer a brief description which incorporates those criteria used by most people when speaking of "stuttering." In this description the terms **clonic** and **tonic** will serve as the focus for identification.

The terms "clonic" and "tonic," used originally in 1829 by a French scholar named Serré d'Alais, were widely used in the field for well over a hundred years. Undoubtedly their continued use reflected their appropriateness in referring to unique kinds of disfluency. In very recent times these words have been "phased out" of the professional vocabulary because they are incompatible with the kind of description preferred by the most prevalent current-day belief—particularly the viewpoint that stuttering is simply a degree of disfluency, not a unique type. Actually, however, these terms happen to denote precisely those features which are the crux of the observational basis for agreement among both lay and trained personnel in their identification of stuttering (Wingate, 1962).

Borrowed from neurology, "clonic" and "tonic" are adjectives used to refer to certain kinds of involuntary muscle function. "Clonus," the noun base, means fairly rapid alternating contraction and relaxation in a muscle or muscle set; "tonus" is the root word referring to steady-state contraction. These meanings were originally applied to stuttering in their literal sense and were used for a long time with that connotation. In fact, for a long time the word **spasm** was frequently used jointly with each of these words. The word "spasm," having a clearly obvious suggestion of neurological deviance, was the first of these terms to be dropped. Thereafter, "clonic" and "tonic" were used largely in a descriptive sense, until they too were eliminated.

In reference to stuttering, clonic means the iteration (repetition) of certain simple movements. Quite clearly, the reference is to the repetition of basic speech elements—sounds and syllables, particularly as part-repetitions of a larger unit. The term "tonic" suggests tautness and immobility; in reference to a form of stutter, it means the unintended protraction of a sound or of a silence.

The principal descriptive features of stuttering are: (1) the repetition of basic elements of speech—sounds and syllables, particularly as word fragments; and (2) prolongations of sounds and the unnatural extension of (normally very brief) silent intervals. There are many sources of evidence that these features constitute the basic observational criteria for the identification of stuttering. There is also compelling evidence that these are the criteria that have been used for a very long time by both trained and untrained observers (Wingate, 1962, 1976).

This description of stuttering can be stated more succinctly: Stuttering is characterized by *audible or silent elemental repetitions and prolongations*. These features reflect a temporary inability to move forward to the following sound. Hence stuttering can be most simply described as a "phonetic transition defect" (Wingate, 1969).

Overall, audible elemental repetitions seem to be the most prominent features of stuttering, and it is particularly in reference to them that the word "stut-

249

tering" so aptly denotes the disorder. "Stuttering" has a quality of **onomatopoeia;** the sound of the word resembles what it refers to. Many words in most languages have this quality. Examples from English are: *whir, thunder, rustle, bang. Stutter* has a staccato sound, portraying the most prominent characteristic. Significantly, the words for stuttering in many other languages also have this onomatopoeic quality. In addition, many of these words also have a derivation which suggests the unique features of stuttering. For example, "stutter" is of Germanic origin, meaning "to knock or push." Here, both the iterative and prolonging characteristics are clearly suggested. The French *begaiement* derives from a Flemish word meaning "chattering." The root word in the Russian word for stuttering means "to hiccough." Thus the names for the disorder provide elegantly simple and compelling evidence of its identifying characteristics.

In any particular case of stuttering, one may observe certain features in addition to the speech characteristics. These vary from slight movements—such as a pursing of the lips, flaring of the nostrils, a brief staring—to more gross movements of the face or head and occasionally of other parts of the body. In some cases these accessory features are quite dramatic and readily observed. However, they do not occur uniformly in stuttering and for a number of reasons must be considered to be of secondary significance. The principal and distinguishing features of stuttering are the speech features.

Etiology

Undoubtedly more has been written about etiology in respect to stuttering than for any of the other speech disorders. That is because the etiology of stuttering is unknown. A vast amount of information has accumulated about variables that may be related to stuttering etiology (Eisenson, 1958; Van Riper, 1971), but the cause of stuttering still remains a mystery. This is probably the major source of the fascination the disorder holds; unfortunately, it also has been the source of excessive speculation and facile explanations of its nature and cause.

The wish to explain stuttering has been as persistent as the presumption of understanding it. As noted earlier, much of the seeming complexity, ambiguity, and contradiction are not inherent in the disorder itself, but in the confusion generated by premature efforts to explain it. A substantial amount of what has been written about stuttering, including much that has been published in modern times, is tied to relevant facts in only a very loose manner or is selective in respect to the facts considered. In a majority of instances, one can discern the directing influence of a favored hypothetical preconception. This is clearly exemplified in the number of extant "definitions" of stuttering which ignore the problems involved in clearly identifying the disorder and instead emphasize a statement of etiology (Hahn, 1958). Examples of such definitions are that stuttering is: "an approach-avoidance conflict" or "a fear hysteria." In effect, such so-called definitions divert attention from the fact that stuttering is primarily a speech disorder. Beyond the matter of the speech features, whatever else may be said about stuttering or stutterers is of subsidiary consideration. Stuttering is not discernible as a type of personality, a network of fears, a set of anticipations, a pattern of avoidances, or anything else of this kind. Stuttering is a unique anomaly of oral verbal expression, manifesed by the features discussed earlier, which reflect an evident difficulty in moving through a sequence of speech acts in a normal manner. The source of this difficulty remains unknown.

A knowledge of the history relating to an area of interest is of value to the student in a number of ways. Beyond the simple fact that such material has a certain amount of intrinsic interest, there are the obvious benefits to be derived from knowing what has been done before. When adequately informed, one is better able to appreciate the scope of the problem with which one is faced. Sometimes there are particular benefits of a very immediate nature. For example, in specific reference to stuttering, even a minimal awareness of the history of stuttering should be sufficient to protect one from accepting the claim (which has been made seriously) that stuttering is a product of modern emphasis on the importance of communication.

There is evidence that stuttering has been recognized for ages, at least since many centuries before the Christian era. Egyptian hieroglyphics of approximately 2000 B.C. contain reference to a speech difficulty that must have been stuttering, especially in view of the onomatopoeic translation of the word "nitit." Ancient Biblical passages (circa 760 and 1200 B.C.) mention a kind of speech disturbance in words that call for translation as "stuttering."

Figures famous in the history of intellectual inquiry and science have contemplated the disorder and attempted to explain it. In ancient times it was discussed by Herodotus, Hippocrates, Aristotle, and Galen. The writings of Aristotle (384–322 B.C.) are of special interest in that his discussion of stuttering includes a descriptive identification of it as "an inability to join one syllable to another sufficiently quickly" (Aristotle; Forrester, 1947). This succinct description is very much like "phonetic transition defect."

Understandably, records of stuttering are few and scattered during the Dark and Middle Ages, but they reappeared with the growth of the Renaissance and thereafter occurred with increasing frequency. Again, famous names were associated with the inquiry into the nature and treatment of stuttering—for example, Mercurialis, Lord Bacon, Hartley, Erasmus, Darwin, Magendie, and Alexander Bell. Interest in stuttering expanded greatly during the nineteenth century, in association with developments in science and medicine. During this period many explanations of the nature of the disorder were advanced, and many different forms of treatment were undertaken, including surgery, suggestion, moral suasion, exercises of many different kinds, habit training, use of appliances, and special regimens of one kind or another involving diet and exercises. Unfortunately, most of the investigation was undertaken without sufficient rigor, objectivity, and care, and the results reported have to be assessed with considerable qualification. Still, there is a great deal to be learned from what is recorded about stuttering during that time.

Interest in stuttering continued to develop actively in the twentieth century. The extent of this interest is best reflected in the fact that since the establishment of the American Speech and Hearing Association in the late 1920s, its journals (described in Chapter 6) have published proportionately more articles on stuttering than any other category of speech defect. In addition, articles on stuttering have appeared regularly in a number of other journals in related fields.

Investigations of stuttering have become proportionately more scientific, following the course of events in other areas of inquiry, particularly those which have come to be known as the behavioral sciences. Even so, a review (Sortini, 1955) of relevant professional journal sources over a 20-year period between 1930 and 1950 revealed that well over half of the published articles on stuttering were not experimental in nature; the writing was still predominantly of the type produced in earlier times.

There are tides of interests and preoccupations which find expression in many areas of human endeavor. Certain areas of science—especially those less closely tied to physical reality—are also subject to fashion and fad. The course of experimental study of stuttering in this century shows patterns of change in focus of interest. In a summary of these events we cannot expect to portray adequately the actual shifts in interest, yet an overview is sufficient to reveal the major trends (Diehl, 1958).

Early investigation was concerned largely with respiratory function in stutterers. Overlapping this was a longer-lasting era in which attempts were made to investigate neurophysiological factors in the disorder. During this time there was a relatively brief interval of exploration of the genetics of stuttering. Then came a period of inquiry into matters of cerebral dominance and laterality. Eventually, by the early 1940s, the focus had shifted heavily to the study of the psychology of stuttering. In the early years of this period some brief attention was directed to linguistic variables in stuttering, viewed essentially from a psychological point of view. This interest waned, then recurred briefly a few years ago, probably as an influence of the developing fields of linguistics and psycholinguistics. However, the major preoccupations of the psychological epoch have been with explaining stuttering as a personality problem or as "learned behavior." During a long phase the dominant emphasis was on personality variables (Goodstein, 1958; Hahn, 1958; Murphy and Fitzsimmons, 1960; Sheehan, 1970). Gradually the emphasis shifted to a preoccupation with the notion that stuttering is learned. In recent years this focus has been expressed in efforts to fit stuttering into the scheme afforded by "operant" notions of learning (Brutten and Shoemaker, 1967; Goldiamond, 1965; Gray and England, 1969; Gregory, 1968; Johnson et al., 1959, 1967; Shames and Egolf, 1976; Shames and Sherrick, 1963; Van Riper, 1971; Wischner, 1950).

Although a focus on stuttering as a psychological problem is the latest effort in the chronological sense of an era, it is not "the latest" in the sense of conceptual development. Unfortunately, too much of the recent literature conveys the impression that the idea of stuttering as "learned behavior" is something new. Actually, the notion of stuttering as "habit" emerged no later than the eighteenth century. And the inference that stuttering is a personality, or emotional, problem is undoubtedly the all-time favorite explanation.

Both of these guesses have their origin and foundation in certain observations made about stuttering. First, many stutterers report and evidence situational variability in the occurrence of their stuttering; they tend to stutter more when they feel stress or pressure and less when they feel relaxed. This is not always the case, but it is reported and observed sufficiently often that the correlation between the two events has been impressive. A second apparently persuasive observation has been that stutterers differ in the gross pattern of their stutter. A third contributing observation is that stuttering is modifiable through conscious processes; that is, some stutterers, at least, can learn to control their stuttering (with or without the aid of a clinician). Although these three observations do not *indicate* that stuttering is a psychologically based disorder, they permit that interpretation.

There is a fourth item which, even though it is not an observation about actual stuttering, undoubtedly has had an influence on the development of ideas of stuttering as a psychological problem, especially the notion that it is learned. This is the fact that stuttering can be intentionally imitated quite convincingly; and anyone can do it. It seems very likely that the prevalent awareness of this fact has suggested, perhaps implicitly, that since the copy so well resembles the real thing, the two must therefore be constructed in the same way. Such analogizing does not carry very far. Anyone who is knowledgeable about cerebral palsy, Parkinsonism, petit mal seizures, or catatonia can produce a convincing imitation of these disorders, yet no one would seriously make much of such apparent similarities.

The notion of stuttering as a psychological problem still rests predominantly on inference and hypothesis. Many of the observations about stuttering, such as those mentioned above, have been woven into patterns of inference which are then presented as adequate explanations of the disorder. However, the value of the basic observations is not increased by such elaborations. For instance, the fact that stuttering occurrence shows some relationship to emotional arousal is simply a finding of partial cooccurrence. It does not indicate that stuttering is an emotional problem, no matter how this relationship is manipulated in conjecture. The cooccurrence must eventually be taken into account in a comprehensive and adequate explanation of stuttering, but the answer is not supplied ready-made in the observation.

Appropriate criticisms of these matters cannot be adequately developed in the limited space available here. In particular, it is not possible to present even an adequate summary of criticisms, reservations, and contradictions relevant to the notion that stuttering is learned; the only alternative is to say simply that the whole superstructure of that conception is balanced on inference and analogy. However, it is feasible to call attention to evidence that very powerfully contradicts the idea that stuttering is a personality problem, since this can be done briefly. At the same time it provides another fact about stuttering.

Views of stuttering as a personality disturbance conceive the observable features of stuttering as "symptoms" that are supposed to be only the surface expression of some underlying, more-or-less covert problem within the individual's psyche or personality. The dimensions of this presumed underlying problem may vary somewhat, depending on the particular version of this kind of theory, but the essential supposition is that there is a common personality type, a personality organization with a typical set of inner "dynamics," a unique pattern of conflicts and modes of adjustment to these conflicts.

A somewhat different view hypothesizes personality problems of stutterers as related to conditions surrounding the development of their stuttering and their reactions to it. From this frame of reference too one should expect to find unique personality characteristics common to stutterers.

Both hypotheses are contradicted by the evidence. A great deal of research has been addressed to the investigation of stuttering as a personality problem, but the findings provide little encouragement for continuing to think of stuttering in any such terms. Careful analysis of extensive research covering a period of over 40 years fails to yield any consistent evidence that stutterers, either as children or adults, have any particular personality pattern or that they are neurotic or even particularly maladjusted. In fact, personality assessments have quite regularly found stutterers to be psychologically more like normal persons than like psychiatric patients (Goodstein, 1958; Sheehan, 1958). The negative findings are especially significant when considered in light of the fact that many of the assessment measures used in these investigations have otherwise been used successfully to distinguish between groups of persons with significant personality problems.

Fear is the emotion most often linked conceptually with stuttering, usually in the sense of fear of stuttering, either in a kind of global sense or as a fear of stuttering in certain situations or "on" certain words or sounds (Brutten and Shoemaker, 1967; Johnson et al., 1967; Van Riper, 1971, 1973). In many writings the claim of stutterers' fears occupies a central position. But there is very good reason to contend that this claim also has been heavily overdone. First, the evidence about fears has come primarily from testimony—and selected testimony at that. Although the literature carries the clear implication that fears are a routine part of stuttering, we have no idea what proportion of stutterers would spontaneously report having such fears.

Statements made about fears come from older stutterers, and it is quite inappropriate to accept their claims as applicable to youngsters, who, after all, do most of the stuttering (Van Riper, 1971, Chapters 1 and 3). Also, we do not see all stutterers, even older ones. Some of them never come to the attention of a speech pathologist, and one of the reasons for this is that their stuttering really doesn't bother them that much. Further, some stutterers who do come for help nevertheless do not fear their stuttering. They may find it annoying, embarrassing, inconvenient, or in some way limiting, but it is not something they fear. Additionally, among those who do mention fear, the extent and nature of the fear vary a good deal. Most often, it seems, these stutterers speak of fears in respect to certain situations; they report being afraid they might stutter in (any number of) situations where they might be sensitive about it, with a reaction ranging from mild embarrassment to mortification. Some stutterers are concerned about a wider range of situations than others. Occasional stutterers do indeed feel this way about very many situations, but this extensive reaction is not common. Certainly one should not be led to believe that the typical stutterer lives in cringing apprehension of stuttering (Wingate, 1976, Chapter 3).

The situational fluctuation of stuttering is one of the interesting observations about the disorder. This would seem to reflect emotional factors, and quite expectedly everyone has interpreted it in this light. But emotion does not automatically produce stuttering; there is some kind of intermediating mechanism that in certain people transduces the aroused emotion into the incoordinations expressed as stuttering.

Although it seems reasonably clear that some stutterers tend to stutter more in some situations than in others, there is still reason to question whether stuttering varies with the situation as much as has been claimed. For instance, it is often stated that in contrast to speaking in "social" circumstances, stutterers do not stutter while speaking when alone. This is a fallacy; it has derived from a naively literal acceptance of stutterers' self-reports. Evidence from several sources of research (Wingate, 1976) reveals that stutterers are not really very aware of many of their stutterings. Most of the individuals studied did stutter when alone, but did not realize it.

Variables

So far, discussion has been directed mainly at an overview of stuttering. In the process of identifying some of the considerable problems extant in the field, certain important facts about stuttering have been brought into focus. In the remainder of this chapter, attention will be directed primarily to some important facts about stuttering. However, in certain cases where an issue is clear, comment on its relevance to the problems in the field will be added.

Age As indicated earlier, most stutterers are children. Stuttering is predominantly a disorder of early childhood. Several sources indicate that approximately 85 percent of cases of stuttering begin well before age five, and most of the remainder before age seven. Although stuttering onset in a small percentage of cases is reported after this age, it is rare to find report of onset after puberty—and such reports are considered questionable (Van Riper, 1971; Wingate, 1976). A claim of stuttering beginning in adulthood, even under such potentially "believable" circumstances as the stress of war experiences, is always suspect. All reports of postpubertal onset carry the suspicion that they are actually precipitated recurrences of earlier stuttering that remitted.

Stuttering is a disorder of childhood not only in the sense that it begins in the early years of life, but also that it is most prevalent during these years. There is substantial evidence that over 40 percent of the youngsters identified as stuttering before five years of age will no longer be stuttering by the time they are about eight years old (Wingate, 1976). Information about remission after age eight is less securely based, but there is ample evidence that recovery from stuttering continues to occur long after age eight (Wingate, 1976). Stuttering remission is an area that deserves much further exploration.

The matter of stuttering remission provides a good example of the stultifying influences of theory in stuttering. The preferred explanations of stuttering, influential for the past 40 years, have conceived of stuttering as a disorder that develops, meaning that it gets worse. Such schemes have chronically omitted readily accessible data showing that stuttering gets better (Wingate, 1976). In particular, they have ignored facts giving evidence of spontaneous remission, that is, that stuttering gets better without therapy. In fact, the occasionally voiced suggestion that some children "outgrow" their stuttering has been vigorously repudiated within the profession. Yet as the facts stand, there is no more reasonable way to account for spontaneous remission than to assume that it reflects changes in the physiology of the growing child.

The notion of the "development" of stuttering is also contradicted by the fact that in the majority of cases in which stuttering persists, it either shows some improvement or remains pretty much the same. There is very adequate evidence to document this (Wingate, 1976); however, it is not necessary to introduce it here. One need simply consider that if stuttering does "develop," at least all adult stutterers should be severe stutterers, and this is certainly not the case.

The presently available estimates of stuttering incidence in the total population are affected by the matter of remission, since the various estimates have been "cross-sectional," based on the number of stutterers counted at some particular time. Most of the estimates made in the United States are based on samples from school-age populations, predominantly grade-school children. This age range of six to fourteen excludes the preschool ages, when most onset and some remission occurs. However, these different estimates agree quite well with one another and, taken at face value, indicate that stuttering will be found in slightly over one percent of the population (Van Riper, 1971).

Culture   Estimates of stuttering incidence have been made in many other nations and cultures, including some "primitive" ones. Always, in such appraisals there are problems about the adequacy of the population samples. However, it is curiously interesting to find that although these incidence estimates show some slight differences, they are all in the neighborhood of one percent. The fact that incidence estimates from so many different cultures cluster around the same value strongly suggests that cultural differences have little to do with the generation of stuttering.

Number   In any large population, such as that of the United States, a percentage figure of one percent represents a considerable number of individuals. This means that there are many persons who stutter and who are presumably in need of some kind of help. At the same time, it should be recognized that one percent is quite a tiny fraction. One is almost forced to acknowledge that whatever the agents that generate stuttering, they do not have a very extensive influence on the human species. Surely one should be led to wonder why stuttering occurs in only about one person in every hundred (or somewhat higher, if only youngsters are to be considered). Particularly if stuttering is due to psychological pressures, which are themselves held to be quite prevalent in a culture, one could very well expect that proportionately many more individuals should be affected with stuttering.

Sex   Stuttering is found much more frequently in males than in females. A best estimate, derived from several sources, would indicate a ratio of four males for every female (Van Riper, 1971). There is some indication that the ratio increases with age; thus there are many more adult male than adult female stutterers. This is consistent with clinical experience. However, the values regarding changes in sex ratio as a function of age have not been worked out very well. Nonetheless, at all ages there are more stutterers among males than among females.

As might be expected, efforts have been made to account for this impressive sex difference in terms of environmental influences that are purported to bear differently on boys than on girls. The typical attempt at explanation claims, of course, that boys are subject to more deleterious pressure of one kind or another than are girls (Schuell, 1946, 1947). Such accounts should raise the question of why there are not, then, even more stuttering boys. In many ways these explanatory efforts are unimpressive. Actually, the evidence indicates that stuttering is somehow related to *physiological* sex, i.e., maleness as contrasted to femaleness, rather than to sex-associated patterns of adjustment and behavior identifiable as masculinity versus femininity. Also, although male and female roles, attitudes, and behaviors differ widely in various cultures, stuttering predominates among males in all of the different cultures studied. This is further evidence of the connection between stuttering and maleness and, as well, its independence of culture.

Heredity   There is compelling evidence of a hereditary factor in stuttering. A great deal of research has indicated consistently that stuttering tends to "run in families." That is, one is much more likely to find other stutterers in the immediate family or family history of a stutterer than of someone who does not stutter (Van Riper, 1971). This does not necessarily mean that all cases of stuttering are determined by heredity; a hereditary factor may seem less likely if a family history of stuttering is not apparent. However, there is good reason to suspect that a substantial majority of cases of stuttering do involve a hereditary component. The appearance of stuttering through generations follows patterns similar to phenomena known to be the expression of hereditary factors—such as appearing in only certain progeny of any particular generation or skipping generations.

The actual extent of hereditary involvement in stuttering is unknown, and the mechanism of transmission has not yet been determined. In short, it is not known whether the genetic agency might be sex-linked, recessive in nature, or conditioned by other genetic action. Much important work remains to be done in this area. As noted earlier, the genetics of stuttering has not been an attractive direction of investigation in this country for some 30 years.

Incidentally, this topic is another instance of the confounding intrusion of theory. The need to explain stuttering in terms of environmental forces has led to the explanation that the tendency for stuttering to recur in family histories is due to imitation, or to anxiety about fluency that is passed from generation to generation. Such explanations cannot credibly accommodate certain clear facts about the pattern of familial occurrence of stuttering. For instance, the observation that stuttering skips generations and also occurs only in certain individuals of any particular generation.

Intelligence   It has often been said that stutterers have above-average intelligence. The sources of this claim are obscure—and biased, for the claim is erroneous. Certainly many stutterers are of above-average intelligence. In fact, thousands of stutterers are college graduates (which presumes above-average intelligence), and many stutterers are to be found in responsible positions in various occupations and professions. Moreover, quite a few outstanding historical figures were stutterers: Charles Lamb; Charles Darwin; the Tudor kings Charles I, Edward VI, and George VI; Aneurin Bevan; Somerset Maugham. But all this presents a very misleading picture. If one looks at the overall picture of the correlation between stuttering and level of intelligence, one finds more stuttering among individuals who are of below-average intelligence. A higher incidence of stuttering is found among children in special-education classes than in regular classes, and there is a very high incidence of stuttering in the mentally retarded (Schlanger, 1953; Schlanger and Gottsleben, 1957). A particularly high stuttering incidence is reported among Mongoloids (Van Riper, 1971). Interestingly, mongolism is now known to have a genetic base.

There are other facts about stuttering which must be taken into account in arriving at an adequate understanding of the disorder and the development of effective means of management. However, appropriate treatment of this material would take us far beyond the scope of an introductory exposure to the field.

Evaluation

There are no tests for stuttering; evaluation is entirely a matter of observation, inquiry, and judgment. The evaluation of stuttering will vary somewhat, depending on the point of view of the person conducting the evaluation. It is not feasible to outline each evaluation format that would be used by representatives of the different viewpoints. However, in overview it can be said that evaluation should include: (1) an adequate appraisal of the symptoms; (2) a history of the problem in the individual; and (3) inquiry into the person's attitude toward the problem.

An adequate description is necessary, of course, in order to specify that the presenting problem is stuttering. Most often a potential difficulty in diagnosis arises only with respect to very young children. Some youngsters tend to speak in a manner that is quite disfluent without, however, constituting a fluency disorder. In contrast, the relatively few disfluencies of certain other children may contain considerable stutterings. Making a distinction between normal and disordered fluency from the pattern of a speech sample is not as difficult as it has been made out to be. In most instances the issue can be resolved through the use of the proper criteria, identified earlier (elemental repetitions and prolongations). It is as important not to misdiagnose normal disfluency as it is to misdiagnose stuttering.

In the case of older stutterers, there is additional reason why adequate description of the symptoms is important. It is surprising how often stutterers are only vaguely aware of the features of their stuttering. They can report gross aspects, such as "getting stuck," but are not able to readily identify many particulars of the stuttering episodes. Specification of the stuttering pattern, in evaluation, is particularly valuable for therapy approaches that work on changing the form of the stutter.

In all cases it is important to obtain history data relative to the course of stuttering and to circumstances and events reportedly associated with changes in the frequency and extent of its occurrence. This information can be of considerable value in management, both indirectly through advice given the parents and directly in therapy with the individual. One is also interested in information about reported onset, although the material must be weighed very judiciously, to avoid the temptation to look so intently for a definitive cause for the disorder that one finds it through the conduct of the inquiry or accepts it from the informant's statement.

The attitude toward the problem maintained by the stutterer and, in the case of children, by the parents can well have a significant influence on the conduct of therapy and the anticipation of its outcome. Stutterers, and parents of stutterers, react in various ways to the disorder, and these variations should occasion different procedures of management.

Management

As might be expected, the management of stuttering varies, depending on the viewpoint maintained by the practitioner. Again, here we can present only a summary statement about this aspect of the problem.

Management procedures for stuttering can be classified as psychotherapeutic or instructional. "Psychotherapeutic" covers a wide range of psychological approaches to the problem. On one hand are what can be called the "purely" psychotherapeutic approaches; the therapy attempts to deal with the conflicts presumed to underlie, and cause, the stuttering. In such approaches the actual stuttering receives only incidental attention. The manner of stuttering, the focus of its occurrence, and variation in frequency are of interest only in the sense that such variables might reveal something about the pattern of conflicts from which they are assumed to originate. Accordingly, the symptoms of stuttering, and even some of the expressed feelings about it, are considered superficial. Resolution of the problem, it is contended, must get to the "real" problem underneath. The conception of this "real" problem varies, although, of course, it always has to do with emotional conflicts of some kind. This form of therapy for stuttering has not been very successful.

Another kind of psychotherapy is tied more closely to the actuality of stuttering. This type of approach attempts to deal with those negative attitudes, feelings, and reactions the individual may have about stuttering and any attendant problems. Psychotherapy of this form also endeavors to alleviate handicapping self-images the individual may have, independent of the matter of the stutter. Some clinicians employ this form of therapy as an independent, or sole, approach to the management of stuttering. More often, however, it is incorporated with an instructional approach to therapy.

The most widely employed approaches to the treatment of stuttering deal directly with the process of speaking. Within the "instructional" classification one can identify three separate forms of therapy. One of these forms is distinct from the other two in that an attempt is made to induce the individual to speak without stuttering. This may be accomplished in several ways, of which the two most immediately effective are: (1) training the person to speak to a rhythm; and (2) inducing the stutterer to decrease speech rate, either by direction of the therapist or with the use of some mechanical device, such as a metronome. Certain methods in this approach have a long and unfortunately notorious history. On the whole, they are rather soundly repudiated within the profession. The remainder of such methods have a dubious status. However, there has been a recent resurgence in the use of these methods; it must be admitted that their value has yet to be assessed judiciously.

The other two forms of the instructional approach attempt to modify stuttering by dealing directly with the stuttering. One of these forms has been for some time the approach to stuttering therapy most widely employed in the United States. Essentially it consists first of training the stutterer to identify what is happening during an instance of stuttering and then teaching the person ways of gradually modifying these acts. The objective is to teach the stutterer not only to speak with less stuttering, but also to effectively control those stutters that may continue to occur. As noted above, the attitudinal form of psychotherapy is usually incorporated into this approach. Many stutterers have evidently received considerable benefit from this treatment form. However, its overall comparative efficacy is unknown.

The remaining form of the instructional approach to dealing with stuttering is the "operant" method. This recently developed technique is an imitation of the training methodology employed in the psychological laboratory. The focus on stuttering is much more specific than in the former method. The stutterer's speech is monitored carefully, and each instance of stutter is followed immediately by some "consequence." These consequences, such as a clinician saying "no" or "wrong" or a brief period of enforced silence, or even a slight shock, are assumed to have a punishing effect. The presumption in this method is that stuttering is a "response" which can be manipulated through consequences it elicits. Exciting claims of the efficacy of this method have been made, but overall the results are suspect because they have not been analyzed with sufficient care.

Cluttering

The section on cluttering will be shorter than the section on stuttering, because there is a narrower base of subject matter from which to present a discussion of this disorder. Cluttering is much less prevalent than stuttering, even though it too has been recognized as a disorder for centuries. Judging from the frequency with which such cases are reported in the literature and professional exchange within the United States, cluttering would actually seem to be rather rare.

The problem has received more attention from European writers, who suggest that cluttering is at least as prevalent as stuttering. However, there are no formal studies of incidence to support this claim. Many authors who write on the subject contend that the prevalence of cluttering is obscured because individuals with this problem are not inclined to seek help voluntarily. However, one could reasonably expect that persons with such a notably distinct speech disorder would quite regularly be referred for evaluation by someone else. In particular, one could expect that at least in school systems such as those typical in the United States, where most children are screened for even less dramatic speech deviations, cases of cluttering would be brought to the attention of someone knowledgeable in the field of speech pathology. Actually, it is difficult to understand how the majority of such cases would escape attention even in school systems having speech remediation programs less well developed than those in America.

Developing a satisfactory general statement about cluttering is also limited by the fact that most of the literature consists largely of case reports. Further, the formal studies that have been undertaken generally have not been done carefully. Therefore, the following discussion will deal essentially with those aspects of the disorder which are mentioned repeatedly in different sources.

Description

The accepted modern technical synonyms for cluttering—**tachylalia** or **tachyphemia,** meaning "fast speech"—identify what is evidently the cardinal feature of this fluency disorder, namely, excessive rate. However, this fast rate is not continuous; the rapid speech comes in "bursts," interspersed with filled or unfilled pauses, interjections, and sometimes with words or phrases in which speech is actually rather protracted. Additionally, a typical feature of the high-rate bursts is that they seem to be initiated with excessive vigor, adding to the overall impression of haste.

Several other features contribute to the typical configuration of this disorder and add to the character so well suggested by the vernacular term "cluttering." These other features are excessive **elision** and omission and transposition of sounds and sometimes syllables. "Elision" means that certain sounds have been slighted in articulation or melded with the sound that follows. Elision is a fairly common feature of normal speech, where it is limited to certain words and expressions that are very familiar and frequently used. For instance, the articles "a" and "the" are usually reduced in connected speech and combined with the succeeding word, e.g., "uhboy" and "thuhboy." When said as a routine form of greeting, "How are you?" is most often produced as "Huhwaryuh?" However, when this kind of reduction and compression are not limited to very familiar words and expressions—which is the case in cluttering—the intelligibility of speech is sharply reduced.

The matter of omission of sounds and syllables needs no explication. "Transposition" of sounds and syllables means that these word elements may be interchanged between different syllables of a word or between words near each other in the speech sequence. Thus "fingertips" is said as "tingerfips," "many Americans" is said as "merry amenicans," and so on. Errors of this kind also occur occasionally in normal speech; in cluttering they happen frequently.

The combination of irregular but predominantly rapid rate, elisions, omissions, and transpositions constitutes a speech pattern distinctively different from the apparent flow and smoothness of normal speech; it sounds "cluttered."

Etiology and Related Variables

The cause of cluttering is unknown, but all writers agree that cluttering must be an organically based condition—a disorder reflecting some integrative anomaly of the central nervous system (Arnold, 1960; Moolenaar-Bijl, 1948; Weiss, 1964). This underlying condition is thought to be constitutional rather than due to some injury or illness, meaning that the individual is born with at least a predisposition to develop the disorder. In view of certain highly suggestive lines of evidence, the condition is believed to be genetic, i.e., inherited.

The nature of this underlying condition is, of course, unknown. There is some reason to think that it might be a kind of defect in the timing for oral expression of speech, in that the impulsion to speak at a rate beyond capability appears to be such a central feature. It might be thought, for instance, that the elisions, omissions, and transpositions are occasioned largely by the excessive rate, inasmuch as speech quality improves when the clutterer is required to slow down. However, most writers believe that the deviances in cluttering are caused by factors beyond the impulsion to speak rapidly. In fact, the claim is frequently made that anomalies of verbal formulation are a regular, though of course less obvious, characteristic of cluttering.

The speech pattern of cluttering is believed to be only one manifestation of a general condition that affects various capacities related to language processes. This broad condition, variously named by different authors, is conceived as a general language disability evidenced in a number of seemingly separate psychological functions, most of which are closely related to language reception and expression. Other problems most frequently mentioned as related manifestations of the hypothesized underlying condition are the following.

1. *Subnormal musical ability*, which is said to be integral with a general facility in language manipulation (Weiss, 1964) and of particular relevance to the adequate development and expression of **prosodic** features of language (such as proper phrasing, intonation, pitch change);

2. *Poor auditory memory*, which is presumed to underlie inefficient regulation of speech, thus leading to confusion in expression;

3. *Defects of concentration and attention span*, which are believed to be necessary to the proper integration of thought processes, also said to be disturbed in clutterers;

4. *Reading and writing problems,* which are viewed as direct expressions of the alleged central deficiency manifested in other dimensions of organized language function.

It should be clearly understood that these problems are not found regularly in clutterers. That much is acknowledged in the literature. More important, it is impossible to make any judgment about either the frequency with which such problems do occur in conjunction with cluttering or the extent of the involvement when it is reported. The reason for this is that so many reports of the existence of such problems do not make clear how these problems were assessed. Careful reading of much of this material forces one to conclude that much of the evaluation was not done adequately.

There are other seemingly related problems mentioned by certain authors as being part of the overall symptom complex, or generalized condition, to which cluttering is thought to be related. These other matters will be omitted from the present discussion not only because of their uncertain status, but also because they do not further illuminate the conception surrounding the issue of cluttering etiology.

Certain authors relate stuttering to cluttering. Some view the two disorders as variants having a common base; others see cluttering as the basic dysfunction out of which stuttering develops. Both viewpoints are essentially conjectural. Actually, the similarity between stuttering and cluttering is presently limited to the fact that explanations for both disorders contain liberal amounts of overgeneralization and the mixing of fact with assumption and guess.

Evaluation

As in the case of stuttering, there are no particular tests appropriate to the diagnosis of cluttering. The essential procedure is observation and judgment based on an adequate sample of the patient's speech. The essential criteria for identification of the disorder are the descriptive features of the disorder.

Some authors emphasize the appropriateness of a neurologic examination to assist in differential diagnosis. They point out that certain kinds of central nervous system disease or injury occasion symptoms of accelerated speech rate. It is also suggested that some cases of dysarthria may occasionally present something of a differential diagnostic problem.

Some writers believe there may occasionally be problems in diagnostic differentiation from stuttering. This concern would seem to be most justifiable for advocates of the view that stuttering evolves from cluttering. Some sources present a list of "signs," other than the speech symptoms, that are purported to be useful in differentiating stuttering from cluttering. Unhappily, these signs are based predominantly on highly questionable "facts" about each disorder.

Actually, there should not often be any particular problem in discriminating the two disorders, in view of the distinctive characteristics of each. As a matter of fact, a number of cases have been reported in which both disorders were manifested by the same individual.

Although evaluation of functions other than speech are evidently not necessary for diagnostic purposes, many writers would undoubtedly contend that other kinds of assessment—for example, of reading and writing skills—should be included in the evaluation for purposes of helping the individual in adjustments beyond that of speech rehabilitation.

Management

The bulk of treatment for cluttering is direct, i.e., working at modifying the speech disorder. As might be expected, the major thrust of treatment is to reduce speech rate. It is found quite routinely that simply reducing speech rate to a level within the patient's capability effects a concurrent improvement in most other aspects of speech. However, helping the clutterer to develop a more appropriate rate requires more than working on rate alone. To this end many other direct techniques are employed, e.g., speaking to rhythm; reading aloud, both in unison with the clinician and alone; exercises in phrasing; **tone support** and **projection; kinesthetic monitoring.** It should be noted that although the treatment approach might seem to focus on elimination of the characteristics of the disorder, the overall procedure actually emphasizes what are really regular processes of normal good speech.

Case Histories

The following material presents two sample cases. Sample cases hardly ever fully illustrate the category they are selected to exemplify; rather, they are simply more or less representative. The first case is a ten-year-old boy who stutters. His case was selected because in matters relative to the boy's attitude and overall adjustment, he is quite representative of many youngsters I have seen. The second sample is of a 27-year-old man whose major fluency problem is cluttering. He was selected because his was the most interesting case of the few available to report as a sample of cluttering. As mentioned in the body of the chapter, cases of cluttering are evidently rather rare.

Case Example 1

Robert was brought to the clinic with a complaint of stuttering. He was a very friendly, personable youngster and conversed readily about his activities and interests. He tended to speak quite rapidly, with frequent instances of stuttering manifested predominantly in silent and audible prolongations, with occasional sound repetitions and use of the verbal feature "I mean." Quite often his prolongations were accompanied by an exaggerated opening of the mouth and a rolling upward of the eyes.

Robert talked freely about his stuttering. He reported being aware of many of his stuttering instances, and he was able to describe the essential character of his accessory features—opening his mouth wider and moving his eyes in an effort to force the sound out. When requested to speak more slowly and to move easily through a block, he was able to speak with considerably less stuttering and essentially no accessory movement. However, he rather quickly reverted to his rapid rate of speech, with the attendant increased instances in stuttering. Consistent with this observation that Robert is able to control his speech more effectively, his father reported that a couple of months ago the boy had improved his speech considerably for a period of a week or so when promised a weekend trip as a reward for doing so. Although his speech was then not completely fluent, it was markedly improved in that stuttering occurred much less frequently and without the accessory symptoms.

Although the parents indicated that Robert started to stutter a year or so ago, a letter from the boy's pediatrician mentioned that the youngster had stuttered as long as the physician had known him, about six years. Evidently the parents were referring primarily to the more dramatic features of Robert's stuttering, saying that this had been more evident as of a year or so ago. All of the children in this family have stuttered for certain periods of time during development, but the rest of them outgrew it. There is a history of stuttering on the father's side of the family.

Robert is described as a fine boy who evidences no particular problems in behavior or adjustment. He gets along well with others and is well liked. His stuttering does not seem to have created any particular problems for him. Although he apparently regards it as a nuisance at times, he does not find it to interfere significantly in his activities at school or socially. At the same time, he is interested in doing something about improving his fluency.

The parents have become concerned because his stuttering has persisted and because they were told that the stuttering would become irreversible after the eighth or ninth grade. They were advised that this is not true, that the success of therapy depends on awareness and motivation of the patient and that in some respects there are advantages to therapy at a later age. It was emphasized to them that Robert already has some useful techniques which he is able to apply to reduce the extent and severity of his stuttering and that he should be encouraged to continue their use in a consistent and diligent fashion. Speech therapy was recommended as a means of assisting and expanding the use of such techniques.

Case Example 2

The second case is presented as a sample of cluttering. This patient does not represent a "pure" case of cluttering, although this is certainly the predominant problem.

This patient was referred for attention to a speech problem described as stuttering. He was referred by the case worker from the local Family Counseling Service, where the patient and his wife have recently been accepted for counseling in regard to problems in marital adjustment. The patient, aged 27, has been married about a year and a half.

The patient was friendly, personable, and responsive, but restless and nervous, as evidenced in a good deal of body movement and quick laughter. At the same time, he did not appear to be psychologically uncomfortable, and he acknowledged that he felt reasonably at ease in this situation.

The patient's speech was characterized by a rapid rate with much imprecise articulation, sound elisions, and omissions. Phrasing was jerky and irregular. He evidenced frequent repetitions of sounds, syllables, and words, and he occasionally prolonged initial sounds. It was necessary to attend carefully in order to consistently understand what he was saying. Sporadically his speech was reasonably intelligible, but much of the time considerable effort was required in order to understand him well.

The patient reported that he has had this speech problem as long as he can remember and that from his own perception and from what he has been told by family members and close friends, there has been little change in it over the years. The patient himself referred to the problem as stuttering and claimed to have difficulty "getting out" some words and phrases. However, he said that he has successfully adjusted to this difficulty by using other words whenever he has such trouble. In spite of this description, the patient's major complaint was that other people have trouble understanding him. He gave several examples of this, the most dramatic of which was that his wife did not understand his full name until after their third date. He indicated that generally he is not particularly concerned about his speech, although there are times when he clearly recognizes that it presents a problem. He cited several situations which are particularly difficult for him—meeting new people, solo recitation in church, and some aspects of his job. In all instances he is reluctant to speak because he anticipates that he will not be readily understood. He said he has no problem with family or close friends, since they have evidently gotten used to his manner of speaking.

The patient received therapy for a brief period while in grade school; he recalled that this therapy consisted primarily of reading aloud. He said that he did not recall that it had been of benefit to him. Other people have frequently suggested to him that he slow down his rate of speech. He claimed that he had tried this, but it does not seem to help. However, when he was required to slow his speech rate during this examination, he showed considerable improvement in both fluency and clarity of speech. He could not maintain this reduced rate for any appreciable length of time; he usually reverted to his former rate after a few sentences. He acknowledged that his speech did seem to be improved when he spoke more slowly, but he protested that it was very difficult to maintain the slower rate.

The patient indicated that he is interested in improving his speech and is willing to initiate therapy; however, he expressed reservation about his ability to effect a substantial change in his speech. I am inclined to agree with the pessimism he expresses in regard to prognosis.

Conclusion

To many people, the disorders of fluency have been the most fascinating of the speech disorders. Undoubtedly, a good part of their fascination reflects the experience that they are phantasmic; their seemingly obvious image appears to blur as we approach them more closely. At the same time, much of their mystery has been created by those who have approached a study of the disorders with too much haste and presumption. The major impediment to a better understanding of these disorders, particularly stuttering, is embodied in the theoretical points of view which ignore important facts that contradict them. The further study of these disorders needs much less conjecture and much more investigation that is truly scientific and objective.

Glossary

Clonic: Adjective form of *clonus,* which means the alternating contractions and partial relaxations of the same muscles.

Cluttering: A fluency disorder of unknown origin characterized by sporadically excessive rate and incomplete and distorted articulation.

Disfluency: A general term meaning simply lack of fluency or lapse in fluency. Equivalent to nonfluency.

Elision: Dropping or only partially pronouncing a sound or syllable of a word or words in sequence.

Filled pause: An interval in the speech sequence occupied by an utterance that is not an integral part of the message.

Fluency: Connected speech proceeding smoothly and without notable discontinuity.

Kinesthetic monitoring: Awareness and control of movement through feedback of sensations of movement.

Nonfluency: A general term meaning simply lack of fluency or lapse in fluency. Equivalent to disfluency.

Normal nonfluency: Kinds of disfluency or lapses in fluency found more or less commonly in the speech of normal speakers.

Onomatopoeia: The sound of the spoken word resembles what the word means (e.g., "plop," "rustle," "thud").

Projection: In speech, energetic but not forceful delivery which emphasizes efficient vocal performance resulting in full and resonant tones.

Prosodic: Aspects of the speech act that constitute its tone pattern or melody.

Spasm: An involuntary and unnatural muscular contraction.

Stuttering: A fluency disorder of unknown origin characterized by elemental repetitions and prolongations.

Tachylalia, Tachyphemia: Speech characterized primarily by rapid rate, but also including other irregularities which impair intelligibility.

Theory: An abstracted set of principles expressing relationships between hypotheses and empirical data.

Tone support: Muscular actions necessary to sustain vocal sound of good quality.

Tonic: Adjective form of *tonus*, which means continuous, prolonged muscular contraction.

Study Questions

1. Does theory help make the fluency disorders comprehensible? In what ways?
2. Can stuttering be "defined" acceptably?
3. Give examples of how certain words can influence, in a general sense, the "understanding" of phenomena such as stuttered or cluttered speech.
4. Why are psychological explanations of stuttering so prevalent?
5. Why is cluttering more likely to be viewed as an organically based condition?
6. Some authorities contend that cluttering is "a functional relative" of stuttering. What bases of support for this contention can you identify?
7. List and discuss several advantages of a historical knowledge of stuttering.
8. Why do you think fear figures so prominently in explanations of stuttering?
9. In what ways might one interpret the finding that stuttering occurs more frequently in males? What explanation contains the best support? Why?
10. Why do we not have any tests for stuttering and cluttering, in contrast to the numerous tests available for other kinds of speech disorders?

Bibliography

ARISTOTLE, *Problemata*, trans. E. Forrester, Oxford: Clarendon Press, 1947, Book XI, p. 30.

ARNOLD, G. E., "Studies in Tachyphemia: I. Present Concepts of Etiologic Factors," *Logos* 3 (1960):25–45.

BLOODSTEIN, O., "Stuttering and Normal Non-Fluency: A Continuity Hypothesis," *Br. J. Commun. Dis.* 5 (1970):30–39.

BRUTTEN, E. J., AND D. J. SHOEMAKER, *The Modification of Stuttering*, Englewood Cliffs, N.J.: Prentice-Hall, 1967.

DIEHL, C. F., *A Compendium of Research and Theory on Stuttering*, Springfield, Ill.: Charles C Thomas, 1958.

EISENSON, J., ed., *Stuttering: A Symposium*, New York: Harper, 1958.

GOLDIAMOND, I., "Stuttering and Fluency as Manipulatable Operant Response Classes," in L. Krasner and L. P. Ullman, eds., *Research in Behavior Modification: New Developments and Implications*, Chapter 6, New York: Holt, Rinehart and Winston, 1965.

GOLDMAN-EISLER, F., *Psycholinguistics: Experiments in Spontaneous Speech*, New York: Academic Press, 1968.

GOODSTEIN, L. D., "Functional Speech Disorders and Personality: A Survey of the Research," *J. Speech Hearing Res.* 1 (1958):358–377.

GRAY, B. B., AND G. ENGLAND, eds., *Stuttering and the Conditioning Therapies*, Monterey, Calif.: Monterey Inst. Speech Hearing, 1969.

GREGORY, H., ed., *Learning Theory and Stuttering Therapy*, Evanston, Ill.: Northwestern University Press, 1968.

HAHN, E. F., *Stuttering: Significant Theories and Therapies*, Stanford, Calif.: Stanford University Press, 1958.

JOHNSON, W., et al., *The Onset of Stuttering*, Minneapolis: University of Minnesota Press, 1959.

JOHNSON, W., et al., *Speech Handicapped School Children*, 3rd ed., New York: Harper & Row, 1967.

MOOLENAAR-BIJL, A., "Cluttering (Paraphrasia praeceps)," in E. Froeschels, *Twentieth Century Speech and Voice Correction*, New York: Philosophical Library, 1948.

MURPHY, A. T., AND R. M. FITZSIMMONS, *Stuttering and Personality Dynamics*, New York: Ronald, 1960.

SCHLANGER, B. B., "Speech Examination of a Group of Institutionalized Mentally Handicapped Children," *J. Speech Hearing Dis.* 18 (1953):339–349.

SCHLANGER, B. B., AND R. H. GOTTSLEBEN, "Analysis of Speech Defects Among the Institutionalized Mentally Retarded," *J. Speech Hearing Dis.* 22 (1957):98–103.

SCHUELL, H., "Sex Differences in Relation to Stuttering: Part I," *J. Speech Dis.* 11 (1946):277–298.

———, "Sex Differences in Relation to Stuttering: Part II," *J. Speech Dis.* 12 (1947): 23–38.

SHAMES, G., AND D. EGOLF, *Operant Conditioning and the Management of Stuttering,* Englewood Cliffs, N.J.: Prentice-Hall, 1976.

SHAMES, G. H., AND C. H. SHERRICK, JR., "A Discussion of Non-Fluency and Stuttering as Operant Behavior," *J. Speech Hearing Dis.* **28** (1963):3–18.

SHEEHAN, J. G., "Projective Studies of Stuttering," *J. Speech Hearing Dis.* **23** (1958): 18–25.

————, ed., *Stuttering: Research and Therapy,* New York: Harper & Row, 1970.

SORTINI, A. J., "Twenty Years of Stuttering Research," *J. Internatl. Council Except. Chldrn.* **21** (1955):181–183.

VAN RIPER, C., *The Nature of Stuttering,* Englewood Cliffs, N.J.: Prentice-Hall, 1971.

————, *The Treatment of Stuttering,* Englewood Cliffs, N.J.: Prentice-Hall, 1973.

WEISS, D. A., *Cluttering,* Englewood Cliffs, N.J.: Prentice-Hall, 1964.

WINGATE, M. E., "Evaluation and Stuttering, Part I: Speech Characteristics of Young Children," *J. Speech Hearing Dis.* **27** (1962):106–115.

————, "Stuttering as Phonetic Transition Defect," *J. Speech Hearing Dis.* **34** (1969): 107–108.

————, *Stuttering: Theory and Treatment,* Chapter 4, New York: Irvington-Wiley, 1976.

WISCHNER, G. J., "Stuttering Behavior and Learning: A Preliminary Theoretical Formulation," *J. Speech Hearing Dis.* **15** (1950):324–335.

Consider a preschooler who doesn't talk at all, a kindergartener with normal hearing who doesn't seem to comprehend, or a second grader who says "Me go home" for "I'm going home." These children exhibit impairments in the use of language, the focus of this chapter. The cause of a language impairment in a child is usually rather complicated. A child cannot be separated from his or her environment; the cause, the child, and the environment all overlap and interact in the development of communication skills.

Various techniques are used to evaluate a child's communicative skills in order to decide if the child does indeed have a "problem" and if so, what should be done about it. The purpose of listening to the child talk, testing vocabulary and comprehension, and interviewing the parents is to make a prediction about what the child will be like in the future. Will communication skills be normal? Will development accelerate in a certain type of training program? This latter question introduces the topic for the remainder of the chapter: language training and habilitation.

There are many ways to approach a child who has difficulty in using language. Some children profit from participating in a nursery school program in which they are given considerable freedom to express themselves as they wish. Others do not

Disorders of Language in Children

learn efficiently in such a situation. They need strong limits on what they are permitted to do so that they can focus on learning a particular skill. We will describe some language-training programs based on knowledge gained from linguistics and psychology, as well as speech pathology. Communication is everybody's game, and the child with a language impairment suffers in school, with friends, and as a person. In this chapter you will meet some of these children and learn how clinicians and teachers are working to help them.

Robert D. Hubbell, Ph.D.
California State University, Sacramento

Introduction

There are many functions of human language, but two are particularly important in considering children with language impairments. First, language is a primary tool for participation in human relationships. People talk to one another, get things from one another, and help one another—all through the medium of language. Second, human beings send and receive specific information, learn and teach, and carry out many other thought-related processes primarily through the medium of language. Obviously, both of these functions are present in much of the talking people do. Thus a major point in considering language disorders in children is that we must think of language as both a cognitive process and a social process.

In addition, we are less concerned with language as an abstract system than with the child's use of language in dealing with the world. In terms of the linguistic concepts introduced in Chapter 2, we are more interested in performance than in competence. All we have to work with is how the child actually behaves —what he or she says and does that demonstrate comprehension. We can speculate about the child's knowledge of abstract linguistic structures, and many clinicians do, but the focus is directly on how the child functions as a communicator. Think of a preschooler who bursts into tears, unable to ask to go to the bathroom; or a second grader who doesn't recite in class, unable to comprehend what is being asked. We are concerned with how children use language to deal with the world. Can they refer to objects? Can they tell people what they want? Can they express ideas? Can they comprehend and make use of what is said? Can they use language to learn, both through understanding what is heard and through asking about things that they do not understand?

Also implicit in this discussion is our concern with both the child's *expression* and *comprehension* of language. In everyday interaction we alternate between speaker and listener roles. An effective communicator must possess skill in both. It is a mistake to think of language skill as primarily a talking skill, although some children clearly have impairments in their expressive abilities. Language usage involves comprehension as well as expression, and many language-disordered children demonstrate problems in both areas.

Language impairment, then, may be defined as significant difficulty in using language, that arbitrary system of symbols described in Chapter 2. This impairment may include both talking and understanding and may have both interpersonal and cognitive aspects. These difficulties are above and beyond those which most people encounter at times in various communicative situations. Thus a child may have problems in encoding thoughts, combining the elements of a sentence appropriately, and comprehending the utterances of others. Further, these difficulties may be very severe or relatively minor. In some children the language impairment is the primary problem. In others, the language impairment occurs in association with other problems such as mental retardation, emotional disturbance, or hearing loss.

Etiology and Related Variables

Several conditions are related to language disorders in children. In some cases one of these conditions is clearly the cause, or **etiology,** of the language disorder. In other cases, no such determination can be made. The etiology of a particular child's language impairment is often quite complicated. Let us begin by considering three views of the causation of developmental problems in children, as described by Sameroff and Chandler (1975).

According to the *main-effect model,* the cause of the child's problem lies in either the child or the environment. Thus the child may have a hearing loss or may be locked in a closet most of the time. The difficulty with this view is that it ignores the possibility of combined effects between the environment and the child. Therefore, a second view, called the *interactional model,* was proposed. This model considers the effects of possible causes in the child and in the environment together. The development of a child with a hearing loss in a home where the parents were neglectful would be different from that of an identical child in a home in which the parents were especially helpful. Similarly, a mentally retarded child with abusive parents would develop differently from some other child with the same parents.

The interactional model is more realistic than the main-effects model, but it assumes that both parents and child remain largely the same during the child's development, which is rarely true. Therefore, Sameroff and Chandler proposed a third view, the *transactional model.* In this model, the child and the environment are seen as mutually influencing each other, much as the influence of the family in normal language development was described in Chapter 2. The child changes the environment and in turn is influenced by that changed environment. Part of the focus of the problem, then, is on the transactions between child and family. An emotionally disturbed child may not talk much, so the parents don't converse much with the child, which further discourages the child from talking.

The transactional model is not meant to imply that there are no conditions in either child or environment which alone can lead to language impairment. Rather, the final outcome is a product of the transactional patterns between child and environment. These patterns are influenced by whatever conditions are present, but the patterns as well as the conditions present determine how the child will eventually function. Several possible etiological conditions have been identified. These etiologies will be discussed briefly.

Hearing Loss

An important part of learning to talk is hearing other people talking and hearing one's own utterances. The child with a hearing loss is impaired in this function. Some types of hearing loss are directly related to the hearing mechanism itself, whereas others are related to neurological processes involved in hearing.

The more severe the loss, the more difficulty there will be in learning language. Many deaf children never develop completely normal language patterns, even through reading and writing.

Mental Retardation

Language is an intellectual process. Clearly, children with intellectual deficits will be impaired in language function. Profoundly retarded children will have little or no usable language. Less severely retarded children may be below age level in their language skills.

Emotional Disturbance

Many children with severe emotional disturbance do not talk normally, if they talk at all. In fact, one of the most common characteristics of emotional disturbance is disturbed or bizarre communicative behavior. Some young emotionally disturbed children do not seem to attempt communication at all. Less severely disturbed children may also show language impairments, such as delayed development.

Autism

Autistic children do not seem to desire any exchange with other human beings. Frequently they do not even engage in eye contact with others. They spend much of their time in solitary activity, often of a ritualistic, self-stimulatory nature, such as rocking, flapping the hands, or simply staring. Autistic children demonstrate severe language problems. They do not show much comprehension or expression of language. Some are echolalic; that is, they parrot the utterances of others exactly, but without showing any understanding of what they are saying. Many experts consider **autism** an emotional disturbance. In recent years, however, it has been proposed that autism may be primarily a severe communication disorder. In either case, the clinician who is able to curtail an autistic child's bizarre behavior is then confronted with a child who uses little language.

Neurologically Based Problems

Neurological dysfunction is related to children's language disorders in a number of ways. First, some cases of brain damage directly affect language skills. Some cerebral palsied children, for example, have poor expressive skills because of problems in controlling the speech mechanism. In addition, because of poor motor skills, they may not have had many of the experiences other children have had. In short, they don't have as much to talk about.

Childhood aphasia is sometimes considered a neurologically based problem. As will be discussed in Chapter 12, aphasia means impairment of language function due to brain damage. The term is usually applied to adults. When applied to children, it refers to disabilities specific to language and not based on such other causes as mental retardation, cerebral palsy, hearing loss, or emotional disturbance. There is considerable debate about the usefulness of the concept of childhood aphasia. For one thing, the term implies the presence of brain damage, but often no such damage can be demonstrated. In fact, a language or learning deficit is often the only evidence of brain dysfunction that can be found. Another problem is that it is difficult to differentiate between children who are aphasic and children who have learning disabilities related to language. These latter children are identified because they are having specific difficulty learning in school. Although there are many reasons for learning disabilities, the two groups of children exhibit many of the same characteristics. To further complicate the picture, language is a major vehicle of learning, particularly classroom learning. At the same time, language itself is learned. Because in many of these children no clear cause can be found, perhaps childhood aphasia should not be considered a statement of the etiology of a particular child's problem, but rather a label which some professionals use to classify certain children.

Finally, some people appear to have a congenital language disability syndrome or central language imbalance. This constellation of difficulties involves many aspects of language, such as grammar, articulation, and rate of speech, as well as other factors. It has been shown to be present in families from generation to generation and is believed to be inherited. As with childhood aphasia, this category may better be considered a classification rather than a cause.

Functional Problems

The term **functional** is sometimes used to mean that there is no physical or neurological basis for a particular problem. However, it often really means that no one knows what the cause of a particular child's language problem is. No clear diagnosis or identification of etiology can be made. Many children who are identified as having delayed language—children who are old enough to talk but aren't doing so—fit into this category. It is sometimes thought that functional delay is caused by poor learning due to an ineffective environment.

Environmental Factors

Environmental differences associated with cultural and social-class groupings are not to be confused with language disorders. Nonstandard speech and language patterns are not necessarily disordered. For example, many black American children don't speak standard English. They speak the variety of English used by their peer group (see Chapter 8). Other differences, such as apparent lack of expressive skills or unwillingness to talk, may be due to cultural mores and stereotypes rather than language disorder. A full discussion of this matter is beyond the scope of this chapter. The point is that the speech clinician should not presume that every child should use standard English.

The paragraph above refers primarily to the influence of the peer group. For the preschool child, the family is the primary language learning environment (see Chapter 2). Occasionally, if there are extreme psychological pressures in the family or if the family members habitually remain silent, the family system itself may be a causal influence for a particular child's language disorder. In any case, a reciprocal influence develops between child and family. The older family members adapt their language usage so the child can understand. As the child's language develops, the other family members will use more elaborate language in their communications with the child. The key is understanding. All family members want to understand one another as they communicate.

The same reciprocal situation applies in families which include a child who is delayed in language development, whatever the etiology of the delay. The family members will work out ways of communicating so they can be understood. The system they develop won't require much talking from the child. Fostering such a system is not to be considered poor parenting. In fact, it is necessary and useful because family members live together and must communicate. The problem is that the methods of communicating the family and child work out together may not do much to encourage more talking from the child. One can see the transactional model at work here. The older family members may talk for the child and anticipate her or his needs. Thus the family may contribute to the maintenance of minimal language development in the child. This problem is not insurmountable. As the child begins to change, usually the parents will change also. In addition, the parents themselves may be trained to communicate in ways that facilitate the child's language development.

In summary, the development of a language disorder in a particular child is almost always a complicated process. It involves whatever etiological conditions may be present in both the child and the environment and the history of transactional patterns between child and environment during development. Some children with severe handicaps do remarkably well, and some children with relatively mild handicaps fare rather poorly.

Evaluation

When a child is brought to a speech clinic, the parents don't often know what the difficulties are in a technical sense. They report simply that the child doesn't talk or can't be understood or something similar. The clinician's first job is to evaluate the child's speech and language. The goals of the evaluation may be represented by the following questions.

1. Are speech and language adequate for the child's age? If the answer is yes, the parents are so informed, perhaps with the suggestion that they bring the child back at a later date if they are still concerned. If the answer is no, there are further questions to be explored.

2. What is the specific nature of the difficulty? Stated differently, what are the child's strengths and weaknesses? At this stage, it is determined whether the child has primarily a language impairment or some other difficulty such as articulation or some combination of factors. A precise description of the child's language skills is made. In addition, a determination is made concerning how adequate the child's language is relative to the human relationship and cognitive functions discussed at the beginning of this chapter.

3. What is the cause of the difficulty? It has already been pointed out that it is often impossible to pinpoint etiology. However, the attempt is worth the effort, because it may lead to a better understanding of the child. In particular, the clinician should watch for signs of etiological conditions such as hearing loss, mental retardation, or emotional disturbance. In addition, an attempt is made to assess the effects of the home environment on the child.

4. What should be done? Depending on the nature and severity of the impairment and the home situation, the clinician may recommend speech and language training, placement in a nursery school or special school, referral to a psychologist or medical doctor, or other forms of treatment.

In summary, the information the clinician considers in an evaluation is concerned with prediction. On the basis of the evaluation, the clinician attempts to predict how the child will progress and what kind of treatment program will be most efficacious.

Reliability and Validity

Before considering evaluation procedures, it is necessary to consider the concepts of **reliability** and **validity.** Briefly, reliability refers to the consistency with which observations are made; validity, to the "truth value" of these observations. These concepts are discussed more fully in Chapter 8. Many of the procedures commonly used to evaluate children's language skills are low in reliability or validity or both. Few rigorous measurement procedures have been developed, partly because of the enormous complexity of language behavior and partly because children's language disorders is a relatively new field of specialization. Hopefully, more sophisticated tests of language skills will eventually become available.

The Importance of Context

As was mentioned in Chapter 2, language is situation-specific; that is, one's use of language varies with the situation or context in which one is talking. Consider your own behavior for a minute. I doubt that you talk the same at home as you do when you're asking a question in a large class. The same is true of children. Children will often talk more when the topic of discussion is of immediate interest to them. They talk differently to peers than to adults, particularly strangers. For example, a story is told about a sociolinguist, William Labov, who once took a group of children who had been identified as using little expressive language into a room in which there was a caged rabbit. He asked the children to take care of his rabbit while he was gone. He said it might be afraid, but if they talked to the rabbit it would be alright. He then left the room. Needless to say, the children talked a mile a minute.

This sensitivity to context in language usage is something that must always be considered in dealing with language-disordered children. In some situations a young child may not even demonstrate comprehension, much less expression. I have worked with children who did not do what I asked, even though they knew what I meant, and they knew I knew they knew what I meant! The teacher or clinician can usually overcome these situational difficulties by trying different activities and giving the child a little time. In fact, context sensitivity can be used to advantage by finding situations which encourage a particular child to communicate (Fig. 11.1). Cazden (1970) has written an excellent review of the effects of context on children's language usage. The point to be made here is that the context of an evaluation will affect both the reliability and the validity of the results.

Evaluation Procedures

The procedures used in an evaluation will be chosen to explore the questions listed earlier. That is, the clinician will want to discover as much as possible about the child's language skills and behavior. If a problem exists, the clinician will want to gather evidence about possible etiologies and influences. Finally, all the information collected will be analyzed with respect to what course of action should be taken.

Parent interview A parent interview is an important part of the evaluation. During the interview, the clinician gains information concerning the nature of the problem as the parents see it. In addition, the parents can supply information on how the child talks and behaves at home, the child's developmental history, and any particular problems she or he has had. The clinician also will want to know what the parents have done about the problem in the past in terms of helping the child at home, ignoring the problem, or taking the child to other specialists. This last matter can be particularly poignant with some severely im-

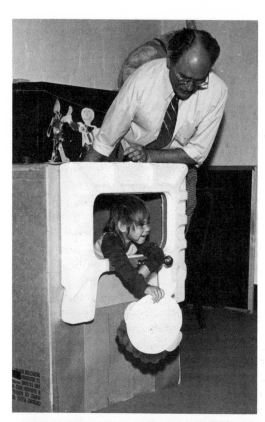

Figure 11.1
Finding activities with intrinsic appeal for young children may enhance their motivation to communicate.

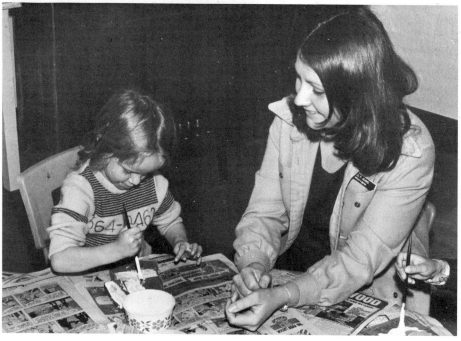

paired children whose etiology cannot be clearly determined. The parents often end up going from expert to expert, seeking some sort of answer.

From the parent interview, the clinician may be able to formulate some ideas about how conducive the home is to the child's language development. Some of this information will have to be inferred, because it is difficult to obtain an accurate picture of family functioning through direct questioning. It is not so much that the parents deliberately present a distorted picture, but that many of the transactional patterns become such deeply ingrained habits that they occur beyond the parents' awareness.

Observation of child's behavior Obviously, the clinician will also see the child during the evaluation. Most clinicians begin an evaluation with play activities and conversation with the child. This gives the child a chance to get used to the situation, and the clinician has a chance to observe the child's spontaneous communicative behavior, comprehension, and general level of maturity. The clinician will note the child's degree of motor coordination and hand preference. One can make suggestions and comments and watch the child's reactions in order to begin to assess comprehension. The child's utterances will be characterized in various ways: Are they intelligible most of the time, only when the clinician knows what the child is talking about, or are they mostly unintelligible? If they are intelligible, do they consist of single words or multiple-word combinations? Do they contain function words as well as content words? Thus the clinician often has some ideas about the child's level of functioning before formal testing is begun. Much of the information picked up during this informal observation can be compared with developmental **norms** for children of the same age and thus contribute to more precise evaluation. Some clinicians also observe the child playing with the parent. In this way the clinician may see the child behaving in a different context. In addition, one may pick up clues about the transactional patterns between child and parent.

Semantics Most evaluations also include specific testing of various aspects of language. The child's semantic functioning is usually evaluated through a vocabulary test. Recognition vocabulary is commonly used because it is relatively easy to measure. In a recognition vocabulary test, the clinician says a word and shows the child several pictures. The child selects the picture that most closely fits the word. This process is repeated with increasingly difficult words. The *Peabody Picture Vocabulary Test* by Dunn (1965) is an example of this kind of test. Comprehension can also be evaluated by giving the child verbal instructions and noting whether they are carried out. Complying with the instructions indicates comprehension; noncomplicity indicates that the child did not comprehend or at least did not cooperate at the moment.

Syntax There is currently great interest in the syntax of language-impaired children. Clearly it is desirable to know as much as possible about the child's language structure, and this structure is reflected mainly in syntax. Most procedures for evaluating syntax involve getting a sample of the child's talking, usually written down verbatim from a tape recording. This sample should contain at least 50 utterances. The child's utterances are then analyzed, either according to the complexity of the sentences the child uttered or by inventorying some of the syntactic structures which are present in the child's speech (Lee, 1974). There are two problems with these procedures, however. First, they are rather time consuming. Second, and more important, they hinge entirely on the clinician's encouraging the child to talk while the recorder is on. Both reliability and the validity of this procedure may be inadequate due to the situational factors discussed earlier.

Tests of syntactic skills have also been developed (Carrow, 1973; Lee, (1969). In evaluating comprehension, these tests are constructed similarly to the recognition vocabulary test. For example, the child may have to choose the correct picture to match the sentence "The boy hit the girl" rather than "The girl hit the boy." These two sentences are identical in construction and vocabulary. If presented a picture of a boy hitting a girl, the only way a child can match it with the appropriate sentence is by knowing the syntactic functions of the subject (the actor) and object (the receiver of the action). Tests of expressive syntactic skills rely mainly on imitation. Frequently children cannot imitate correctly a grammatical construction that they do not generate spontaneously in their own talking. Another method of evaluating syntax is to note the kind of structures, pronoun usage, and other linguistic elements that the child uses and compare them with developmental norms, such as those published by Gesell *et al.* (1940). Another common technique is to note the average length of the child's utterances.

Articulation   The evaluation frequently includes some testing of the child's articulation. In some cases it turns out that the child's problem is more in the area of articulation than language. That is, although language structure and vocabulary are adequate, the child can't be understood. Assessment of articulation was discussed in Chapter 8.

Psycholinguistic skills   It is sometimes appropriate to evaluate various **psycholinguistic skills.** As mentioned in Chapter 2, the term "psycholinguistic" refers to psychological processes in language use. In memory, for example, one must remember not only vocabulary items, grammatical rules, and the like, but also the beginning of a sentence by the time the end of it comes around; otherwise, the sentence will be meaningless. Sequencing, or keeping things in order, is another example of such a skill. The two combined form sequential memory, a psycholinguistic skill necessary to produce or interpret sentences properly. The importance of this skill is readily seen in the sentence "Mary introduced Jan to Betty." It is through the skills of memory and sequencing as they interact with knowledge of syntax that one knows who did the introducing and who was introduced to whom.

Another example of a psycholinguistic skill is auditory discrimination, or the ability to hear the differences between various sounds. It is difficult to test auditory discrimination precisely, because the testing always involves other skills, such as comprehension and vocabulary, not to mention hearing acuity.

The most widely used test of psycholinguistic skills is the *Illinois Test of Psycholinguistic Abilities* (Kirk, McCarthy, and Kirk, 1968). This test attempts to measure a number of skills, both in receptive functioning and expressive functioning. It was originally designed for use with retarded and learning-disabled children. Because of the test's emphasis on language-related skills, it is widely used by speech pathologists. The primary purpose of the test is not to obtain an overall score, but to compare various psycholinguistic abilities within the same child. That is, the test consists of several subtests which produce a profile of the child's skills so that comparisons can be made between auditory and visual reception, vocal and gestural expression, and automatic, overlearned language skills versus language usage involving more active cognitive processing.

Hearing   A hearing screening test must always be included in a language evaluation. Hearing assessment is of basic importance because hearing is so important in language acquisition. If the results of the screening indicate any possibility of a hearing loss, a full audiological evaluation is done. Hearing assessment was discussed in Chapter 5.

Other procedures   In some cases the child will not respond to any tests; the child is "untestable." Frequently such children are extremely immature or uncooperative. They may have a short attention span or fatigue easily. Sometimes activities such as playing with clay will help the child adjust to the situation, or perhaps the child will have to return another day. With such children, the clinician's first goal will be to encourage communicative behavior.

Some children are enrolled in a clinical program in which the emphasis is on careful observation over time. In such a program, the clinician uses a variety of procedures and activities designed to help understand the child's communicative difficulties and experiment with ways of fostering speech and language development.

An evaluation always ends with the clinician summarizing the findings to the parents and making recommendations. On some occasions, if elaborate testing was done or if the child was unusually uncooperative, it may be necessary for the clinician to ask the parents to return another day. The important point is that the parents should leave knowing more than they did before and with some concrete ideas of what to do next.

From the discussion above, it is obvious that an evaluation can be very extensive. It is doubtful whether a clinician would ever use all the procedures mentioned above with the same child. In selecting tests and procedures, the clinician should choose only those that can be justified as providing necessary information for a particular client. The most necessary information is that which will provide a basis for making predictions and decisions about that particular client.

If there is any evidence of mental retardation or emotional disturbance, the clinician will make an appropriate referral. Such evidence might be slow developmental history, low functioning in many different areas during the evaluation, bizarre or unusual behavior, or evidence of possible brain injury. It is not ethical for a speech pathologist to make the determination that a child is retarded or disturbed. This identification should be made by specialists. The same is true if the clinician suspects neurological dysfunction.

Because of the intimate relationship among language impairments, mental retardation, and emotional disturbance, it is very difficult to identify the primary problem or combination of problems in some children. The younger the child is, the more this is true. Evaluation by an interdisciplinary team is perhaps the best solution. The team should include a speech pathologist, an audiologist, a pediatrician, and a psychologist or psychiatrist. Other specialists, particularly educators, are often involved. Sometimes home visits are incorporated in the evaluation. The team approach is beneficial, obviously, because the various experts can evaluate the child together, thus looking at various possibilities at the same time.

Treatment

There are several different strategies for working with language-impaired children. The selection of a particular strategy depends partly on the clinician's personal preferences, but mostly on the kinds of difficulty the child is having.

Developing Language Behavior

In order to talk, it is necessary to have something to talk about. For some children, the deficiency lies primarily in this area. They lack the conceptual development that normal children have had. Retarded children and children who have lived in a very restricted environment often fall in this category. These children need a lot of stimulation, a lot of new experiences. This need can be met by work in a speech clinic or parent training or often simply placement in a nursery school or similar environment (not merely a babysitting service) (Fig. 11.2). As a part of this program of general stimulation, the child should hear a lot of talking. Someone can put into words whatever is happening, describe what the child is doing, supply the names of things, and provide vocabulary input for

Figure 11.2

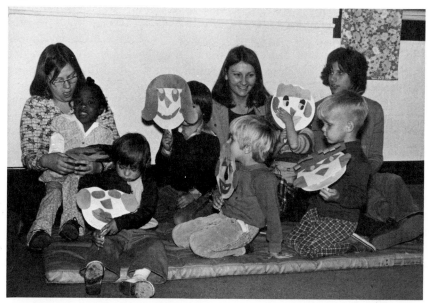

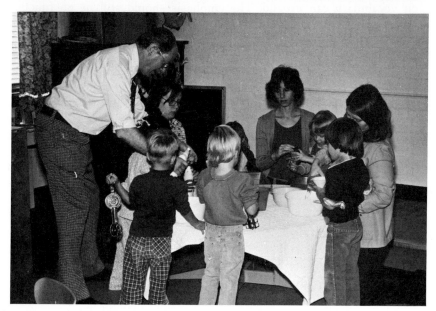

Group activities may be used to facilitate communicative behavior.

the child in other ways. Such a program should be designed so that the child participates actively rather than as a passive recipient. Merely bombarding the child with stimuli is not enough. The child needs to develop ways to process the stimuli received. There are special materials that have been developed for this kind of language and conceptual stimulation. The *Peabody Language Development Kits* by Dunn, Horton, and Smith (1965, 1966, 1968) are examples of these materials.

If a child's repertoire has sufficient concepts in it, the emphasis should be on developing language skills. With a child who is mostly nonverbal, building vocabulary will be an early goal. Out of the universe of English words, the question is where to begin. The best answer seems to be to select words or expressions that will be immediately useful to the child. These early expressions will be more at the relationship than the cognitive level, although the two are never entirely separate. They will be ones that help the child express needs and generally deal with the people in the environment. These expressions might be called "functional communication." Any understandable utterance is accepted at this stage. The fine points of grammar and articulation can come later. The point is to give the child some expressions that can be used at home. Successful use of these expressions will encourage more talking and foster in other family members the expectation that the child will talk. As the child's talking increases, work on vocabulary can expand. The emphasis should still be on functional, useful items, though. It makes little sense to teach children to name six colors if they can't ask to go to the bathroom.

An inescapable fact in language training is that the clinician can never teach a child everything necessary to speak the language. There are too many vocabulary items and too many grammatical structures. At some point, the child must take over. Nobody knows how this process occurs, but it's a good bet that practice is a crucial element. The more the child talks, the more language development will occur. For this reason, most clinicians encourage parents to converse with the child, encourage talking, accept that talking without correcting it, and in general emphasize the fact that the child is communicating through language. This process helps to develop more facilitative transactional patterns between child and parents. In other words, once they get started, many children will move along on their own if they have an appropriate environment. The process is accelerated as they learn that speech is useful to them.

Structured Language Training

Some children, however, need training and structure beyond that just discussed to develop adequate language skills. This need may be particularly keen in children of the aphasic learning-disability group and children with profound handicaps such as emotional disturbance, mental retardation, and severe hearing loss. Structured language training leans more toward the cognitive aspects of language than the social ones. Vocabulary development is often a primary focus. As the child's vocabulary increases, the emphasis may shift to grammatical skills. Let us begin by considering comprehension and expression.

Comprehension It is interesting that most work with language-impaired children focuses on expression, with the assumption that the comprehension can't be far behind. Perhaps the reason for this situation is that the child does not seem to do very much when listening. There are few behaviors to work with, compared with expression, where successes and failures are much more obvious. For the same reason, the major complaint expressed by parents usually is that the child is having difficulty with talking, not comprehending. It may be, however, that a child can learn a word and its meaning easier through comprehension than through expression. Olson (1970) has suggested that comprehension is basically a recognition process and therefore requires less specific information than expression does. One can often get the meaning of an utterance without attending to all its details, whereas to produce that same utterance requires knowledge of every detail. Typically, a speaker will have to make more linguistic decisions in the production of an utterance than a listener will in comprehending that utterance. This relative simplicity suggests that one should begin with comprehension training. This training should be based on more than merely hearing language—it should require the active participation of the child. That is, the child should be required to do things while listening, to make responses to what is heard, so that the skills needed to process the information are indeed learned. Recently, Winitz (1973) discussed just such a program for training grammatical structures through comprehension, based on what he refers to as problem solving. Winitz suggests that this kind of training can be done and that it may well be more efficient than concentrating on expression.

Several other factors are related to training comprehension. The first is attention. The child won't comprehend much without paying attention to the appropriate stimuli. This statement seems obvious, but it is remarkably difficult to get some children to attend to what you have in mind. They may find other things in the situation much more appealing. Second, there is a limit to the child's information-processing span. That is, the child can comprehend utterances only up to a certain length. Children may behave appropriately even when they hear utterances that are too long for them to comprehend, because they read the whole situation. Thus an adult may assume that a child can comprehend much more than is actually the case. For example, you might say, "Billy, would you please get up and turn on the light for me," while looking at the light switch and perhaps gesturing to it. The child needs to comprehend very little of this relatively long sentence in order to comply.

This situation leads to a third factor; it is often very difficult to determine just how much a child does comprehend (see Chapter 2). Comprehension is an internal process. We infer comprehension when we see appropriate behavior following an utterance, but we can never actually see comprehension itself. This fact limits much comprehension training to certain types of utterances, such as commands, suggestions, and questions, which can elicit some behavior or talking from the child. These factors need not impede comprehension training, however. They merely emphasize the need of working with care and precision so that you know just what the child is attending to and comprehending.

Expression Expressive language may be approached in various ways, depending on how specific the training goals are. A clinician attempting to elicit a particular word or grammatical construction from a child will structure the situation very highly and actually limit the child's verbal output (ideally) to that particular item. The clinician may ask the child to complete a sentence with a word or phrase or perhaps to imitate an utterance. The importance of imitation in normal language acquisition has generated considerable debate. Whitehurst and Vasta (1975) have presented an interesting review of this material.

Regardless of this debate, concerning normal processes, imitation has been frequently used in clinical language training for an obvious reason. It presents a simple method to get a child to produce a particular utterance. I have two cautions regarding imitation training. First, the clinician must make sure that the child comprehends what he or she is imitating. Otherwise, the child is not truly learning language. Second, when first training a child to imitate, the clinician should simultaneously be planning how to teach the child to stop imitating when the time comes. Imitation should be viewed as a first step in expression. Children must learn to generate their own utterances as soon as possible.

This last sentence suggests an interesting question: Can a child be taught to talk spontaneously? Spontaneous talking is usually defined as talking on one's own volition in response to one's own thoughts and perceptions. In language training, the child's talking is usually directed; thus it is not truly spontaneous. The degree of spontaneous talking a child uses is intimately tied up with the sensitivity to context discussed earlier. I worked with a child once who had good comprehension skills but absolutely wouldn't say a word in the clinic, but when I ran into him on the sidewalk one day, he talked in whole sentences! It may be that for some children at least, the more structured the training is, the less conducive it is to the child's spontaneous talking. A reasonable solution to this problem is to train specific skills first and then move to less structured situations to encourage more spontaneous talking.

As was mentioned earlier, the relationship between comprehension and expression is complicated. There is some disagreement about whether it is more efficient to concentrate primarily on one or the other. To me, this may be one of those questions that will never get satisfactorily answered. For one thing, it may vary from child to child. It makes sense to assume that comprehension and expression are related through some sort of feedback process, so that each enhances the other. From this perspective, language training should involve both comprehension and expression.

Language Training Programs

Training in syntactic skills raises a parallel question to that raised in vocabulary training: Out of the great number of grammatical forms, which should be taught first? Further, once a starting place is established, a logical sequence is needed in which to present other language forms. One approach in answering these questions has been the development of structured language programs. In simplest form, such a program consists of a set of language skills, laid out in sequence from start to finish. All the steps are specified in considerable detail, building from simpler structures to more complicated ones. Several such programs are now available in published form. In the discussion that follows, I will be concerned primarily with the rationale for each program rather than the detailed training sequence; the focus will be on the principles on which each program is based.

One of the earlier programs was presented in *Teaching Disadvantaged Children in the Preschool* (Bereiter and Engelmann, 1966, Chapters 5–8). This program was designed for use with disadvantaged preschoolers, and there is considerable debate about its appropriateness for such children. The debate centers on the fact that the program is based on middle-class English, a dialect that many disadvantaged children do not use. Aside from this issue, the program has been used in working with language-impaired children. It is designed for teaching language as a logical tool. There is little emphasis on traditional vocabulary building. Rather, the focus is on the little words, the logical operations such as "is, not, but, and, if . . . then." The program is based on two sentence types and develops to more elaborate forms one step at a time. The children use complete, fully formed sentences, although, of course, early in the program these sentences are very simple. Again, the program is designed to help children use language as a tool for logical thought, to learn to reason with language. It is therefore much involved in cognitive stimulation as well as language.

The Bereiter and Engelmann program is based on an adult assessment of what's important in language. Another approach to language programing is to follow the normal sequence of children's grammatical development. A program of this type is presented by Eisenson (1972, Chapter 9). The program begins with various kinds of two-word combinations and gradually builds to more complex forms that increasingly approach the standard form of adult grammar.

A third approach is to develop programs for training children to use various basic adult sentence types as described by linguists. Thus the children are trained through a series of steps to use declarative sentences, questions, and other sentence types. One such program is reported in *A Language Program for the Nonlanguage Child* by Gray and Ryan (1973).

At the present time, there is no way to tell whether any one of these programs is more effective than the others. Comparisons among them center on whether to base a program on cognitive content, on the sequence of children's grammatical development, or on adult sentence forms. It does seem that some sort of program is useful in prolonged language training because it helps establish an order among the many aspects of language that need attention.

The emphasis on programing and teaching things in sequence lends itself to the application of **operant conditioning** principles. Operant conditioning is a training system based on building toward a goal through many small, controlled steps. It was developed as a general training strategy, not expressly for language or speech pathology. The individual's behavior is controlled through reinforcement, the presentation of positive or negative **stimuli** immediately following performance. The behavior of interest is described very precisely, and careful records of that behavior are kept over a period of time. The child moves through a series of graded steps, directed by the stimuli given, and motivated by the positive reinforcements received. The reinforcements are also used in ways that guide the child toward the behavior desired by the clinician. At the same time, the clinician knows exactly what progress is made because of the emphasis on precise record keeping. Operant conditioning can be combined with the training programs mentioned above rather nicely. In fact, the Gray and Ryan program is constructed in just this way.

At the present time, more sophisticated programs are being developed which attempt to combine insights from linguistic theory, developmental psychology, and learning principles. In addition to grammatical development, these programs place more emphasis on such things as the functions of language. That is, by analyzing what language can accomplish for the child, such as asking for things, the program can be designed to train the child to use words for these functions rather than using nonverbal communication. This goal is not very different from the "functional communication" mentioned earlier, but the training is through a formal program. Another trend is to focus on cognitive prerequisites for language—the skills that a child must already have before he or she can learn language. For example, a young child must come to realize that objects still exist even when they are out of sight. Otherwise, symbolization loses much of its power. Interesting discussions of current efforts in programed language training will be found in McReynolds (1974) and in Schiefelbusch and Lloyd (1974, especially sections VI and VII).

Psycholinguistic Skills

Some children have particular deficits in specific psycholinguistic abilities. From the profile of the child's psycholinguistic skills that was mentioned earlier, the clinician has a picture of the child's strengths and weaknesses. Training can be planned, then, to make use of the child's strengths and to improve areas of difficulty. Thus the focus is on skills underlying language, such as sequential memory and auditory discrimination rather than on language usage itself, as in most of the programs mentioned above. The assumption is that language skill in general will improve as these particular skills improve.

Working with Parents

To be most effective, the clinician must work with the parents as well as with the child. Parents can often learn ways to stimulate and talk with their child. It is often helpful for parents to understand better specifically what the child's difficulties are. Sometimes parents and child are given regular daily assignments in addition to the child's clinic sessions. It is important in these cases to keep close contact with the situation to give the parents appropriate guidance and encouragement. Remember that the child spends many more hours per week with the parents than with the clinician.

Some parents and children, however, are not very comfortable when the parents take on a direct teaching role with the child. This situation may arise if, for example, the parent doesn't have a knack for teaching or if direct teaching violates too many of the transactional patterns the family has already established. Work with such parents can focus on changing some of these transactional patterns in ways that foster more communication from the child without requiring that the parent act as a teacher. This strategy is similar to that discussed in Chapter 7 regarding parental questions and commands. An example of this strategy appears in Seitz (1975).

Another area of great importance in working with parents is helping them with their feelings about their child and themselves. For example, parents of a severely language-disordered child may fear that the child is retarded or has emotional problems. These fears are best handled by giving the parents plenty of support but at the same time telling them the facts. Frequently, parents feel that they have done something wrong which has caused the child's problems. I remember one mother of a four-year-old child who told about an accident in which boiling water was spilled on the child when he was a little less than two years of age. She was sure that this accident had caused the child's difficulties, because it happened right when he was beginning to talk. My approach in such situations is to help the parents put the focus on the present. There is nothing

293

they can accomplish by dwelling on the past, but there are things they can do now to help their child develop. This emphasis on the positive helps the parents to see themselves as competent people and thus helps provide the emotional support that they need.

Conclusion

Various approaches to working with children's language impairments have been presented. Obviously, not all approaches will be used with the same child. The clinician is encouraged to experiment, try various strategies, find what is most effective with different kinds of children. Patience and flexibility are virtues to be cultivated. It often seems that we learn more than the children do. Working with language-impaired children is both fascinating and challenging.

Glossary

Autism: A severe childhood disorder involving minimal efforts at contact with other human beings; often includes ritualized, repetitive activities or bizarre behavior; usually includes significant language impairment.

Childhood aphasia: A label used to categorize certain children who demonstrate severe language impairments, but without identifiable sensory or intellectual deficits; usually implies the presence of neurological dysfunction, although proof of any such condition may be lacking.

Etiology: The specific cause of a particular disorder in an individual.

Functional: In describing the causes of various disorders and conditions, "functional" means either that there is no organic pathology or that the cause cannot be determined.

Norm: Typical or average performance at a particular age level in some aspect of human behavior.

Operant conditioning: A system for changing an individual's behavior whereby consistent use of rewards and punishments is used in conjunction with a graded series of steps through which the individual's behavior is changed in small increments.

Psycholinguistic skill: A psychological skill thought to be necessary to comprehend or express language; based on human information-processing skills.

294

Reliability: Consistency in the measurement of human behavior.

Stimulus; Stimuli: Anything that excites receptors, such as objects, odors, or sounds.

Validity: The relative truth value of a measurement of some aspect of human behavior.

Study Questions

1. Define children's language impairment in your own words. Make your definition inclusive enough that it is not related to only one etiology, but specific enough that it does not include problems in areas other than language.

2. List several possible causes of language impairment in children. Explain in detail how the transactional model of causation might apply in each case.

3. Some experts have stated that emotional problems and intellectual deficits are primarily problems in communication and language. In what ways might these claims be true? How might they be false?

4. Supposing a four- or five-year-old has good comprehension skills but almost no expressive language skill. Is this child likely to have more difficulty learning about the world than a normally developing child? Why?

5. Tests have many functions. College students often think of grading as a primary function. Have you ever taken any tests, in or out of school, where the major purpose was prediction? What sorts of tests were they? Is there a parallel between this kind of prediction and that discussed in the section on evaluation? How might grading have a predictive function?

6. Some young children have impairments in both expressive language and articulation. That is, they don't have much to say, and what they do say is unintelligible. Which should you work on first? Start your thinking with the idea of functional communication.

7. We have mentioned auditory sequencing and auditory discrimination as examples of psycholinguistic skills. Describe at least three other psycholinguistic skills. Don't worry about whether or not the skills you think up are the same as the ones in some book or test. Try to understand what processes are involved in comprehending and expressing language.

8. It has been pointed out that much language training for children focuses almost entirely on expression. Is this strategy appropriate with all language-delayed children? Why might training comprehension be more efficient in some cases?

9. Why are well-developed formal tests desirable? Are there situations in which they should not or cannot be used? What does one do then?

10. This chapter included a section on the importance of context. What is meant here? How might this apply in the classroom? In the clinic? What strategies might be employed to deal with such situations?

Bibliography

BEREITER, C., AND G. ENGELMANN, *Teaching Disadvantaged Children in the Preschool*, Englewood Cliffs, N.J.: Prentice-Hall, 1966.

CARROW, E., *Test for Auditory Comprehension of Language*, Austin, Texas: Learning Concepts, 1973.

CAZDEN, C. B., "The Situation: A Neglected Source of Social Class Differences in Language Use," *J. Social Issues* **26** (1970):35–60.

DUNN, L. M., *Peabody Picture Vocabulary Test*, Minneapolis, Minn.: American Guidance Service, 1965.

DUNN, L.M., K. B. HORTON, AND O. S. SMITH, *Peabody Language Developmental Kits, Levels #P, #1, #2*, Circle Pines, Minn.: American Guidance Service, 1968, 1966, 1965.

EISENSON, J., *Aphasia in Children*, New York: Harper & Row, 1972.

GESELL, A., *et al.*, *The First Five Years of Life: A Guide to the Study of the Pre-School Child*, New York: Harper, 1940.

GRAY, B., AND B. RYAN, *A Language Program for the Nonlanguage Child*, Champaign, Ill.: Research Press, 1973.

KIRK, S. A., J. J. MCCARTHY, AND W. D. KIRK, *Illinois Test of Psycholinguistic Abilities*, rev. ed., Urbana: University of Illinois Press, 1968.

LEE, L. L., *Northwestern Syntax Screening Test*, Evanston, Ill.: Northwestern University, 1969.

———, *Developmental Sentence Analysis*, Evanston, Ill.: Northwestern University, 1974.

MCREYNOLDS, L. V., ed., *Developing Systematic Procedures for Training Children's Language*, ASHA Monographs, 18, Washington, D.C.: American Speech and Hearing Association, 1974.

OLSON, D. R., *Cognitive Development: The Child's Acquisition of Diagonality*, New York: Academic Press, 1970.

SAMEROFF, A. J., AND M. J. CHANDLER, "Reproductive Risk and the Continuum of Caretaking Casualty," in F. D. Horowitz, ed., *Review of Child Development and Research*, Chicago: University of Chicago Press, 1975.

SCHIEFELBUSCH, R. L., AND L. L. LLOYD, *Language Perspectives: Acquisition, Retardation, and Intervention*, Baltimore: University Park Press, 1974.

SEITZ, S., "Language Intervention: Changing the Language Environment of the Retarded Child," in R. Koch, F. de la Cruz, and F. Menolascino, eds., *Downs Syndrome: Prevention and Management*, New York: Bruner-Mazel, 1975.

WHITEHURST, G. J., AND R. VASTA, "Is Language Acquired through Imitation?" *J. Psycholinguistic Res.* **4** (1975):37–59.

WINITZ, H., "Problem Solving and the Delaying of Speech as Strategies in the Teaching of Language," *ASHA* **15** (1973):583–586.

CHAPTER 12
Overview

Sometimes adults suffer brain damage from a stroke or accident. Extensive damage to the left cerebral hemisphere of the brain may cause a loss or reduction of language abilities (aphasia). Descriptions of the several kinds of aphasia are given in this chapter, along with descriptions of some of the physical symptoms which aphasic patients may also suffer, such as paralysis of the arm and leg, loss of vision, and reduction of intelligence. The language evaluation of adult aphasic patients is described as the preliminary step toward speech and language rehabilitation. Both individual and group speech-remediation sessions are described as part of the speech pathology services offered the patient. Some examples are given of adults who acquired brain damage with resulting aphasia and who then received intensive speech remediation.

Daniel R. Boone, Ph.D.
University of Arizona

Disorders of Language in Adults

Introduction

Whereas children may experience developmental language impairment (Chapter 11), adults sometimes acquire language disorders. The primary language disorder we shall discuss in adults is **aphasia**, a loss of language function. Language function (see Chapter 2) includes such *decoding* skills as understanding what is said and what one reads and the *encoding* skills of speaking and writing. Aphasia, then, is an impairment of these language functions after one has suffered brain damage from a stroke or other brain trauma. Since most adults who acquire aphasia still retain partial language functions, the term *dysphasia* (reduction of language function) is often used to describe the language loss; however, because of the word confusion with the word *dysphagia* (swallowing difficulty), the term *aphasia* is more widely used. We shall look at the problem of aphasia in an effort to understand what it is, what causes it, and what kind of associated problems exist, the evaluation of the disorder, and its management.

Description

Aphasia has been studied by diverse specialists—neurologists, psychologists, linguists, and speech pathologists. The early neurologists' conceptualization of aphasia in terms of a sensory-motor dichotomy has influenced neurological thinking up to the present day. That dichotomy is based on the observation that posterior portions of the spinal column and brain generally serve sensory functions (Chapter 5), whereas anterior portions are concerned more with motor functions (Chapter 3). This sensory-motor model led to a viewpoint termed neurological **localization;** physiological and cognitive processes were believed to be controlled by rather discrete segments of the brain. In keeping with that viewpoint, early neurologists introduced the concept of receptive aphasia (language-decoding problems) and expressive aphasia (language-encoding problems).

The classical concept of language localization probably began with a paper by Broca in 1861 in which he presented two cases at autopsy, each of which had a lesion in the third convolution of the left frontal lobe. Broca argued that the lesions were responsible for almost purely expressive disorders from which the patients suffered before their deaths. This was the first acclaimed paper asserting that a specific lesion in an area of the brain could cause a specific deficit. Further support for localization was found in the work of Wernicke, who in 1874 demonstrated that lesions to the left posterior temporal lobe could produce devastating problems in understanding spoken language. These two papers by Broca and Wernicke are classically cited as landmarks in the study of cerebral localization; in addition, verbal **apraxia** was frequently called "Broca's aphasia," and receptive problems were sometimes called "Wernicke's aphasia."

Although modern localizationists may still attribute particular functions to particular brain areas, there is far greater recognition today of the interplay among all parts of the brain as a requisite for normal functions, a view long advocated by the nonlocalizationists. Penfield and Roberts (1959) presented both localization and nonlocalization viewpoints; they found by electrostimulation of the left cerebral hemisphere during brain surgery that different areas within the dominant hemisphere seemed to demonstrate control of various functions of language. Anterior areas of the brain seem to have much to do with the planning and execution of language, as seen in speaking and writing. Posterior areas of the brain appear to have definite roles in recognition and comprehension of language. Figure 12.1, of the left cerebral hemisphere, shows anterior and posterior brain areas with their designation of language function.

Prominent among the early nonlocalizationists was Hughlings Jackson, who preferred to think of generalized cerebral function rather than of discrete areas of the brain having discrete functions. Marie followed Jackson, with his 1901 devastating critique of the early Broca work, and it then became popular to take a gestalt, or whole-brain approach, rather than assigning particular aphasic defi-

Figure 12.1

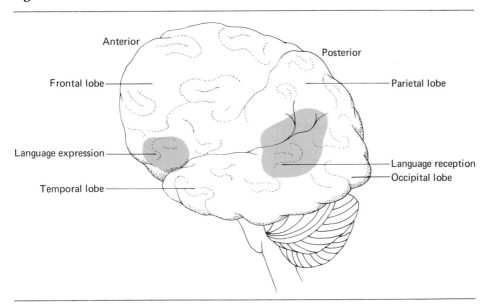

The left cerebral hemisphere is divided into four lobes: frontal, parietal, temporal, and occipital. Anterior areas of the hemisphere vital for language expression and posterior areas which have been found to be essential for language reception are identified by the shaded areas.

301

cits to certain areas of the brain. The history of localization and nonlocalization is well reviewed by Schuell (Schuell, Jenkins, and Jimenez-Pabón, 1964).

Disturbances in recognition may be called **agnosia**, a term introduced by Freud in 1891. Patients with visual agnosia cannot recognize what they see; those with auditory verbal agnosia cannot understand the words they hear. Disturbances in verbal expression have had such neurological labels as *oral verbal apraxia*, the terms used to describe impaired volitional ability to say words with automatic functioning normal; for example, a patient who could not repeat after the examiner the word "dam" could profanely say "damn" as an automatic verbal response. Another expressive problem is **dysarthria;** the patient has slurred, uncoordinated, imprecise speech due to motor dysfunction of various parts, as presented in Chapters 2 and 8, of the speech-voice mechanisms.

Cerebral dominance is the term used for hemisphere lateralization for language, and its relationship to handedness has received much investigation by psychologists. Nevertheless, most aphasic patients seem to have lesions in the left cerebral hemisphere regardless of which hand they previously used. That is, there appears to be only a loose relationship between handedness and cerebral dominance for language. Some persons who use their left hands almost exclusively may be right-brained for language, but it seems safe to conclude that most adults who acquire aphasia have had lesions in the language areas in the left cerebral hemisphere.

The discipline known as neuropsychology has done much to measure and study the effects of neural lesions on behavior. Much is known today about the general lowering of intellectual functioning in patients who acquire brain lesions, regardless of the hemisphere involved. In fact, right-hemisphere lesions tend to have greater deleterious effects on intelligence than left-hemisphere involvement does. The right hemisphere appears to play a vital role in the individual's ability for spatial organization and response. The cerebral lesion, regardless of its location, may have the effect of lowering the individual's overall intellect. Among some aphasic patients, psychologists have found a greater concreteness and lack of ability to abstract, a slower reaction time, a reduced body image and self-concept, perseverative behavior, and greater frustration levels in coping.

Linguists are relatively late in the chronological history of the study of aphasia, but their present influence is important. Using the linguistic term "decoding" for receptive language and the term "encoding" for expressive language, the linguist is less interested in the study of lesion effects than on the disordered input and output processes of language. Spreen (1968) has taken a linguistic view of aphasia and developed a hierarchy for looking at language behavior: abstractness, frequency of usage, age at acquisition, phrase length, and grammatical class. Frequency of usage was thought by Spreen to be a useful way to look at the abstractness of a word, with the least frequently occurring words the hardest ones for the aphasic patient to recall.

Chapter 2 suggested a linguistic model for looking at language in its phono-logic (speech sounds and voicing patterns), syntactic and morphologic (gram-mar), and semantic (meaning) dimensions. Wepman and Jones (1961) developed the following classifications of aphasia:

1. *Pragmatic aphasia.* The patient conveys very little linguistic meaning to the listener, but does maintain relatively good melody flow of speech. This person may use meaningless words, with little self-awareness of errors. A 51-year-old marine engineer developed pragmatic aphasia secondary to a cerebral thrombo-sis. Although he had no unilateral weakness of arm or leg, he did demonstrate this kind of speech, typical of pragmatic aphasia: "I were when I was a little boy many years afloat with the country's problems with crospen. We could kepp the turtens going on a very small budget."

2. *Semantic aphasia.* The patient has a great difficulty remembering familiar and substantive words, employing various pauses while trying to recall the spe-cific word. The least frequently occurring words are the ones the patient has most difficulty recalling. A 32-year-old secretary had a long history of rheumatic heart disease, which led to a cerebral **embolus,** which left her with a right-sided hemi-paresis, right hemianopsia, and semantic aphasia. Six months after the embolus, this recording was made of her speech: "I see the ———, the ———, oh, here we go again. It is a ———, no, I mean a ———. I love the green uh ———, the uh ———, the green ———. Oh, I don't know what it is. I do but I can't find the word. It's a green ———, uh, a green, eh, ———."

3. *Syntactic aphasia.* The patient omits many function words, such as articles and conjunctions, and speaks telegraphically, with little normal melody flow re-tained in speech. The patient often demonstrates better facility for recalling less frequently occurring words than for frequent and familiar words. A 23-year-old pipe fitter experienced a devastating head wound in the left temporal area, with resultant right hemiphegia and syntactic aphasia. Four months after the onset of aphasia, he was observed to speak this way: "Car race. Blue car. Green car ahead. Finish line soon. Victorious green."

4. *Jargon aphasia.* The patient generally has severe auditory impairment, with problems in auditory comprehension. Many of the patients are so severely in-volved auditorally that they cannot hear or monitor their own jargon. Although the melody flow of speech resembles normal, the phonemes are jumbled into original words or neologisms. A 62-year-old insurance executive experienced a stroke of a thrombotic type which left him with a severe jargon aphasia. He ex-perienced no weakness of limb or other symptom, but his speech was similar to this: "Well, the cresh tisde of the jinishto when corruth groms the battish. There's no question about sconish the corruth."

5. *Global aphasia.* The patient is severely involved in both the decoding and encoding of language. Although unable to follow what others say, the patient

may well look as if she or he is understanding. The patient's own verbal response is generally perseverative, repeating the same senseless sounds or words over and over again: "Ba ba ba ba ba chee. Uh-huh. Ba ba ba ba chee."

Speech pathologists have been active in the study, classification, and management of the aphasic adult primarily since World War II, when a number of veterans were found to have aphasia as a result of head injuries. Consequently, a number of service and veterans aphasia rehabilitation programs were established. The typical speech pathologist who works with aphasics today utilizes a blend of information from speech pathology, learning psychology, and neuropsychology and uses treatment programs peculiar to his or her training and experience.

Etiology and Related Variables

Stroke

Aphasia in adults is generally the result of some kind of acquired insult to the brain. The most common kind of brain insult is the CVA (cerebrovascular accident), or stroke. A stroke is a medical emergency characterized by an impairment of blood flow to or within the brain, requiring immediate medical treatment. Unfortunately, most CVA's are not predictable, and they usually strike their victims without much warning. There are basically three types of CVA's: thrombus, embolus, and hemorrhage.

Thrombus A thrombus is a blood clot that forms within a blood vessel, obstructing the flow of blood. In a CVA, a cerebral artery is blocked because of the thrombus, and brain cells beyond the thrombus block do not receive their needed arterial blood. Without sufficient blood to nourish them, these brain cells die or become damaged, causing various kinds of symptoms, such as aphasia.

Embolus An embolus is a blood clot that forms somewhere in the body and travels to an artery, eventually obstructing the flow of blood within that artery. In a CVA, the embolus obstructs a cerebral artery, impeding the flow of blood to certain brain cells. Brain cells without adequate blood supply become damaged or die, producing various symptoms.

Hemorrhage A third form of CVA is a hemorrhage. Sometimes blood vessels have ballooned, weakened walls (aneurysms) which sometimes spontaneously rupture. If a ruptured aneurysm occurs in the brain, it may well produce severe and sudden symptoms. Other forms of hemorrhage may be related to severe and prolonged hypertension (high blood pressure), which eventually may lead to cerebral artery hemorrhage.

Other Causes

Besides CVA, other possible causes of injury to the adult brain include the result of tumor or the surgical access to such a tumor. Severe trauma, such as gunshot wounds, may cause severe and dramatic aphasias. The veterans' hospitals and military hospitals serve numerous veterans who have sustained head wounds in war and war-related accidents, many of whom have aphasia and dysarthria. Younger patients and those relatively free of vascular disease have a better prognosis for physical and language recovery. For this reason, the younger traumatic patient probably presents a better prognosis than the older patient with vascular disease. However, patients of all ages are often responsive to language therapy; therefore, age and type of injury do not necessarily have strong prognostic implications.

The following symptoms may be caused by the same lesion which causes the aphasia: hemiplegia or hemiparesis, hemianopsia, seizures, cardiovascular instability.

Hemiplegia or hemiparesis A left hemisphere lesion will frequently produce a right-sided paralysis (hemiplegia) or right-sided weakness (hemiparesis). A lesion to the left hemisphere motor cortex or descending motor tracts will affect the opposite extremities (arm and leg), trunk, and face. Since aphasia is basically a left hemisphere disease, the aphasic patient with hemiplegia will have right hemiplegia. Generally, the leg is slightly less involved than the arm, and it is usually possible for the hemiplegic patient to learn to walk again. Through the cooperative efforts of physical therapy, occupational therapy, and perhaps vocational rehabilitation, the hemiplegic patient will learn to ambulate, be independent in self-care activities, and perhaps be vocationally competent as well.

Hemianopsia The visual field of each eye may be cut in half because of the patient's cerebral lesion(s). The optic impulses from the left half of each retina go to the left cerebral hemisphere, and those from the right half go to the right cerebral hemisphere. The curvature of the eyeball and its lenses are such that the left half of each eye sees off to the right side. Therefore, a patient who has a left hemisphere lesion, such as most aphasic patients do, runs the risk of having right hemianopsia, an inability to see the right visual field in each eye (due to the left hemisphere damage). Aphasic patients with right hemianopsia, for example, may not see people or things in their right peripheral vision. Because of the relatively high incidence of right hemianopsia among aphasic patients, it is necessary that the patient be evaluated thoroughly for these visual-field defects. Once diagnosed as having this defect, it is relatively easy for the patient to compensate for the visual loss by learning to move the head from side to side in order to see the lateral environment.

Seizures Some aphasic patients, particularly those with traumatic head injuries, develop epileptic seizures. *Grand mal* (major muscle contractions and sometimes loss of consciousness) and *petit mal* (minor spasms, short in duration) are the two primary types of seizures observed in these patients. Today, seizures can generally be prevented and controlled with some form of anticonvulsant medication.

Cardiovascular instability   Often the same vascular problems which caused the patient's CVA are still present and continue to bother the patient to some degree. Psychological lability, hypertension, and mood shifts are frequently observed; some of these problems may be related to medication irregularity and some to the general physiological instability of the patient. Most CVA patients take some medication for their vascular systems, and some of these medications alter the patient's overall responsiveness. Other patients may be taking anticonvulsant medications or tranquilizers. Each of these types of medications might have systemic effects which influence the patient from time to time.

Evaluation

The focus of the aphasia evaluation is to discover the residual language skills of the patient in order to plan a suitable rehabilitative program. Immediately after the onset of aphasia, the typical patient begins to improve. This **spontaneous recovery** period is most rapid the first few months after onset and gradually ends near the end of the sixth month after onset. Evaluation and therapy should not be deferred during this time, but begun as soon after onset as the patient's physical condition permits. Spontaneous recovery is basically physiological. The period during which spontaneous recovery occurs is an excellent time to stimulate the recall of existing or residual language. The relatively rapid success experienced motivates the patient toward language therapy. In working with the aphasic adult, the speech pathologist hopes to teach the patient nothing new, but instead to stimulate the recall and utilization of past competencies.

Evaluation begins with the first contact with the patient and his or her family. The speech pathologist observes how well the patient understands what is said in social conversation and may also give a few simple spoken commands to follow to sample the patient's auditory comprehension. Observing how the patient formulates language and speaks will provide much information about the type of condition (receptive aphasic or apraxic, for example) the patient has, whether or not the patient demonstrates oral verbal apraxia or dysarthria. An early contact with the family will tell the clinician much about the members' coping abilities, how they will relate to the patient, how they will relate to the environment, and the effect of the illness on them. Since very few families understand much about aphasia, they should be given something to read about aphasia, such as *An Adult Has Aphasia* (Boone, 1965). Such reading materials make good background reading for the family prior to counseling. The family is most important in aphasia rehabilitation; in fact, the family frequently plays the most critical role in the patient's total rehabilitation.

Several different evaluational-diagnostic batteries may be used for testing the aphasic patient. Sometimes the most functional evaluation of the aphasic adult is a series of short tasks administered to determine the patient's decoding function in understanding spoken and written language and encoding functions of speaking and writing. Simple baselines taken in these areas will often allow the perceptive clinician to tailor a program specific to the patient's residual language skills. Commercially available tests which help relate the patient's particular scores to the typical scores of other patients, aiding both in establishing recovery prognosis and in planning early therapy procedures, can also be used. Several evaluative instruments that may be useful in evaluating the residual language competencies of adult aphasics are listed below.

1. *Boston Diagnostic Aphasia Examination* (Goodglass and Kaplan, 1972). This test, which takes about 60 minutes to administer, determines the patient's language competence in five areas: conversational and expository speech, auditory comprehension, oral expression with focus on identifying oral apraxia, reading, and writing. This test provides the clinician with a thorough psycholinguistic analysis of the patient's residual language and relates this information well to the neuropathological status of the patient.

2. *Functional Communication Profile* (Taylor, 1963). This scale allows the clinician to evaluate the patient's functional communication abilities without directly testing the patient. The examiner observes the patient directly in functional situations or asks the family and staff how the patient performs. These general areas are tested: movement (nonverbal activities), speaking, understanding (auditory comprehension), reading, writing, and arithmetic.

3. *Minnesota Test for Differential Diagnosis of Aphasia* (Schuell, 1965). This comprehensive test takes approximately 60 minutes to administer to the average aphasic patient. Since the testing tasks are primarily in the aural input/oral output areas, the test has much immediate relevance to the clinician who wants to determine how well the patient understands and speaks. This test has much therapy relevance, as seen in Schuell's statement: "Careful description of aphasia impairment provides a guide for treatment, since therapy must deal with the disabilities that are present."

4. *Porch Index of Communicative Ability* (PICA) (Porch, 1967). This innovative examination requires about 60 minutes to administer. It is composed of 18 subtests: eight nonverbal, four verbal, and six graphic. It looks at decoding abilities by evaluating response, measuring specific level of output ability with which a good clinician may make inferences about the patient's input language. Scoring is on a graded scale of 1–16, with 16 representing a perfect performance and all values less than that representing some diminution of performance. Because of the difficulty in using graded scoring on the PICA, the examiner must have intensive training in PICA administration before using it with a patient.

5. *Sklar Aphasia Scale* (SAS) (Sklar, 1966). The SAS requires only 30 minutes to administer and provides the clinician with a measure of the patient's language abilities in listening, speaking, reading, and writing. The SAS is often used as a language screening device because of its relative brevity of administration time. Although it identifies gross language impairment well, the SAS does not have enough difficult items to give an accurate language profile of the mildly involved patient.

Although other aphasia evaluation instruments may be used, it is important that testing of the patient be done judiciously and selectively. In most testing situations, the patient is forced into response-failure situations; that is, we continue testing until the patient experiences some degree of failure. Unfortunately, the adult aphasic is a relatively fragile personality, and his or her low tolerance for test failure may cause a real distaste for further encounters with the clinician.

It is sometimes necessary to evaluate the present intelligence of the patient. Because of the verbal limitations imposed by the aphasia, we get the most valid look at the patient's overall intelligence by using a nonverbal intelligence test. For example, the *Progressive Matrices* (Raven, 1962) yields a performance mental age which is determined by the patient's ability to match one of four foils of a cutout to a visual design or pattern; the test is strictly visual-motor performance and requires no verbal instruction by the examiner and no verbal response by the patient. The performance section of the *Wechsler Adult Intelligence Scale* (Wechsler, 1955) does not handicap the verbally impaired patient too much and will give a rough estimate of the patient's "performance" intelligence.

Hearing tests to determine how well the patient hears are often given. Tests of auditory discrimination or sequencing which require only pointing responses to picture stimuli are useful. The degree of apraxia, explained in Chapter 8 on disorders of articulation, which may prevent the patient from saying what she or he wants to say, might be assessed. Oral verbal apraxia, once carefully identified, can often be minimized in its effects; however, oral verbal apraxia is always a poor prognostic sign, and patients who have this disorder do not very often make significant expressive language recoveries. Dysarthria may be assessed, perhaps by making a tape of the patient's speech for further analyses of voice quality and pitch, articulation, respiration, prosody, or rhythm.

Management

Finding activities that will enable the patient to make a language recovery is only one aspect of the total management needs of the aphasic patient. Physical recovery will remain in the hands of the physician, who will employ the physical therapist and the occupational therapist, among others, to aid the patient in learning to walk and to become independent in self-care. The clinical psychologist and the medical social worker may play primary roles in helping the patient adjust to his or her altered life situation. Intensive counseling efforts may be initiated with the family.

Many and varied kinds of language therapy have been tried with aphasic patients, each with varying degrees of success. No one approach seems to have distinct advantages over the others. We shall list and describe some various approaches to treatment and then select and combine some of them into a typical plan of aphasia therapy.

Programed Instruction

Programs consist of sequences of stimuli for presentation to the patient, who must respond correctly to a given stimulus to advance to the next stimulus in the program. If an error is made, a mechanism is provided to take the patient back to an earlier step and to provide the experience necessary to success at an advanced level. A program may be presented by a clinician or an aide, but more commonly is presented by a teaching machine which the patient can operate. Teaching machines used with aphasic patients can present both visual and auditory stimuli. Few speech pathologists would recommend programed instruction to the exclusion of other treatments. Rather, programed instruction is often used as a self-practice tool to supplement other individual and group language therapy that the patient may be receiving. Self-practice appears to be particularly effective for the more mildly involved patient.

Traditional Individual Therapy Approach

Most individual therapy for aphasic patients falls under this heading. Some clinicians work directly in the area of the patient's language deficit; for example, if the patient has a problem in naming, drill work is done in naming. An opposite approach would be to work with the patient's residual language skills. Identifying residual "can do" behaviors is a prelude for exploiting these behaviors in therapy; if the patient cannot name well but can repeat well, therapy focuses on extending the length of the patient's repetitions (maybe from one word at first to a span of six words), with no direct work on the naming deficit. The rationale for the "can do" approach is that the purpose of individual therapy is to stimulate the patient's utilization of past language competencies rather than to "teach something new."

Most individual therapy utilizes the presentation of some kind of stimuli and the request that the patient make some kind of verbal response. The reinforcement of the patient's correct responses lacks any kind of fixed interval, as compared with the programed approach. In effective therapy the clinician presents material that the patient can generally do successfully. Recent quantification of success in therapy seems to require that the patient be successful 65 to 80 percent in his or her responses (Boone and Prescott, 1972). This means that whatever the clinician asks the patient to do in therapy, the patient better be able to perform correctly about three-fourths of the time. If the patient's success rate is lower than this, the clinician must decrease the complexity of the therapy material.

Individual Stimulation Approach

Many patients seem to profit as much from the social interaction with the clinician as they do from the formal therapy materials. For example, I observed the opening of a rehabilitation hospital in a facility that had for 20 years been a custodial nursing home. Many of the patients had been domiciled there for years, and most of them showed the symptoms of neglect: muscle contractures from the lack of proper physical therapy, verbal perseverations (saying the same nonsense utterance over and over), and shyness from years of social isolation. When given the stimulation of systematic visitation by the speech clinician and his aides, many of these people made dramatic improvements in their overall functional communication. They were treated as human beings and were expected to talk. In response, they made efforts to speak, and the more they talked, the better they talked.

Wepman (1972) has taken a critical look at traditional and programed approaches in speech therapy for the aphasic. He wrote that perhaps the most important thing is to present a stimulating environment in which the patient will think and try to communicate. Wepman comments on the "shutter principle," likening the vacillations in attentiveness which the patient demonstrates to the opening and closing of the camera shutter. When the shutter is open, it is important for the patient to have some human stimulation. This kind of therapy is generally an affective one, allowing the patient and the clinician to express feelings about things. Perhaps the most successful aphasia clinicians are those who have a high regard for the aphasic patient as a person and are not hesitant to interact with the patient, regardless of the therapeutic approach one might use.

Group Therapy for the Patient

Group therapy has long been used in the treatment of aphasic patients. Some groups are didactic in nature; specific content is taught to the patients, almost as a teacher would teach a small class. The patients might meet daily for instruction in naming, sentence formulation, reading, writing, and arithmetic. A totally different type of group would be the social-group experience, with the patients talking about holidays, problems, movies, television, and sports. The format of the group is loose, and the group clinician must provide as much socialization opportunity for each patient as possible. When such a social group is really successful, there is much horizontal interaction among the members of the group, with only minimal direction from the clinician.

A middle-ground group would be one that does some work on language (such as structuring what one would do in a restaurant) and some spontaneous interaction about feelings (perhaps stimulated by a recovered patient who comes back and talks about his or her aphasia). From the clinician's standpoint, group therapy with aphasic patients is difficult, requiring the clinician to know the language levels of all of the patients, their general backgrounds, and their present medical status; furthermore, the group clinician must afford all patients the opportunity to participate (difficult to do with the severely involved expressive patient) and not allow one or two patients to "take over" the group.

Family Group

Since the survival of the patient as a social human being is a primary consideration in aphasia rehabilitation, it is essential for the speech pathologist to work closely with the patient's family. Many times this work with the family is facilitated by working closely with the medical social worker. The various family members should meet as a group at least once a week. Not only can important answers be given to their common and separate questions, but they also derive much psychological support from one another. For example, how one family copes with the patient's despondency may serve as a model for other families, or just as important, it may serve to illustrate how *not* to manage such a situation. If observational facilities are available, it is good for the families to observe the patient group with the clinician. Observation of the patient group, however, should generally be done only with the supervision of the clinician, who can do some interpretation when it is needed.

Patients who receive language therapy should be scheduled, whenever possible, for a two-hour block of time daily. To provide a two-hour block of language therapy requires disciplined use of staff time, utilization of electronic teaching aids, and trained volunteers or aides. The use of all five therapy approaches mentioned above is recommended, perhaps on the basis of the following kind of time sequence.

1. *Thirty minutes.* The patient receives individual therapy with the speech pathologist. A baseline is taken of a particular language ability, and instruction begins at that "can do" point. Whatever is presented by the clinician must be met with a general 75 percent success rate; if the patient is not this successful, the work is simplified. If success is much higher than 75 percent, the complexity is increased. Perhaps ten minutes are spent in individual stimulation. Any topic of legitimate interest to the patient may be pursued. At this time, mention is given to such things as prognosis, eventual vocational goals, family situation, and financial problems.

2. *Thirty minutes.* The patient will perhaps practice with programed instruction, self-practice using a teaching machine, or drill with a volunteer or therapy aide. Generally this kind of practice can be self-directed by the patient, but a fairly high level of response success must be maintained. For example, the typi-

cal aphasia program would require that the patient maintain a success rate in excess of 90 percent; the patient does not move on to the next sequence of the program unless he or she has previously experienced success. Perhaps the patient needs practice in oral formulation, requiring something like a cassette tape recorder, with previous models recorded by the clinician. Sometimes it is good to have a volunteer or an aide present to help the patient with these formulations. At other times, the patient may be better off working alone. This practice-drill experience may well be the type of activity that the patient will also be able to practice at home.

3. *One hour.* Patients with various types of aphasia (semantic, syntactic, jargon) may well be placed together in a group that meets almost an hour daily. The optimum size for such a group appears to be from three to eight patients, plus the clinician and perhaps a volunteer or aide. Different topics and teaching materials may be used for each session; for example, a wall map of the United States may well be a catalyst for a group discussion about who has lived or visited where or about relative climates. The patient with limited encoding ability can often participate in such a map discussion by pointing to specific locales and gesturing regard for that area. Birthdays of group members, holidays, elections, entertainers and sports figures, shopping, and dining are all topics well suited to adult group discussion. Some time with the group should be allowed for the patients to interact with one another, commenting on such things as their symptoms, hope for the future, or confidence in their families. Care must be taken to allow all patients to vent their feelings and not to permit a particular patient (often a jargon type) from monopolizing the group discussion. Patients appear to have high regard for aphasia group therapy, frequently insisting that their families bring them to therapy even in the most adverse weather.

The families also benefit from the group experience. Perhaps once weekly, the family members should meet concurrently when the patients are in their group. Social workers or clinical psychologists often combine well with the speech pathologists in conducting the family-type group. Frequently, a particular topic can be introduced by the group leader to initiate discussion; a short, formal presentation of the topic area may be followed with an informal group discussion. Or, the group may prefer to develop its own topics, requesting only occasional "answers" or help from the group leader. On occasion, it has been found to be particularly beneficial for the collective family members to observe the group of patients in therapy. Often the family can develop real insights by watching other patients as they relate to one another.

Histories of Two Aphasic Patients

C. W., a 31-year-old priest, received a head injury in an automobile accident which left him with semantic aphasia, right hemiplegia, right hemianopsia, and epileptic seizures. Brain surgery was performed within three hours after the accident by a neurosurgeon who found an extensive laceration of "superficial cortical areas of the temporal and parietal lobes of the left hemisphere." Five days after the operation, the patient was evaluated with the *Boston Diagnostic Aphasia Examination* (Goodglass and Kaplan, 1972), which found him to have moderate difficulties in auditory and visual verbal recognition, with marked problems of word recall in both speaking and writing. He was subsequently started in a rehabilitation program which included daily physical therapy and two hours of speech rehabilitation daily. Six months following the accident, most of the patient's hemiplegia had resolved, and a marked reduction of his aphasia was noted. He continues to receive intensive daily individual and group speech remediation. Counseling and vocational rehabilitation have begun, with hopes of helping C. W. return to some pastoral capacity in his local church.

M. H., 56 years old, experienced a severe CVA 17 years ago which left her with right hemiplegia and a severe oral verbal apraxia. As a mother of three children and wife of a miner, she stayed in the home as homemaker rather than move from an outlying small town to the rehabilitation facilities in a large city. Consequently, she never received speech remediation for her aphasia for the 17 intervening years between onset of aphasia and the present time. A recently administered speech and language evaluation found the woman to have severe oral verbal apraxia with relatively normal verbal reception. On all comprehension items on the *Porch Index of Communicative Ability* (Porch, 1967), she displayed normal function. Her score on the *Progressive Matrices* (Raven, 1962) examination of intelligence showed her to be within normal limits of intelligence. She could say nothing in imitation after the examiner, and her only spontaneous speech was the perseverative words, "Oh, boy." She said this repeatedly with various inflectional meanings and was able to indicate feelings of approval, despair, hope, and "no" by the sound of her voice by saying the "Oh, boy" utterance.

The remediation focused on producing sets of monosyllabic words, all beginning with the same speech sound. Daily speech remediation was initiated along with intensive family counseling. The patient began working at home with a young adult daughter, practicing the speech material she was learning in the speech clinic. At the time of this writing, she has learned some 300 words and can use them functionally. Considering her 17-year history with no speech, her progress after receiving speech pathology services has motivated the patient to receive additional speech remediation on a twice-daily basis.

Conclusion

Aphasia in adults is a language disorder the patient acquires after any one of several kinds of brain trauma. The aphasic language problem typically includes problems in understanding what is said, in reading, in speaking, and in writing. Interest in these language disorders has led to many studies of brain functions in language, and specialists in neurology, psychology, linguistics, speech pathology, and other fields have contributed to our present knowledge of aphasia. The speech pathologist, concerned with the language recovery of the aphasic patient, begins contact with the patient by observing how well the patient speaks. After language testing is completed, language therapy is initiated. Language therapy for the adult aphasic patient includes programed instruction, individual instruction, stimulation therapy, group therapy, and group family therapy. Although the speech pathologist's focus is on the patient's language, considerable effort in counseling is also given to both the patient and his or her family.

Glossary

Agnosia: Impairment of recognition (auditory, visual, tactual) as a result of damage to the central nervous system.

Aphasia: A loss or reduction of language functions following brain damage. Patients may show impairment in verbal understanding of what they read and hear, with associated problems in language formulation (writing and speaking).

Apraxia: An inability to execute voluntary motor movements; involuntary and automatic movements are normal. Apraxia is the result of central nervous system damage.

Cerebral dominance: The term used for cerebral hemisphere lateralization for language.

Dysarthria: An impairment in articulation, voice, and speech rhythm as a result of central nervous system damage.

Embolus: A traveling blood clot that eventually lodges in an artery, obstructing the flow of blood within that artery.

Hemiplegia: Weakness or paralysis of one side of the body, such as the left leg and left arm.

Localization: The neurological specification of cerebral function, such as performing arithmetic or speaking, to particular cortical areas of the brain.

Spontaneous recovery: The period of time, usually within the first six months after the onset of aphasia, when aphasic patients experience some return of language function with or without the need for formal language therapy.

Thrombus: A blood clot that forms within an artery, eventually obstructing the flow of blood within that artery.

Study Questions

1. What is aphasia?
2. What is the difference between localization and nonlocalization of cerebral function?
3. What are the five types of aphasia presented by Wepman and Jones? Make up examples how patients with each of these five types of aphasia would talk.
4. What are the typical causes of aphasia?
5. What is the purpose of a language evaluation for patients with aphasia?
6. Develop a comprehensive language remediation program for an adult with aphasia.

Bibliography

BOONE, D. R., *An Adult Has Aphasia*, Danville, Ill.: Interstate Printers, 1965.

BOONE, D. R., AND T. E. PRESCOTT, *Application of Videotape and Audiotape Self-Confrontation Procedures in Training Clinicians in Speech and Hearing Therapy*. Final Report, U. S. Department of Health, Education, and Welfare, Office of Education (BEH), #OEG-0-70-4758-607, University of Denver, 1972.

GOODGLASS, H., AND E. KAPLAN, *The Assessment of Aphasia and Related Disorders*, Philadelphia: Lea and Febiger, 1972.

PENFIELD, W., AND L. ROBERTS, *Speech and Brain Mechanisms*, Princeton, N.J.: Princeton University Press, 1959.

PORCH, B. E., *Porch Index of Communicative Ability*, Palo Alto, Calif.: Consulting Psychologists Press, 1967.

RAVEN, J. C., *Progressive Matrices*, New York: Psychological Corp., 1962.

SCHUELL, H., *Minnesota Test for Differential Diagnosis of Aphasia*, Minneapolis: University of Minnesota Press, 1965.

SCHUELL, H., J. J. JENKINS, AND E. JIMENEZ-PABON, *Aphasia in Adults*, New York: Hoeber (Harper and Row), 1964.

SKLAR, M., *Sklar Aphasia Scale*, Los Angeles: Western Psychological Corp., 1966.

SPREEN, O., "Psycholinguistic Aspects of Aphasia," *J. Speech Hearing Res.* **11** (1968): 467–480.

TAYLOR, L. L., *Functional Communication Profile*, New York: New York Medical Center, 1963.

WECHSLER, D., *The Wechsler Adult Intelligence Scale*, New York: Psychological Corp., 1955.

WEPMAN, J. M., "Aphasia Therapy: A New Look," *J. Speech Hearing Dis.* **37** (1972): 203–214.

WEPMAN, J. M., AND L. JONES, *Test for Aphasia*, Chicago: Education-Industry Service, 1961.

CHAPTER 13
Overview

In this chapter the types and causes of hearing disorders are considered. The characteristics of conductive, sensorineural, and mixed types of disorders are explained. Hearing loss may be congenital—present at birth—or acquired later in life. These problems may be hereditary, may originate prenatally because of maternal viral infection, or may be associated with complications occurring near the time of birth. Childhood viral or bacterial infections may cause hearing loss, and some of these losses may be temporary or correctible, whereas others are permanent. Some medicinal drugs are dangerous to hearing. Noise-induced hearing loss is a real problem in our culture. Hearing loss frequently occurs in elderly people.

The evaluation of hearing is explained. Measurement of auditory sensitivity—the ability to detect sound—and auditory discrimination ability—the ability to differentiate sounds—is explained. Various auditory tests are used to elicit this information from children, adults, or those who are difficult to test. There is a discussion of how test results are interpreted.

Disorders of Hearing

Management of hearing loss is presented briefly in terms of medical treatment. In more detail, management is covered from an audiologic viewpoint. Hearing conservation in infants, schools, and noisy industries is considered. There is a discussion of the advantages and limitations of hearing-aid use, as well as the process of learning to use amplification. Sample audiograms and case histories illustrate details of hearing-aid use. Finally, speech and language problems associated with hearing loss are discussed, as well as speechreading and auditory training.

William R. Hodgson, Ph.D.
University of Arizona

Introduction

Disorders of hearing occur when **auditory sensitivity** (ability to hear sounds) or **auditory discrimination ability** (ability to differentiate sounds) is poorer than normal. Sensitivity and discrimination ability are related, but as you will learn later in this chapter, some hearing disorders cause a large problem with one and only a small problem with the other.

Description

Definitions

The terms "deaf" and "hard of hearing" are useful in talking about hearing disorders because they classify people into two groups who behave differently because of their hearing disorder. "Deaf" means that hearing is not functional for everyday purposes. It does not mean that the person may not have some remaining hearing, because most deaf people do. "Hard of hearing" means defective hearing which is functional with or without the use of a hearing aid. The distinction is important for another reason. Deaf children require different educational procedures than do children who are hard of hearing. Many people with hearing disorders fall into a borderline area, and decisions about educational needs are sometimes made on the basis of nonauditory influences, such as intelligence or the kind and extent of training the person gets. Later in this chapter, I will comment more about the distinction between deaf and hard of hearing. The term "hearing impaired" describes people who are either deaf or hard of hearing.

Types of Hearing Loss

Hearing losses are divided into three types: conductive, sensorineural, and mixed. A **conductive** disorder results when something impedes the movement of acoustic energy through the outer or middle ear. For example, a buildup of wax that occludes the ear canal reduces the effective energy reaching the inner ear, and a conductive hearing loss results. Since the inner ear is normal, a conductive loss causes primarily a loss of hearing sensitivity.

If damage to either the inner ear or auditory nerve causes a hearing disorder and the sound-conducting parts of the ear remain normal, the result is a **sensorineural loss.** Damage to these sound-analyzing parts of the ear causes a loss of both hearing sensitivity and auditory discrimination ability. Sensorineural losses are permanent, whereas conductive losses are potentially reversible.

The third type of loss, **mixed** loss, occurs when there are problems in both the sound-conducting and sound-analyzing parts of the ear. In other words, a conductive and a sensorineural loss are both present in the same ear. Mixed

319

losses reduce both sensitivity and discrimination ability, but since part of the loss is conductive, discrimination ability will be reduced less than in a pure sensorineural loss of equal magnitude.

These three types of disorders are caused by problems in the peripheral auditory mechanism—the part outside the central nervous system. The central auditory nervous system can also malfunction. The resulting disorder is usually subtle, such as a reduction in auditory discrimination in difficult listening conditions (when listening in noise, for example). Reduction in auditory sensitivity ordinarily does not result from damage to the higher parts of the brain. A term sometimes used, central deafness, does not appropriately describe the disorder, nor is the term "hearing loss" appropriate. Problems associated with damage to the central auditory nervous system are referred to as "central auditory disorders" (Berlin and Lowe, 1972).

Etiology and Related Variables

The cause of a hearing loss cannot always be determined. Most of the time, however, a probable reason can be found. If the origin of the loss is before or around the time of birth, the loss is called *congenital*. If the loss develops later, it is called *acquired*. This distinction is important because losses acquired after the development of language and speech are less devastating. A severe congenital loss interferes with normal language and speech development and necessitates special teaching methods. Some common causes of hearing loss are discussed below.

Hereditary Factors

Hearing disorders of genetic origin are a common cause of congenital deafness, but not all hereditary losses are congenital. In many cases, the hereditary defect does not manifest itself until years later. There are many kinds of hereditary losses, and they range in severity from slight to complete (Proctor, 1967; Pashayan, 1975). Both parents of a genetically deaf baby may have normal hearing but be carriers of the trait, and that deaf baby may grow up to have children with normal hearing. In most inherited deafness, the person is otherwise normal, but there are many **syndromes** which include deafness as only one of the abnormalities. For example, the manifestations of Waardenburg's syndrome include congenital sensorineural loss and the following characteristics. There is displacement of the fold of skin at the inner corner of the eyes, giving the appearance of a broad nasal base and eyes that are set wide apart. The eyes may be of different color, e.g., one blue and one brown. There may be a "white forelock," or streak of white in the hair above the forehead. These symptoms, including the hearing loss, are variable, not all appearing in a given individual.

Treacher Collins syndrome provides an example of congenital conductive loss with other hereditary anomalies. The external ears may be deformed or absent, and the external ear canal may be partly or completely unformed. The middle ear may be abnormal. There are deformities of the eyelids and an underdeveloped mandible which give the face a characteristic appearance. Cleft lip and cleft palate may also occur. Since the inner ear is usually normal, hearing may be improved by surgery.

Maternal Rubella

German measles is a mild disease. It is dangerous, however, when the disease occurs in the early stages of pregnancy. The rubella virus then may retard development of fetal organs, being especially likely to cause sensorineural hearing loss, visual and cardiac problems. Rubella is a cyclical disease, and major outbreaks in the United States have resulted in the birth of thousands of multiply handicapped or hearing-impaired infants. A vaccine to prevent rubella has been developed, and control of this problem appears possible.

Perinatal Hearing Losses

Prematurity or birth trauma may lead to complications, such as **anoxia** from failure to initiate normal breathing. Hearing loss may result. The incidence of hearing loss associated with prematurity and anoxia is not clear. There is one well-known cause of neonatal hearing loss—complications arising from Rh incompatibility. This condition can develop when there are incompatible aspects between fetal and maternal blood. Antibodies developed by the mother destroy components of the infant's blood, and brain damage and hearing loss may result. Athetoid-type cerebral palsy is another possible consequence. Therefore, hearing loss should be suspected in all athetoid persons.

Treatment to prevent damage in cases of Rh incompatibility has been developed. Exchange blood transfusions are used to remove antibodies from the infant's system, and immunization techniques can prevent development of maternal antibodies. Hopefully, these medical advances will reduce the incidence of this problem.

Otitis Media

This disorder is especially common in children, but also occurs in adults. Sometimes the Eustachian tube (see Chapter 5) fails to aerate the middle ear. In a cold, for example, the swollen membrane of the throat may prevent entrance of air at the nasopharyngeal port of the Eustachian tube. When this happens, some of the existing air in the middle ear is absorbed by the tissues that line the middle-ear cavity, and a partial vacuum results. The greater atmospheric pressure in the ear canal, pushing against the eardrum, may cause pain. Fluid may be pulled from the middle-ear tissues, resulting in a condition called *serous otitis*, or middle-ear effusion. Some conductive hearing loss results. The fluid in the middle ear is not caused by bacterial infection, and if the condition preventing Eustachian tube function passes (the person recovers from the cold, for example), everything, including the hearing, may return to normal.

Recurrent serous otitis, possibly allergenic, is a problem with some children. In persistent or recurring cases of Eustachian-tube malfunction, the otologist may insert a tube through an opening made in the eardrum, providing a substitute channel for equalizing middle-ear air pressure.

An infection may develop as bacteria enter the middle ear via the Eustachian tube either in conjunction with serous otitis or in the absence of earlier middle-ear problems. This disorder is known as *purulent*, or *suppurative, otitis media*. The result is pain, fever, and if enough pus is generated in the middle ear, rupture of the eardrum. *Myringotomy*, or surgical incision of the eardrum, is occasionally necessary to provide drainage of the middle-ear cavity and prevent the less desirable spontaneous rupture. Myringotomy may also be done to remove the effusion of serous otitis media. Possible complications of untreated otitis media are: (1) mastoiditis (intrusion of the infection into the bone of the skull in the area behind the ear); (2) labyrinthitis (invasion of the inner ear, with resultant sensorineural hearing loss); (3) meningitis (invasion of the tissues that cover the brain, a disease that can be fatal); or (4) the acute stage may subside, and a chronic otitis may gradually erode and destroy the eardrum or middle-ear contents.

Serous otitis may either precede or follow an ear infection. Antibiotic treatment may suppress the infection but leave fluid in the middle-ear cavity. Over time, this residue may thicken and adhere to the ossicular chain, reducing its motility. This condition, *adhesive otitis media*, results in damage to the ossicles and progressive conductive loss. Obviously, the possible complications of middle-ear infection dictate prompt and thorough medical treatment.

Meningitis

The *meninges* are the covering layers of the brain and spinal cord. Infection in this area is often fatal unless treated quickly. The infection may invade the inner ear, destroying its function. Although the expected result is complete hearing loss, milder and even unilateral sensorineural losses occur. For example, an eight-year-old girl came to our clinic after recovering from meningitis. She had obviously suffered a hearing loss. The parents were almost apologetic for bringing the child. They had been told that meningitis causes complete hearing loss, but they wanted to explore every possibility. As expected, the girl had no measurable hearing on one ear. However, on the other ear she had a flat 70 dB loss.

We tried a hearing aid on that ear. The girl ran to her parents, saying, "Mama, they made me hear again!"

Other bacterial infections, such as diphtheria and typhoid fever, may cause hearing loss. However, these diseases now are rare in the United States because of widespread immunization.

Viral Diseases

Of the viral diseases common in childhood, sensorineural hearing loss has been attributed to measles, mumps, chickenpox, influenza, and the common cold. Of these, measles (not rubella) is a recognized cause of sensorineural loss in children. Mumps also causes hearing loss, ordinarily in one ear only. In both children and adults, viral diseases which are usually innocuous sometimes cause sudden, bilateral sensorineural losses of varying magnitude.

Ototoxic Drugs

Some medicinal drugs damage the ear if taken in large enough doses. Overdoses of aspirin or quinine can cause hearing loss, although recovery of hearing is common. Some antibiotics can cause permanent sensorineural loss; dihydro-streptomycin, neomycin, kanamycin, and streptomycin are examples. These drugs are particularly dangerous in patients who have poor kidney function, which fosters retention of the drug. Use of these drugs is carefully controlled, and doses dangerous to the ear are given only if necessary to save the patient's life.

Otosclerosis

A common cause of hearing loss in adults, *fenestral otosclerosis,* is a slowly progressive conductive loss—usually bilateral, but not necessarily bilaterally equal. *Labyrinthine otosclerosis* causes a sensorineural loss. Otosclerosis a hereditary disorder. The loss is usually first noticed when individuals are in their teens or twenties. The problem results when the bone surrounding the inner ear changes in composition and grows. The otosclerotic growth affects the bone surrounding the footplate of the stapes, as well as the stapes itself. The mobility of the ossicular chain is reduced, and the result is a conductive loss (fenestral otosclerosis). Intrusion of the bony growth into the inner ear causes a sensorineural loss (labyrinthine otosclerosis).

The loss caused by fenestral otosclerosis is surgically correctible by replacement of the diseased stapes with a prosthesis. Because the loss is slowly progressive, the individual may not initially identify the problem as a hearing loss. According to one patient with advancing otosclerosis, over a period of months he had the developing awareness that something was wrong. He seemed unable to get the point of conversations or to get all the details exactly straight. He could tell by the strange looks he received that he didn't always respond appropriately. He was afraid, he said, that he might be losing his mind, and his family shared his concern. Then one day he noticed he could no longer hear a particular sound which had previously been audible. He realized he had a hearing loss. Happily, it was correctible.

Noise-Induced Loss and Acoustic Trauma

As described in Chapter 6, exposure to intense noise causes a temporary **threshold** shift of hearing sensitivity. Exposure to sufficiently intense noise will result in permanent sensorineural loss. Noise-induced loss is the term for the slowly progressive loss associated with long-term noise exposure. Acoustic trauma results from exposure to sound, such as an explosion, sufficiently intense to do immediate damage to the ear through physical destruction of inner ear tissues. Noise-induced loss is usually attributed to noisy working environment (boiler maker's deafness), but motorcycles and snowmobiles may be noisy enough over long exposure to induce permanent loss. Estimation of dangerously high noise levels is complicated by the fact that individuals vary considerably in their susceptibility to noise damage. Some indicators of noise levels high enough to be dangerous to your ears with sufficient exposure are: (1) trouble hearing others because of the noise; (2) **tinnitus** (ringing of the ears); or (3) temporary hearing loss noticeable on emerging from the noise. Protective earplugs or muffs, properly used, reduce the danger of noise-induced loss.

Noise-induced loss progresses slowly as exposure continues. Sensitivity for only the higher frequencies is affected at first. These frequencies contribute little to the perceived loudness of speech, but are important for intelligibility. Since the change is so gradual and is mostly in the perceived clarity of speech instead of loudness, a person may not pinpoint the problem until after a handicapping noise-induced loss has already developed.

I once talked to an audience which contained many people with long-term noise exposure. I carefully pointed out the insidious nature of the problem and how its effects might not be realized. Afterwards, an old fellow commented, "Doc, you've got it all wrong. If you just learn to shut the noise out, it won't bother you. I've been working in noise for 20 years, and I've learned to shut it out so well that now two people can be talking five feet away from me, and I don't even hear 'em!"

Meniere's Syndrome

Usually unilateral, this hearing disorder is characterized by progressive hearing loss, tinnitus, and episodes of vertigo and nausea. These symptoms are caused by development of excess fluid pressure in the membraneous parts of the inner ear, affecting its hearing and balance functions. If medical treatment is not successful and the discomfort is severe, the inner structure of the pathologic ear is sometimes destroyed by surgery to relieve the symptoms. This action may be necessary because the vertigo may be incapacitating. Once when my wife and I were eating dinner in a restaurant, we saw through the window a man walking at an odd angle and obviously about to fall. "That poor fellow is having an attack of Meniere's disease," my wife said. "You must go out and help him." I did. You've probably anticipated the fact that I found myself in the street holding up a drunk. However, the reverse can happen. During an attack, people with Meniere's disease are sometimes mistakenly thought to be intoxicated.

Acoustic Tumor

These slow-growing benign tumors of the auditory nerve variously cause hearing loss, tinnitus, vertigo, and in later stages facial paralysis. An untreated tumor results in death from increased internal cranial pressure. Typically, acoustic tumors cause greater reduction in auditory discrimination ability than would be expected relative to the loss of hearing sensitivity. Surgical removal of the tumor ordinarily causes complete loss of hearing in the operated ear.

Presbycusis

Hearing loss in old age, in the absence of other observable causes, is called *presbycusis*. Presbycusis is associated with degeneration of sensory cells in the cochlea and with atrophy of other vital cochlear structures. The effects of aging on the vascular and central auditory systems add to the complexity of the disorder. The typical patient presents a mild, bilaterally equal sensorineural hearing loss somewhat greater for high frequencies. Auditory discrimination ability is often poorer than the loss of sensitivity would suggest, and a special term, *phonemic regression*, is used to describe the situation. Individuals with phonemic regression may not benefit much from additional intensity of speech. They understand better if speech is clearly and slowly articulated.

The problems discussed above are among the most common causes of hearing loss. There are other known causes, and, no doubt, some causes that remain as yet unknown.

Evaluation of Hearing Loss

Hearing tests have several purposes: (1) to measure hearing sensitivity and auditory discrimination ability; (2) to determine the type of hearing loss; (3) to help differentiate one auditory disease from another; (4) to determine degree of handicap; (5) to aid in deciding educational placement; or (6) to answer questions about hearing-aid use. Auditory function and measurement were discussed in Chapters 5 and 6. Clinical application of hearing measurement to evaluate hearing disorders is discussed below.

Pure-Tone Audiometry

The purpose of this basic hearing test is measurement of auditory sensitivity as a function of frequency. Figure 13.1 illustrates the basic features of a pure-tone audiometer. This instrument electronically generates simple signals of known frequency and controllable intensity. These signals are called "pure tones" because each is supposed to have energy present at only one frequency. The tones sound like those produced by a tuning fork. Most audiometers can produce

Figure 13.1

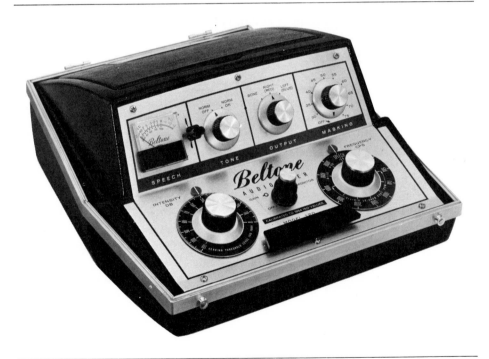

Pure-tone audiometer. The hearing-loss dial controls output intensity, and the frequency selector determines test frequency. (Photograph courtesy Beltone Electronics Corporation, Chicago, Illinois.)

tones of 125, 250, 500, 750, 1000, 1500, 2000, 3000, 4000, 6000, and 8000 Hz. Recall that Hertz, abbreviated Hz, stands for cycles per second and describes the frequency of the signal. Thresholds are ordinarily determined only at octave intervals from 250 through 8000 Hz unless markedly uneven thresholds call for additional information.

In cooperative adults or school-age children, the usual procedure is to place earphones on the individual being tested and ask the person to say "yes" or to raise a hand each time a tone is heard. Then, by varying the intensity of tonal presentation, threshold is determined for each frequency in each ear.

Thresholds are plotted in decibels. Special procedures are used to determine thresholds of uncooperative individuals and younger children. Auditory testing should be done in a quiet room. Otherwise, noise may prevent audibility of low-level test signals and cause invalid results. Sound-treated rooms that reduce the intensity of outside noise and provide a quiet test environment are commercially available.

The graph on which thresholds are plotted is called an *audiogram* (Fig. 13.2). Right-ear thresholds are designated by a red circle; those of the left ear, by a blue X. Zero dB approximates normal sensitivity, and progressively greater hearing loss is indicated by thresholds recorded "farther down" on the audiogram. The presentation of stimuli through earphones is called air-conduction testing. Pure-tone air-conduction thresholds are a measure of overall sensitivity. Bone-conduction thresholds are ordinarily obtained only when a hearing loss is found. These thresholds generally reflect the sensitivity of the inner ear, which must be presumed normal if air-conduction thresholds are normal. Bone-conduction thresholds usually are obtained by placing a vibrator on the mastoid area of the skull behind the ear and stimulating the inner ear "directly." Since the signal "bypasses" the outer and middle parts of the ear, bone-conduction testing can reveal defects of the inner ear. We use arrows or brackets to indicate bone-conduction thresholds (blue < or] for the left ear and red > or [for the right ear). Frequency-response limitations of the vibrator limit testing to the range 250–4000 Hz.

Comparison of air- and bone-conduction thresholds permits classification of a loss as conductive, sensorineural, or mixed type. Figure 13.3 shows the audiogram of Larry F., an 11-year-old with recurrent middle-ear problems. He has a conductive loss. The normal bone-conduction thresholds indicate that the inner ear is undamaged. Note that the discrimination scores are normal bilaterally. The conductive disorder is reducing the effective intensity of sound reaching the inner ear, causing abnormal air-conduction thresholds. This disparity between air- and bone-conduction thresholds in the same ear is called an *air-bone gap* and is the audiometric indicator of a conductive loss. Larry needs a medical examination, and treatment may follow. Successful medical treatment may close the air-bone gap and restore hearing sensitivity to normal.

Figure 13.2

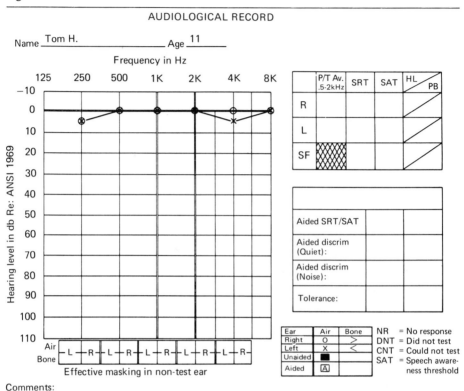

AUDIOLOGICAL RECORD

Name Tom H.   Age 11

Pure-tone audiogram. Most audiogram forms provide space for pure-tone thresholds, other test results, and pertinent information. The auditory thresholds shown here illustrate normal sensitivity.

Recall that masking was discussed in Chapter 6. Clinically, masking involves introducing noise into the nontest ear to prevent its participation. The rules governing masking are complex and beyond the scope of our discussion. However, masking was necessary for obtaining the results shown in Fig. 13.3 and in some of the audiograms shown in subsequent figures.

Figure 13.4 shows the audiogram of Margaret H., age 62, who has a sensorineural loss. Thresholds obtained by air conduction (measuring the response of the entire peripheral auditory mechanism) and by bone conduction (measuring sensorineural function only) are the same. The audiometric indicator of a pure sensorineural loss is essentially equal air- and bone-conduction thresholds. Mrs. H. was examined by an **otolaryngologist** who found no medically treatable basis for her hearing loss. She complained of difficulty hearing faint speech. Her audi-

Figure 13.3

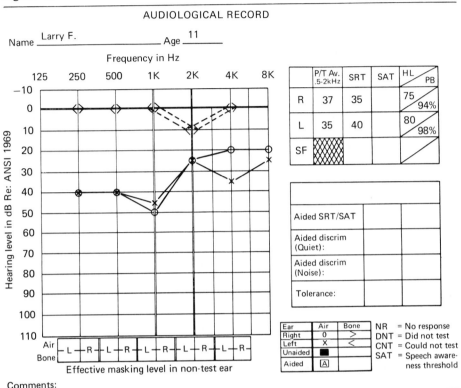

AUDIOLOGICAL RECORD

Name  Larry F. _____ Age ___11___

Frequency in Hz

	P/T Av. .5-2kHz	SRT	SAT	HL / PB
R	37	35		75 / 94%
L	35	40		80 / 98%
SF				

Aided SRT/SAT		
Aided discrim (Quiet):		
Aided discrim (Noise):		
Tolerance:		

Ear	Air	Bone
Right	O	>
Left	X	<
Unaided	■	
Aided	Ⓐ	

NR = No response
DNT = Did not test
CNT = Could not test
SAT = Speech aware-
ness threshold

Effective masking level in non-test ear

Comments:

Audiogram showing conductive hearing loss. Normal bone-conduction thresh-olds reflect the intact inner ear on either side. Reduced air-conduction thresholds indicate that the hearing loss is caused by a conductive blockage. The air-bone gap, or difference between air- and bone-conduction thresholds, indicates the magnitude of the conductive loss. As noted in the text, masking was used as necessary in this and subsequent audiograms to ensure that the nontest ear was not participating in the response.

tory discrimination ability is reduced, but remains fairly good. Later in this chapter, some rehabilitative measures for Mrs. H. are discussed.

Figure 13.5 shows a mixed loss on the right ear of Harriet L., age 60. The left ear has a sensorineural loss. On the right ear, the amount by which the bone-conduction thresholds are reduced from normal represents the magnitude of the sensorineural loss. The size of the air-bone gap indicates the conductive component. Mrs. L. has excellent discrimination on the right ear and very poor discrimination on the left. She was referred to us by an otolaryngologist for a

Figure 13.4

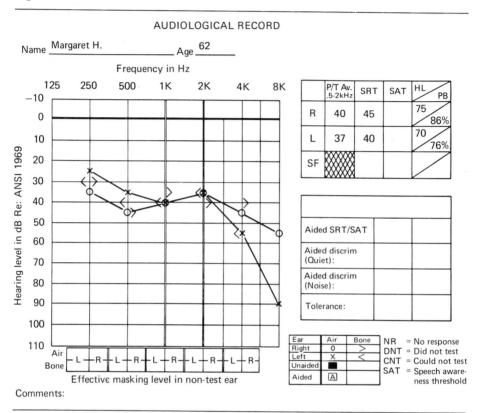

AUDIOLOGICAL RECORD

Name Margaret H.   Age 62

Frequency in Hz

	P/T Av. .5-2kHz	SRT	SAT	HL / PB
R	40	45		75 / 86%
L	37	40		70 / 76%
SF				

Aided SRT/SAT			
Aided discrim (Quiet):			
Aided discrim (Noise):			
Tolerance:			

Ear	Air	Bone
Right	0	>
Left	X	<
Unaided	■	
Aided	Ⓐ	

NR = No response
DNT = Did not test
CNT = Could not test
SAT = Speech aware-
    ness threshold

Effective masking level in non-test ear

Comments:

Audiogram showing sensorineural loss. Reduced bone-conduction thresholds, equal to air conduction, indicate that the origin of the loss is probably in the inner ear or the auditory nerve.

hearing-aid evaluation. The results and recommendation are described later in this chapter.

Play Audiometry

Young children may find responding to pure tones abstract and uninteresting. Better responses may be obtained by incorporating into a game some specific motor response to pure-tone stimuli. Typically the child is asked to drop a block in a box or place a peg in a pegboard each time the tone is heard. Correct responses are reinforced with verbal or tangible rewards. Figure 13.6 illustrates play audiometry: (a) the **audiologist** gets the child to listen for the signal; (b) the

Figure 13.5

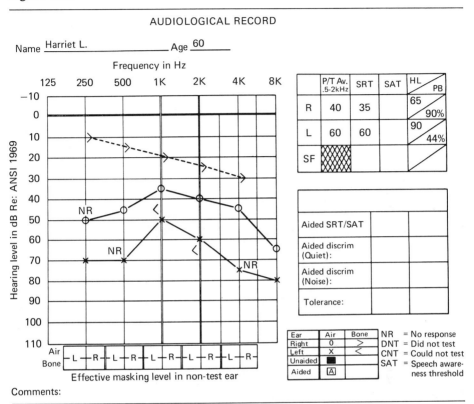

AUDIOLOGICAL RECORD

Name Harriet L. _____ Age 60 _____

	P/T Av. .5-2kHz	SRT	SAT	HL / PB
R	40	35		65 / 90%
L	60	60		90 / 44%
SF				

Aided SRT/SAT			
Aided discrim (Quiet):			
Aided discrim (Noise):			
Tolerance:			

Ear	Air	Bone		
Right	0	>	NR	= No response
Left	X	<	DNT	= Did not test
Unaided	■		CNT	= Could not test
Aided	Ⓐ		SAT	= Speech aware-ness threshold

Effective masking level in non-test ear

Comments:

Audiogram showing mixed loss on the right ear and sensorineural loss on the left. On the right ear the sensorineural component is represented by the reduction in bone-conduction thresholds, and the conductive component is indicated by the air-bone gap.

child hears the tone; (c) she responds by placing a wooden ring on a post; and (d) she receives praise for her response. Play audiometry may be appropriate for children between two and six years or for older retarded children (Hodgson, 1972).

Speech Thresholds

Although the pure-tone audiogram gives a sensitive measure of hearing, it is an indirect answer to the question of greatest interest, namely, the amount of hearing loss which exists for speech. To obtain a direct measure and to confirm the results of pure-tone testing, speech thresholds are routinely obtained when a

331

Figure 13.6

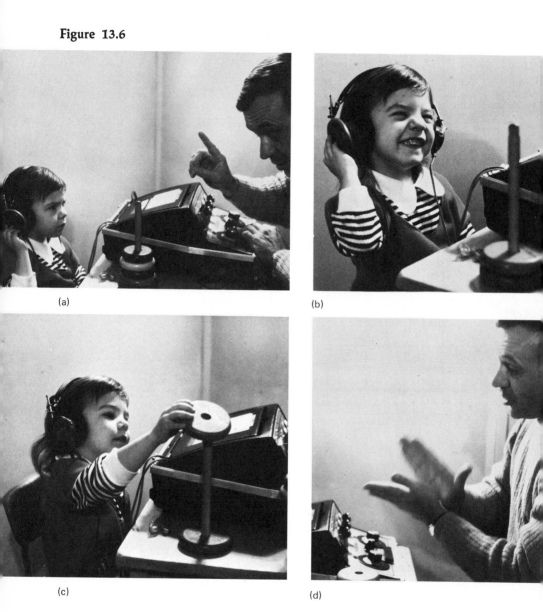

(a)

(b)

(c)

(d)

Play audiometry with a three-year-old child. (a) Examiner prepares the child to listen; (b) she hears the tone; (c) she responds; (d) response is reinforced.

hearing loss is found. A speech audiometer has controls similar to the pure-tone instrument described earlier, but delivers a speech signal instead of tones. A speech audiometer usually makes provision for both live-voice testing, in which case the examiner speaks test words into a microphone, or for recorded tests, which originate from a tape recorder or phonograph. Live-voice testing requires a two-room facility; the examiner and patient are in separate rooms so that the patient hears the signal through the calibrated system rather than directly.

Words used to determine the threshold for speech should be highly intelligible and equally intelligible. **Spondee words** (two-syllable words with equal stress on both syllables, for example, cowboy, birthday, airplane) meet these criteria and are commonly used. As the person being tested repeats the words presented, the intensity of presentation is varied until the level is found at which he or she can repeat about 50 percent of the words. This speech-reception threshold, expressed in dB, should agree with the average of pure-tone thresholds for the frequencies 500, 1000, and 2000 Hz (or the two best of those three thresholds in the case of markedly uneven sensitivity across this speech range). Refer to the speech thresholds shown in Figs. 13.3, 13.4, and 13.5 to examine agreement between speech and pure-tone thresholds.

Testing Auditory Discrimination Ability

Speech-discrimination tests evaluate how well a hearing-impaired person can differentiate among sounds once speech is made loud enough to overcome the effects of loss of hearing sensitivity. This testing is usually done with phonetically balanced **(PB) lists.** These PB word lists usually contain 50 one-syllable words which reflect the frequency of occurrence of speech sounds as they occur in ordinary usage of the language. These lists are presented through a speech audiometer (live voice or recorded) at an intensity sufficient to elicit the best possible response. The person being tested repeats each word heard, and each response is scored correct or incorrect. Results are recorded in percent correct.

Objective Auditory Tests

Sometimes patients cannot or will not respond reliably to auditory stimuli presented in the ways we have described. In these cases, audiometry using standard procedures is not possible. Objective techniques have been developed, wherein behavioral responses by the patient are not necessary. Details of these procedures are beyond the scope of this book, but some general information is presented below.

The objective procedure most common in clinical use is impedance audiometry. The impedance audiometer measures the acceptance of energy by the middle ear. The ability of the middle ear to accept sound energy is different in normal ears and those with conductive hearing loss. It also varies among conductive disorders. Therefore, impedance measurements are useful diagnostically. They help differentiate conductive and sensorineural loss and give information about the cause of conductive losses. There are even procedures to estimate auditory threshold by impedance testing (Jerger *et al.*, 1974).

Sound energy introduced into the cochlea gives rise to electrical phenomena in the peripheral and central auditory system. The measurement of these sound-evoked auditory potentials may give information about hearing status. One measurement procedure is called electrocochleography. An electrode in place near the inner ear permits recording of the response of the auditory nerve. Observation of the intensity of sound necessary to elicit a response permits estimates of auditory sensitivity (Glattke, 1977).

Similar procedures can detect sound-evoked responses in the central auditory nervous system. This technique developed from the observation that changes in the electrical activity of the brain, as monitored by electroencephalography, occurred when auditory stimuli were presented. Auditory assessment of this sort is called evoked response audiometry, or electroencephalographic audiometry. Early investigators had difficulty differentiating the auditory-evoked response from other stronger ongoing electrical activity. The use of computers was found to be helpful. These specially designed instruments help to prevent recording of random responses and enhance the auditory-evoked responses of interest. Computers are necessary in electrocochleography also. In spite of these advances, many problems remain in the clinical application of electrophysiological techniques (Skinner, 1972).

Special Auditory Tests

The tests described above (pure-tone air- and bone-conduction thresholds, speech thresholds, and speech-discrimination testing) are those routinely performed in the audiological evaluation of a hearing-impaired person. There are a number of other auditory tests, some of which have the purpose of supplementing or validating the tests discussed above. Additional tests, called special auditory tests, provide information for the otologist which helps in the diagnosis of ear disorders. The purpose of these tests is locating the site of lesion.

Interpreting Test Results

Auditory tests can provide considerable information about the hearing-impaired individual and his or her handicap. They cannot predict with unfailing accuracy the auditory behavior of each person, because people with hearing loss remain individuals and retain individual differences. Other information, such as intelligence, motivation, training, and attitudes, has to be considered in interpretation of auditory test results.

Classification of Loss

Hearing loss is usually classified according to loss of sensitivity in the better ear. Since this classification is based on magnitude of loss, it does not take into account the amount of discrimination deficit. In other words, it is a comment about only part of the hearing loss. However, generalizations about discrimination deficit are also possible. Table 13.1 shows a commonly used system for classifying hearing loss. Thresholds in dB are either pure-tone averages for the speech range or speech-reception thresholds. Hearing losses are classified as slight, mild, moderate, severe, or profound. Comments are made about expected behavior in each class if the loss is congenital or if it is acquired. "Congenital" in this instance is used broadly to mean hearing loss originating before the development of language and speech. "Acquired" means hearing loss occurring after the acquisition of speech and language. Comments about discrimination ability in Table 13.1 assume a sensorineural loss. If the loss is conductive, discrimination remains quite good up to the maximum conductive loss, about 70 dB.

The individual with good auditory sensitivity for low frequencies and a high-frequency loss presents a special case of hearing disorder. In children, this loss is frequently detected late or may be misdiagnosed as mental retardation, emotional disturbance, aphasia, or learning disability. In older school-age children, the loss even if detected is frequently not understood and its severity underestimated. High-frequency loss constitutes a common configuration in the hearing disorders of adults whose complaint is, "I hear you, but I don't understand you." The following comments describing the hearing loss shown in Fig. 13.7 generalize more or less to all high-frequency losses. Because hearing is near normal to 1000 Hz, there is no great overall loss of hearing sensitivity. This fact is illustrated by the nearly normal speech-reception thresholds. However, because of the distortion associated with sensorineural loss and the reduced ability to hear weak, high-frequency consonants, auditory discrimination ability is sharply reduced. The individual is able to follow simple speech of normal intensity when listening in quiet. These conditions place relatively small demands on the impaired discrimination. But if the speech becomes faint, more complex, or especially if noise is added to the listening condition, the ability to understand disintegrates. These facts explain why the person with high-frequency loss can do so well when chatting with a friend and so poorly when listening to a lecture in a noisy classroom or when trying to communicate among a group of people. Hearing aids designed to amplify only high frequencies can be helpful, but people with high-frequency loss are problem hearing aid candidates, requiring careful audiological evaluation, training, and patience to achieve successful hearing aid use.

Table 13.1   Classification of hearing loss.

THRESHOLDS IN BETTER EAR*	CLASSIFICATION	EXPECTED PROBLEMS AND NEEDS
0–25 dB	Functionally normal	People near the bottom of this range may have occasional difficulty understanding faint speech or speech in noise. However, they ordinarily do not feel that they have a hearing loss.
26–40 dB	Slight loss	If the loss is congenital, language and speech development are a little slower than normal. In school, the child needs preferential seating, as do all children with hearing loss. Additional help with language arts may be required. There is a little difficulty with faint or distant speech, but discrimination is good to excellent. Trouble understanding in noise may be reported. Depending on how critical demands on listening are, part-time hearing-aid use may be needed as loss approaches 40 dB.
41–55 dB	Mild loss	Mild congenital loss causes significant delay of language and speech. Language instruction is needed. Articulation problems are likely. People with mild loss understand normal conversation in closeup, one-to-one situations, but miss a lot in class or groups. Auditory discrimination is good; but deteriorates in noise; the person may get along better without an aid in some noisy places. Speech-reading instruction may be helpful.
56–70 dB	Moderate loss	Moderate congenital loss causes severe retardation of language and speech development unless special training is provided. Children need preschool training, and most will need to start school in special classes for the hard of hearing. They may move to regular classes later, at least for some subjects. Alternatively, children may attend regular classes and receive additional individual tutoring as needed. Severe articulation

* Thresholds are in dB according to 1964 ISO (International Standards Organization) standards, based on sensitivity in better ear (pure-tone averages across the speech range or speech-reception thresholds).

THRESHOLDS IN BETTER EAR*	CLASSIFICATION	EXPECTED PROBLEMS AND NEEDS
		problems are likely. Voice disorders may be present. If loss is acquired, there may be some deterioration of language and speech for this and subsequent classifications (Penn, 1955). Essentially full-time hearing-aid use is indicated, with substantial benefit, since discrimination is expected to be fairly good. Speechreading is necessary to supplement hearing.
71–90 dB	Severe loss	Severe congenital loss causes delay in learning consistent response to audible sounds. Only rudimentary language and speech develop without special training. Children need preschool training and special-class placement, but may eventually attend regular class, at least for some subjects. Full-time hearing-aid use is needed. The aid makes speech audible, but poor auditory discrimination may limit its effectiveness. With training, the use of hearing and vision may permit reasonably effective communication.
91 plus dB	Profound loss	Congenital profound loss prevents learning consistent response to sound or development of language and speech without special training. Children should be in full-time educational programs for the deaf. Those who have hearing in the upper part of this class, and auditory responses across the speech range, may use a hearing aid to supplement visual clues for speech. Those with fragmented audiograms and no response for frequencies higher than 500 or 1000 Hz receive only gross auditory clues and have extremely poor auditory discrimination.

Audiologic Management of Hearing Loss

Most conductive losses are potentially correctible; almost all sensorineural losses are not. Medical and surgical treatment of hearing disorders was mentioned briefly earlier in this chapter. The following is a discussion of the habilitation or rehabilitation of persons with hearing loss.

Figure 13.7

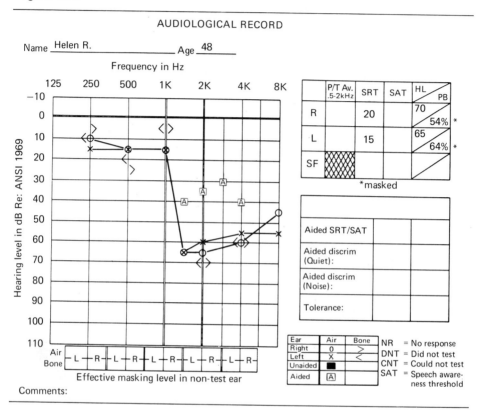

AUDIOLOGICAL RECORD

Name Helen R.   Age 48

High-frequency hearing loss. Audiogram shows bilaterally equal hearing with close to normal sensitivity to 1000 Hz and a sharply falling high-frequency configuration.

Hearing-Conservation Programs

The most desirable management of hearing loss is prevention. To this end, there are hearing-conservation programs in noisy industries, in schools, and in other settings. Experimental programs to detect hearing loss in neonates are being evaluated with the goal of detecting hearing loss during the first days of life, while infants are still in the hospital nursery.

Hearing-conservation programs in schools aim to detect children with losses sufficient to impede educational progress. The hope is to secure for these children medical or surgical remediation when possible, and when not, to minimize the effects of the loss through appropriate audiological and educational procedures.

Hearing-conservation programs conducted where people spend time in noisy surroundings attempt to prevent or minimize noise-induced loss. Analysis of noise levels and spectra is the first step in such a program to determine which noise levels are dangerous. Damage-risk criteria have been developed to serve as a guide to maximum safe intensity levels and limits of time exposure. Another important step consists of obtaining preexposure audiograms to serve as baselines for comparison with tests obtained at later dates. When possible, dangerously high noise levels are reduced, or exposure of personnel to these levels is limited. Sound-protective devices, such as earplugs or muffs properly fitted and worn, significantly reduce the danger of noise damage. If in spite of these precautions, individuals are found to be acquiring a permanent threshold shift over time, they may be removed from the noisy environment or compensated for the damage to their hearing.

Counseling

Hearing loss is a poorly understood problem, even by those who suffer from the disorder. People with hearing loss, their relatives, and friends need counseling to help them understand the effect of hearing loss on language and speech, on listening, and on personality. They need realistic information about the possibilities and limitations of habilitative measures. They need practical advice about improving everyday communication. Particularly, parents of children with congenital impairment need to learn about hearing loss and how to accept and assist the handicapped child. Teachers should understand the problems of their hearing-impaired students. Preferential classroom seating is important for all children with hearing disorders. They must be seated near the teacher and their seating arranged so they can see the teacher's face well. If at the same time, classroom noise is reduced as much as possible, the resulting favorable **speech-to-noise ratio** will improve the child's ability to understand. Classroom noise reduces the intelligibility of speech more for hearing-impaired children than for those with normal hearing (Watson, 1964; Ross and Giolas, 1974). If the child has better hearing in one ear or is wearing an at-the-ear hearing aid, seating should be arranged to orient that ear toward the teacher so the child will not have to listen in the sound shadow of his or her own head **(head shadow effect).** The progress of the hearing-impaired child who remains in the regular classroom must be watched carefully, and the child may need individual help or placement in a class for hard-of-hearing children.

Hearing Aid Use

A hearing aid is commonly described as a miniature public address system. As such, it has the power to make sounds louder, but not any clearer. Therefore, people with a primary loss of hearing sensitivity get significant help from hearing aids. As auditory discrimination ability decreases, however, the likelihood of satisfactory hearing aid use also decreases. Despite this limitation, the vast majority of hearing aid wearers have sensorineural loss. The hearing aid overcomes the loss of sensitivity, enabling the person to utilize whatever auditory discrimination ability remains.

At-the-ear aids are preferable for mild, moderate, and some severe losses. An at-the-ear aid is shown in Fig. 13.8(a). For some severe and for profound losses, more powerful body-worn aids are appropriate. Such an aid is shown in Fig. 13.8(b). Body aids should be worn outside the clothing; otherwise, sounds may be obscured and noise added from clothing movement in contact with the grill covering the microphone. Outside the clothing, body aids are accessible for adjustment, a procedure necessary for good hearing aid use. Figure 13.9 shows a child wearing a body aid in a cloth carrier.

When hearing aid use is being considered, audiological evaluation is important. The evaluation determines if an aid is needed, the amount of help that can be expected from an aid, and the kind of aid that will deliver comfortable, useful amplification.

Most people need a good deal of help learning to accept a hearing aid and use it effectively. They also need psychological support. People commonly do not understand what an aid can and cannot do. Therefore, their expectations may be unrealistic, and without counseling may become disappointed and reject the hearing aid. Most new hearing aid users are bothered by the audibility of sounds that they have not been accustomed to hearing. They complain that the hearing aid is noisy. Many need guidance while becoming accustomed to amplified sound. They may begin by wearing their aid only in quiet places with gradual exposure to more demanding situations. The typical new hearing aid

Figure 13.8

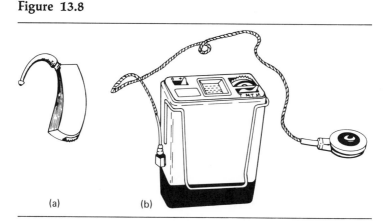

(a)   (b)

(a) Behind-the-ear hearing aid; (b) body-worn hearing aid.

Figure 13.9

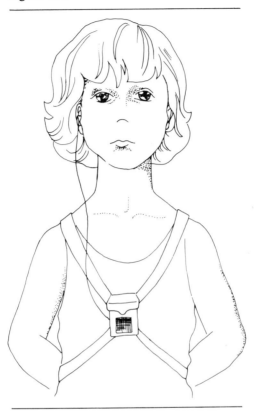

Child wearing a body-type hearing aid in a cloth carrier.

owner, without instruction, may eagerly try the aid in the difficult listening situation where he or she has the most trouble. Unaccustomed to operating the aid and listening to amplified sound, the new user may be bitterly disappointed.

The new hearing aid user needs help learning about the care and operation of the aid. The user must learn how to put it on and remove it, when and how to replace batteries, and how to clean the earmold. This person must be advised about the listening situations in which the greatest help can be expected. Some persons, because of the nature of their loss, are properly part-time aid wearers and should be so informed. Most important, the individual must learn to adjust the volume control of the aid to get optimum amplification for different listening conditions. Specifically, the volume control should be turned up to achieve comfortable loudness in quiet listening situations and turned down in noisy places. Without training, the wearer may use one volume control setting all the time.

341

This setting is likely one that is comfortable in noisy surroundings, but inadequate in quiet circumstances. Because learning to use a hearing aid is a complex and difficult procedure, support and instruction from the audiologist are important. The following paragraphs present hearing-aid recommendations for patients whose auditory disorders were discussed earlier in this chapter.

Mrs. H.'s audiogram is shown in Fig. 13.4. She works in a quiet office where people tend to speak with low intensity, and sometimes she needs to hear speech originating from some distance. For these reasons part-time use of a hearing aid seemed indicated. We recommended the right ear for amplification, because discrimination ability via that ear may be a little better. With minimal assistance, Mrs. H. learned to use her aid effectively. She always wears her aid at work, as well as in some other quiet places where people talk softly.

To solve the amplification problems of Mrs. L. (Fig. 13.5) and Mrs. R. (Fig. 13.7), different applications of a special type of hearing aid were made. The aids are known by the generic name of CROS (Harford and Barry, 1965). CROS aids were first used for people with unilateral loss. These individuals had normal or near-normal hearing on one ear and hearing too poor on the other ear to benefit from hearing aid use. People with unilateral loss usually report that they have trouble locating the source of sound and that they have difficulty when people speak from the side of their poor ear during difficult listening conditions. The second problem occurs because the good ear is in the sound shadow cast by the head, and the effective level of speech is thereby reduced.

CROS aids, usually built into eyeglasses, work as follows. A microphone is placed in the temple bar of the glasses on the side of the poor ear. It picks up sound from that side of the head, converts it to an electrical signal, and carries it via a wire in the glasses over to the side of the good ear. There the rest of the hearing aid is located. The signal is amplified slightly, changed back to sound energy, and carried to the good ear via a plastic tube. This tube is held in the ear canal by an *open earmold*, which is quite different from a standard earmold. Both types are pictured in Fig. 13.10. An open earmold does not plug the ear canal. Therefore, the person with unilateral loss, using a CROS aid, hears signals which originate from the side of the good ear directly via the open ear canal. The person hears via the hearing aid and, with slight amplification, signals originating on the side of the poor ear. Thus although hearing all sounds in the good ear, the person is hearing from both sides of the head, and the harmful effect of the head shadow is eliminated. Most people with normal hearing in one ear require quite critical demands on their hearing to justify use of a hearing aid. However, for unilateral patients who need to hear as well as possible, the CROS aid has been helpful.

Mrs. L., whose audiogram is shown in Fig. 13.5, has a complex problem, and a version of the CROS aid was recommended to help solve it. She has a slight loss on the right ear, with excellent discrimination, and a moderate loss on the left ear, with poor discrimination. In fact, her left-ear discrimination ability is

Figure 13.10

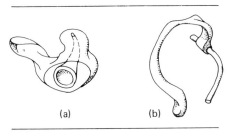

(a)   (b)

(a) Standard earmold; (b) open ear-mold.

probably too poor to permit appreciable benefit from amplification on the ear. In this case a BICROS aid was recommended. BICROS is a special aid that picks up signals from each side of the head and delivers them to one ear. There are two microphones, usually one located in each temple bar of the patient's glasses. The signal from both microphones is amplified and delivered to one ear. In the case of Mrs. L., the signal was delivered to the right ear. This type of amplification prevents Mrs. L. from being forced to listen with her head in the way. That is, signals originating on her left side are carried around her head electrically, amplified, and fed to her better ear. Signals originating on the right are fed directly to that ear. This arrangement reduces the appreciable effect of the head shadow on the audibility and intelligibility of speech.

Whereas an open earmold is used with most CROS arrangements, a standard mold is usually employed with BICROS. There are two reasons. First, sounds from both sides of the head are amplified, and there is no need for an unoccluded ear canal through which sounds can pass directly. Second, an open earmold leaks a lot of sound. When amplified sound emitting from a hearing aid receiver (earphone) reenters the aid's microphone and is reamplified, the result of this feedback is a high-pitch squealing sound. Therefore, with BICROS, a standard earmold is usually used to reduce feedback problems.

A CROS arrangement was also recommended for the patient whose audiogram is shown in Fig. 13.7, but for a different purpose than in the case above. In this case, the head shadow was utilized rather than eliminated. To explain, an open earmold was desirable in this instance. As sound moves into the ear canal through an open mold, much of its low-frequency energy is dissipated to the outside air. Its high-frequency components, however, travel on to the eardrum. This effect on frequency response of the open earmold is desirable in cases of high-frequency loss. With near-normal low-frequency sensitivity to 1000 Hz and a sharply falling high-frequency loss, Mrs. R. is a problem hearing aid candidate. Although hearing aids can be tailored to high-frequency emphasis, success of a conventional aid in reducing the hearing imbalance without tolerance

343

problems is unlikely. In this case an open earmold assisted. With this arrangement, Mrs. R. gets amplification of high-frequency sounds for which she has a hearing loss. Yet without amplification she hears naturally and comfortably those low-frequency sounds for which she has normal hearing. That is, these sounds enter the unoccluded ear canal through the open earmold. The CROS arrangement, called HICROS in this instance, is used to separate the hearing aid microphone and receiver. By placing the head between these **transducers,** the head shadow is utilized to permit use of an open earmold without feedback problems.

Language Instruction

Congenital hearing loss is associated with language retardation. All of the developmental language skills described in Chapter 2 are affected. There is a positive relationship between the severity of the loss and the degree of retardation. The child who is born deaf acquires no verbal language without specific and extended instruction. Even a slight congenital loss, however, often results in measurable language retardation. Language-training procedures for children are discussed in Chapter 11. For children with severe loss, the primary concern of early training programs is language development.

There is controversy about the kind of language that should be learned by those with congenital hearing impairment. Some educators, aware that deaf people live in a hearing world, recommend instruction in verbal language, speech, and speechreading for all hearing-impaired children. Others, citing the many failures resulting from such attempts at oral education, prefer a system of manual communication for the hearing-impaired. The dilemma is obvious. Verbal language for the deaf is overwhelmingly preferable but overwhelmingly difficult. Manual language, conversely, is learned easily by the deaf, but permits communication only with other deaf and the few hearing people who know it. Because of their biases, advocates of both systems sometimes lose sight of the needs and abilities of individual children.

One of the most unfortunate aspects of the oral versus manual controversy is the erroneous decisions that are made. The child who fails in an auditory-oral program may be without adequate language and communication ability for a long time, or forever. Therefore, an additional dilemma is how to decide which children are capable of learning verbal language and speech. Downs (1974), concerned about the many children she had seen fail in auditory-oral educational programs, presents the way to a possible solution. She suggests a scale, the Deafness Management Quotient, by which she hopes to predict the probability of success in an oral training program. Several factors contribute to the scale. The amount of remaining hearing is one. Other factors are intelligence, freedom from brain damage, support to be expected from the family, and socioeconomic situation. The more favorable each of these factors, the higher the deafness management quotient and the greater the probability of success in an oral training program.

For those children in whom probability of success seems low, Downs recommends a Total Communication training program. This procedure incorporates manual communication with the use of amplification, auditory training, and instruction in speechreading. That is, the goal is communication through all possible inputs and development of both manual and verbal language ability.

Speech Instruction

The child who cannot hear well requires assistance to learn to talk. This child has a poor auditory model for speech production, and even with instruction, his or her speech is likely to be grossly distorted. All aspects of vocal production are affected: pitch, intensity, quality, rate, and articulation. Remediation in these areas, discussed elsewhere in this text, is variously necessary in persons with congenital hearing loss, depending on the severity and configuration of the loss. Experimental devices are available which give visual feedback about adequacy of the vocal qualities mentioned above, to help make up for reduced auditory function (Nickerson, Kalikow, and Stevens, 1976).

Speechreading Instruction

Individuals who cannot hear all or part of what is said must rely on visual clues for assistance. The hearing-impaired person must learn to watch the lips and facial expression of the speaker. Of course, knowledge of verbal language is prerequisite to speechreading ability. Stated differently, the individual must know the meaning of the words he or she attempts to receive visually. Therefore, speechreading instruction for the congenitally impaired is part of a larger training program incorporating language and speech instruction. For those whose hearing becomes impaired after the acquisition of language and speech, speechreading instruction may be conducted as a separate skill.

The effectiveness of speechreading as a means of communication is sharply reduced by the fact that many of our speech sounds cannot be seen clearly. For example, /h/ has no visually observable characteristics at all, whereas /k/ and /g/ have characteristic tongue placement so far back in the mouth that they usually cannot be seen. In fact, only lip movements and positions may be sufficiently distinct to offer visual clues, and the other articulators contribute little or nothing. Speechreading is also made more difficult by the fact that many speech sounds which sound different look alike. For example, there are almost no visual differences between /b/, /p/, and /m/. Therefore, the words "ban," "pan," and "man" are most difficult to differentiate visually. Speech readers have to depend on contextual clues to resolve this dilemma.

In spite of the limitations of speechreading, it can be particularly helpful to individuals who learn to supplement their defective hearing with speechreading

345

skill. For people with auditory discrimination too poor to benefit from amplification through listening alone, combined listening and looking may improve discrimination ability enough to justify hearing-aid use.

Auditory Training

Normal-hearing listeners in most conversations receive more information than the minimum amount necessary for comprehension. Because of this redundancy, the person with normal hearing can be a little lazy while listening, but the hearing-impaired listener must learn to concentrate on every clue available. Goals of auditory training are to improve ability to differentiate acoustically similar signals and to help people structure conversational situations advantageously. The former goal is based on the belief that practice in differentiating minimally different signals will lead to improved ability to do so. An example of instruction associated with the latter goal is teaching an individual with unilateral loss to orient the good ear toward the talker in difficult listening conditions. In short, auditory training attempts to teach the hearing-impaired person to listen more efficiently and effectively. For a fuller discussion of habilitative audiology, see O'Neill and Oyer (1973).

Conclusion

Everyone faces the possibility of hearing impairment. There is increasing concern about traumatic hearing loss in our noisy environment. With advancing age, the probability of significant hearing loss increases. Hearing loss results from many causes. Some of the disorders are a threat to life, whereas others limit their damage to the hearing mechanism. Some are correctable; others are permanent and irreversible.

The handicap of hearing loss extends beyond the obvious inability to hear or differentiate signals. Congenital loss is a barrier to language and speech development and isolates the individual from the sounds of everyday life. Acquired loss may cause personality changes and introduce practical problems relating to communication, occupation, and life-style. The profession of audiology has an important role in the detection, evaluation, and prevention of hearing loss as well as in the habilitation and rehabilitation of hearing-impaired individuals.

Glossary

Anoxia: Absence or lack of oxygen.

Audiologist: Audiology is the science of hearing. An audiologist is an individual professionally trained in the field of audition and in the assessment and remediation of problems resulting from hearing disorders.

Auditory discrimination ability: The ability to differentiate among sounds. Discrimination scores are expressed in percent correct.

Auditory sensitivity: A measure of the sound intensity required for audibility. Sensitivity is measured in decibels.

Conductive hearing loss: The type of loss caused by deficits in the sound-conducting mechanism of the ear, which reduces the effective intensity of sounds reaching the inner ear.

Head shadow effect: The reduction in intensity of a sound reaching an ear on the opposite side of the head from a sound source. The overall head shadow effect on speech has been established at about 6 dB.

Mixed hearing loss: A loss with conductive and sensorineural components in the same ear.

Otolaryngologist: A physician who specializes in disorders of the ear, nose, and throat.

PB list: Fifty monosyllabic words in which the frequency of occurrence of individual speech sounds approximates that of those sounds in the language. PB lists are used in discrimination testing.

Sensorineural loss: Hearing loss caused by a disorder in the inner ear or auditory nerve.

Spectrum (plural, spectra): The distribution of energy across frequency in a complex acoustic signal.

Speech-to-noise ratio (or signal-to-noise ratio): The difference in dB between the level of a desired signal (speech) and an interfering noise. Plus SNR's indicate that the speech is more intense than the noise; Minus SNR's indicate that the noise is more intense than the speech.

Spondee words: Two-syllable words spoken with equal emphasis on each syllable. These words are used to determine speech thresholds.

Syndrome: A group of symptoms which occur together in a disorder and are useful in identifying the disorder; or, a disorder characterized by a specific group of symptoms.

Threshold: The lowest level at which response occurs for a specified fraction of trials. Fifty percent response is the usual criterion for threshold.

Tinnitus: Ear noises which are not attributable to external stimuli.

Transducer: A device that changes energy from one form to another. Common examples are microphones and earphones.

Study Questions

1. Differentiate between the terms "deaf" and "hard of hearing."
2. What are the three types of hearing loss?

3. What are common causes of congenital hearing loss? Of acquired hearing loss?

4. What are some ototoxic drugs?

5. What are three subjective indicators of a noise level which may be intense enough to damage the ears through long-term exposure?

6. What are the automatic indicators of the three types of hearing loss referred to in question 2 above?

7. Describe the play audiometry process used with young children.

8. Briefly describe three objective auditory tests.

9. Name three purposes of a hearing-conservation program.

10. What are the major advantages of hearing-aid use? What are the major limitations?

11. Describe the Deafness Management Quotient.

12. What are the advantages and limitations of lipreading skills?

Bibliography

BERLIN, C., AND S. LOWE, "Temporal and Dichotic Factors in Central Auditory Testing," in J. Katz, ed., *Handbook of Clinical Audiology*, Chapter 15, Baltimore: Williams and Wilkins, 1972.

DOWNS, M., "The Deafness Management Quotient," *Hearing and Speech News* **42** (1974):8–9, 26–28.

GLATTKE, T., "Electrocochleography," in J. Katz, ed., *Handbook of Clinical Audiology*, rev. ed., Baltimore: Williams and Wilkins, 1977.

HARFORD, E., AND J. BARRY, "A Rehabilitative Approach to the Problem of Unilateral Hearing Impairment: The Contralateral Routing of Signals (CROS)," *J. Speech Hearing Dis.* **30** (1965):121–138.

HODGSON, W., "Testing Infants and Young Children," in J. Katz, ed., *Handbook of Clinical Audiology*, Chapter 26, Baltimore: Williams and Wilkins, 1972.

JERGER, J., P. BURNEY, L. MAULDIN, AND B. CRUMP, "Predicting Hearing Loss from the Acoustic Reflex," *J. Speech Hearing Dis.* **39** (1974):11–22.

NICKERSON, R., D. KALIKOW, AND K. STEVENS, "Computer-Aided Speech Training for the Deaf," *J. Speech Hearing Dis.* **41** (1976):120–132.

O'NEILL, J., AND H. OYER, "Aural Rehabilitation," in J. Jerger, ed., *Modern Developments in Audiology*, 2d ed., Chapter 7, New York: Academic Press, 1973.

PASHAYAN, H., "The Basic Concepts of Medical Genetics," *J. Speech Hearing Dis.* **40** (1975):147–163.

PENN, J., "Voice and Speech Patterns with the Hard-of-Hearing," *Acta Otolaryng.* Suppl. 124, 1955.

PROCTOR, C., "Understanding Hereditary Nerve Deafness," *Arch. Otolaryng.* **85** (1967): 45–82.

ROSS, M., AND T. GIOLAS, "Effect of Three Classroom Listening Conditions on Speech Intelligibility," *Amer. Ann. of Deaf* **116** (1974):580–584.

SKINNER, P., "Electroencephalic Response Audiometry," in J. Katz, ed., *Handbook of Clinical Audiology*, Chapter 22, Baltimore: Williams and Wilkins, 1972.

WATSON, T., "The Use of Hearing Aids by Hearing Impaired Children in Ordinary Schools," *Volta Rev.* **66** (1964):741–744, 787.

AUTHOR INDEX

SUBJECT INDEX

355

v